**The Halstead-Reitan
Neuropsychological Battery:
A Guide to Interpretation
and Clinical Applications**

To my friend and colleague - Van -

Best of luck in your re-newed Neuropsychology

studies

Warm regards

Jeff

The Halstead-Reitan Neuropsychological Battery

A Guide to Interpretation and Clinical Applications

Paul E. Jarvis, Ph.D.
Jeffrey T. Barth, Ph.D.

PAR Psychological Assessment Resources, Inc.
P.O. Box 998/Odessa, Florida 33556/Toll-Free 1-800-331-TEST

Chapter 12 (Forensic Issues) is designed to provide accurate and authoritative information in regard to the subject matter covered. The reader should understand, however, that neither the authors nor the publisher is engaged in rendering legal or other professional service. If legal advice or other expert assistance is required, the services of a competent professional should be sought.

The neuroanatomical illustrations (Appendix C) were produced by the Medical Illustrations Department of the University of Virginia.

Library of Congress Cataloging-in-Publication Data

Jarvis, Paul E., 1931-
 The Halstead-Reitan neuropsychological battery: a guide to interpretation and clinical applications/ Paul E. Jarvis, Jeffrey T. Barth.
   p.   cm.
 Includes bibliographical references and index.
 ISBN 0-911907-13-0
 1. Halstead-Reitan Neuropsychological Test Battery. 2. Brain damage—Diagnosis. I. Barth, Jeffrey
   T., 1949- . II. Title.
 [DNLM: 1. Neuropsychological Tests. 2. Brain Damage, Chronic—diagnosis. WL 354J38hb 1994]
 RC386.6.H34J373   1994
 616.8'0475—dc20
 DNLM/DLC
 for Library of Congress   93-23601
                                                                                                    CIP

9 8 7 6 5 4 3 2 1   Printed in the United States of America   Reorder #RO-3043

TABLE OF CONTENTS

PREFACE

This book was developed as a result of the response to our earlier work, *Halstead-Reitan Test Battery: An Interpretive Guide* (Jarvis & Barth, 1984). That book had as its goal the teaching of a systematic method of interpretation of data generated by the Halstead-Reitan Neuropsychological Battery (HRB). We have been gratified by the favorable reception it received over the past 9 years and appreciative of the feedback we have received from psychologists, interns, and graduate students who have used the book in their study of neuropsychology.

Advances in the neurosciences and related changes in the clinical practice of neurology and neuropsychology during the past decade have been, in some areas, dramatic. The impact of Magnetic Resonance Image (MRI) scans is but one example. Clinical research on the HRB has also had significant implications for interpretation of test data. The normative data for the HRB and other tests provided by Heaton, Grant, and Matthews (1991) have made comparisons of patient performance to groups of neurologically normal subjects of the same age, gender, and education level practical for the first time. This results in more accurate diagnosis and treatment planning. Similarly, studies such as those by Thompson, Heaton, Matthews, and Grant (1987); Long and Hunter (1981); and Ross, Thrasher, and Long (1990) require a revision of several key hypotheses described in our earlier book (Jarvis & Barth, 1984). These developments, by themselves, dictated a need for significant revision of the Interpretive Guide.

In addition, users of our earlier book frequently asked for practical information about clinical applications: How do you incorporate interpretive inferences into a report of a neuropsychological evaluation? What are the implications for everyday functioning and neuropsychological rehabilitation? What should be the role of the neuropsychologist in the newly opened forensic arena? We have attempted to respond to those questions in this current book.

We initially started out to revise the earlier Interpretive Guide (Jarvis & Barth, 1984) to incorporate the newly available information about interpretation. As we began our attempt to respond to the requests from users of the earlier book for information about clinical applications, we realized that we were going so far beyond such a revision as to produce a different book. It is our hope that the current volume is successful in both updating the systematic method of interpretation and providing useful guidelines to clinical applications.

Paul E. Jarvis
Denver, Colorado

Jeffrey T. Barth
Charlottesville, Virginia
October, 1993

INTRODUCTION

This book has two general purposes: 1) To teach a systematic method of interpretation of data generated by the Halstead-Reitan Neuropsychological Battery (HRB) and certain other tests in order to answer questions about cerebral dysfunction that are frequently asked of clinicians, and 2) to illustrate some of the clinical applications that are most important for neuropsychologists today. The 14 chapters and 3 appendices are divided into three general sections.

Section 1, which contains chapters 1 through 9, presents the method of interpretation. Chapter 1 gives a brief rationale for the use of the Halstead-Reitan Battery (HRB). In chapter 2 the tests of the battery and certain other widely used neuropsychological tests are described, including the requirements for successful performance of them. The reader should note that the descriptions provided are not sufficient to enable one to administer the tests. Proper administration of the battery requires considerable training and practice and is not within the scope of this book. An understanding of the material in this chapter is, however, essential for adequate interpretation of the data.

Chapter 3 is the heart of this section. In this chapter, the methods of interpretation are described. These methods are essentially the same as those described earlier by Jarvis and Barth (1984). There is, however, one significant change. In the earlier volume, the use of a profile adapted from Russell, Neuringer, and Goldstein (1970) was recommended. Since then, corrections for age, education, and gender have become available for scores from the HRB and certain other tests (Heaton et al., 1991), and profiles of *T* scores, which incorporate those corrections are used in this book. Readers should keep in mind the *Caveat* at the end of this chapter regarding the limitations of blind interpretation of test data whenever they apply these interpretive methods in their clinical work.

Chapters 4 through 8 present a number of hypotheses regarding brain-behavior relationships pertinent to the data derived from the battery. Many of these hypotheses have long been widely accepted by neuropsychologists. In those instances, only one or two citations to the relevant literature are provided for each specific hypothesis, although others would have been equally appropriate. Some of those citations refer to original empirical studies regarding the hypotheses; others refer to secondary sources in which the clinical use of the hypotheses has been described. Secondary sources include works on interpretation of the HRB published by Reitan (e.g., Reitan & Davidson, 1974; Reitan & Wolfson, 1985), Golden (e.g., Golden, 1978; Golden, Osman, Moses, & Berg, 1981), and others as well as materials that have been widely used in training workshops presented by Reitan (e.g., Reitan, 1959a, 1972, 1979b). Finally, there are some hypotheses for which no specific citations are provided. Some of these, such as those regarding certain aspects of brain anatomy, are so basic and widely acknowledged that specific citations would be redundant. Others, a distinct minority, are ones that appear intuitively obvious, but for which specific supporting data are not yet available. Several examples of this last category are found in chapter 8.

The hypotheses presented were chosen on the basis of their utility in both clinical work and in teaching this method of interpretation. As such, the reader is cautioned to regard them and use them strictly as hypotheses, not as *rules*. This is particularly important for many of the hypotheses regarding implications for everyday functioning in chapter 8. Prediction of everyday functioning, sometimes called *ecological validity*, is a topic which is receiving a great deal of attention today, but the base of empirical data still needs expansion.

Many of the hypotheses in chapters 4 through 7 are the same as those described earlier by Jarvis and Barth (1984); others are new or are modifications of older ones based on recent research. The work of Thompson et al. (1987) on the effects of hand preference, age, sex, and education on performance on certain tests, for example, resulted in several important changes.

The reader will note that many of the hypotheses are repeated several times across chapters, as they were in Jarvis and Barth (1984). This redundancy is intentional and serves two purposes. The first, for the reader who is relatively unfamiliar with the field, is a mnemonic one. Reading the same hypotheses over and over again will help fix them in memory and begin to clarify the relationships between factors such as test data, location of lesions, neuropathological processes, and so on. The second is a reference aid for the user of the Guide who is proceeding through the steps in the method of interpretation. This redundancy ensures that the relevant hypotheses will be encountered at each step as one proceeds through them.

Chapter 9 presents sample cases, which illustrate the method of interpretation described earlier. The illustrative interpretations are, for the most part, based on only the test data and certain demographic information. This is done to demonstrate both the potential value of blind interpretation and its limitations. The cases in this chapter are presented only for the purpose of teaching the methods of interpretation that are described in the earlier chapters; they are *not* clinical reports of neuropsychological evaluations. It is stressed that blind interpretation is *never* appropriate in actual clinical situations.

Section 2, which includes chapters 10 through 13, illustrates some important clinical applications. Chapter 10 describes the types of data other than test scores that are essential in any clinical application. Chapter 11 presents an overview of the field of neuropsychological rehabilitation, which is one of the fastest growing areas of neuropsychology today. Chapter 12 provides an introduction to the forensic arena, which neuropsychologists are frequently entering today. Chapter 13 presents an approach to the preparation of reports of neuropsychological evaluations that integrates the information on interpretation and clinical applications described in earlier chapters; two sample reports are also included in this chapter.

Section 3, which includes chapter 14 and the appendixes, provides additional information that is intended to assist psychologists who lack experience in medical settings to understand certain important aspects of cases they may encounter in clinical neuropsychological practice. Chapter 14 describes neurological examination procedures, including neuroimaging, to which many patients are exposed. Appendix A is a glossary of important neuropsychological and neurological terms. Appendix B is a list of widely used abbreviations of medical terms that will be frequently encountered while reviewing medical records. Appendix C consists of illustrations of certain important features of brain anatomy.

It is hoped that this book will serve as a blueprint and reference in guiding the beginning student of neuropsychology through the complex process of clinical application.

SECTION 1
INTERPRETATION

Chapter 1

Selection of Instruments for Neuropsychological Assessment

Single Tests Versus Batteries of Tests

Jarvis and Barth (1984) summarized the history of a search for "a single test for organicity." Although there will undoubtedly be "promising new single tests for brain damage" proposed in the future, the complexity of the human brain and the variety of behavior that is dependent on it make it certain that no single test will be able to reveal the richness of the brain-behavior relationships that are the subject of clinical neuropsychology.

Even when the only question asked of a neuropsychological evaluation is whether there is "brain damage," single tests are inadequate. Reitan (1975) pointed out the problem of the high false negative rates produced by single tests, and Russell (1975) and Jarvis and Barth (1984), for example, described cases of patients with severe cerebral impairment who were misidentified by several commonly used single tests. Today, however, the questions asked of neuropsychological evaluations are more complex and sophisticated. For example, surveys of neuropsychologists have indicated that most referrals today request treatment recommendations (Hamlin & Jarvis, 1987; Jarvis, 1988a), and forensic evaluations, which neuropsychologists are increasingly being asked to provide, pose their own complex questions. It is clear that a competent neuropsychological evaluation requires a battery of tests.

Choice of a Battery

A neuropsychological test battery should provide for the examination of a broad spectrum of behaviors ranging from sensory input and perceptual integration, to motor output, and a variety of "higher-order" cognitive functions such as memory, concept formation, and problem solving. Some, including Lezak (1983) and Walsh (1985), have argued for the use of "flexible" batteries or a "process" approach, designed for individual patients, and the supports for that approach were summarized by Jarvis and Barth (1984). More recently, Benton (1992) has suggested what might be called a "flexible-fixed" battery composed of a very short list of "fixed" tests, supplemented in each case with additional tests chosen on the basis of the unique aspects of the case.

There are two major problems with these approaches:

1. Frequently, patients have problems that will be missed because they are not apparent from information provided by either the referral or the patient. For example, what is described as a problem with reading comprehension may be due to a visual scanning deficit.

2. Since evaluations based on the flexible battery approach tend to focus on problems or deficits, they provide little of the information about patients' strengths, which are important for treatment and rehabilitation planning. The use of a standard battery minimizes both of those problems.

Because of these problems, and because of a lack of research evidence supporting the use of a flexible battery or pure process approach, the use of a fixed battery and a more empirical approach is indicated.

There are a number of fixed batteries available today, the Halstead-Reitan Battery (HRB) being the most thoroughly validated one; a discussion of the others is outside the scope of this book. The use of the HRB provides a number of important advantages:

1. It provides for the assessment of many of the major domains of behavior that are dependent on adequate functioning of the brain.

2. It allows the application of multiple methods of inference in interpretation of data.

3. It is supported by the largest base of research data of any neuropsychological test battery.

4. There are normative data available from Heaton et al. (1991) which provide corrections for certain important demographic factors.

5. It allows for administration by trained technicians, freeing the time of the neuropsychologist for such functions as interpretation, treatment planning, and research. Some have argued that this deprives the neuropsychologist of the opportunity to observe the patient's behavior. The trained technician, who is more skilled at test administration than most psychologists who administer their own neuropsychological tests, however, may actually be better able to observe and record important aspects of the patient's behavior than a psychologist administering the tests. Most neuropsychologists will also conduct their own interviews with patients in addition to having them tested.

Additional Considerations

One of the advantages of the HRB is that it has been administered to thousands of people, using the same standard procedures. Consequently, the tests should always be administered in the standard manner. Under those conditions, however, a few patients are unable to perform some of the tests. When that happens, the examiner should note the nature of the patient's difficulty and attempt to determine the reasons for it. Sometimes patients are unable to perform certain tests because of peripheral sensory or motor deficits, rather than impairment of brain functioning. Other patients may be unable to perform some tests because of emotional problems such as anxiety about the blindfold required for the Tactual Performance Test (TPT). Any such difficulties and the apparent reasons for them should be noted. Following that, test procedures may be modified in an attempt to determine whether the patient can accomplish the task in a different way. When this is done, the interpretation of the data will necessarily be more tentative, but the additional information may have implications for both diagnosis and treatment.

Another modification of standard procedures that may be useful with some tests is what Lezak (1983) has called "testing the limits." On a time-limited test such as the Block Design subtest of the Wechsler Adult Intelligence Scale–Revised (WAIS-R; Wechsler, 1981), for example, the examiner may allow the patient to continue working on a test item beyond the "cut-off" time, noting what was achieved by the end of the standard time limit. If the patient then completes the task, which had a 60-second cut-off time for credit in 120 seconds, one can calculate two scores: a "standard score" and a "maximum possible" score.

When this is done, it is possible to differentiate between the person who is able to complete the task if given sufficient time and the person who is completely unable to perform it under any condition. It is also frequently possible to determine whether the problem interfering with performance of the task is due to motor, cognitive, emotional, or other deficits. This, again, may have implications for both diagnosis and treatment.

A final consideration is the administration of additional tests to supplement the HRB. Heaton et al. (1991) have provided normative data for several tests, which are added to the HRB in many settings. Descriptions of the supplemental tests used in the cases discussed in this book are provided in chapter 2.

Chapter 2

Description of the Halstead-Reitan Neuropsychological Battery

Halstead (1947) originally employed a battery of 27 measures in his study of cerebral functioning and biological intelligence. From these he eventually selected 10 measures, which contributed to the Halstead Impairment Index. Reitan (1955) later discarded three of these measures, which were based on the Time/Sense Test and the Critical Flicker Frequency procedure, since he found they did not contribute significantly to the discrimination of brain-damaged from intact patients. The Halstead-Reitan Neuropsychological Test Battery today consists of eight tests, which will be described below. The complete instructions for administration of these tests are given in Reitan and Wolfson (1985, 1993).

Category Test

The first of these measures is the Category Test. For this test the patient is seated in front of an opaque glass screen on which 208 stimulus slides are serially projected. Located below the screen are the patient's response keys, which consist of four numbered lights with a spring-loaded switch below each light. The patient is told that he/she will see a series of slides on the screen and that each slide will remind the patient of a number between 1 and 4. The patient is instructed to push the switch corresponding to the number that he/she is reminded of and that a correct response will result in a positive reinforcement (a bell). On the other hand, when the patient presses the switch corresponding to an incorrect answer, he/she hears a noxious-sounding buzzer. The test is divided into seven subtests, and the patient is told that there is a common principle or idea that governs the determination of the correct response in each subtest. The first subtest has a very simple principle: The patient is required only to match the Roman Numeral, which appears on the screen with the Arabic Numeral on the response unit. In the second subtest, the patient is required to give a response corresponding to the number of items (circles, squares, etc.) appearing on the screen. As the subtests progress, the stimuli and the principles determining the correct answers become more complex. For example, stimuli may differ along several dimensions such as size, shape, color, position, and solidness of the figure (see Reitan & Davison, 1974, for a more complete description of the stimuli in the more complex subtests). The seventh and final subtest is different in that the correct answer is not determined by any single principle; instead, this subtest repeats items from the first six subtests. Therefore, it introduces a memory component, rather than requiring new concept information.

This test is a complex test of new problem solving, judgment, abstract reasoning, concept formation, and mental efficiency. It requires a number of higher-order functions such as the ability to note similarities and differences in the stimuli and to formulate hypotheses regarding the principle that determines the correct answer. It is also a test of learning ability utilizing nonverbal material. Finally, there is a memory component to the test that not only requires the patient to remember which principle was correct in determining the answer to an individual problem item, but also in subtest 7, requires a longer recall of previously learned correct responses.

The "General Instructions For The Halstead Category Test" (Reitan, 1959, 1979) stress that it is important for the examiner to "elicit the best performance of which the subject is capable." To ensure this, examiners are urged to provide extensive "prompts" or suggestions to patients who are making repeated errors without, of course, ever telling them what the principles underlying any of the subtests are. For example:

> Some patients need to be told repeatedly to observe the items carefully (in some instances they should be asked to describe the figures before being permitted to answer), or to state the reason for selecting a particular response.

> ...with subjects who are extremely impaired in their ability to form concepts, it may become necessary to urge them to study the picture carefully, to ask for their descriptions of the stimulus material (followed by questions directed to the subject such as, 'Does that give you any idea of what might be the right answer?'), to urge them to try to notice and remember how the pictures change since this often provides clues to the underlying principle, and to try to think of the possible reason when a correct answer occurs. (Reitan, 1959, 1979, p. 26; see also Reitan & Wolfson, 1985).

There are relatively few pitfalls in the administration of the Category Test; however, some patients will attempt to make a second response when the first response to a stimulus is incorrect. Patients should be told that this is not allowed and if the patient shows a tendency toward this behavior, the examiner should anticipate this and make every effort to prevent the patient from making a second response following an incorrect one.

Subtest 3 is radically different from and more difficult than the first two subtests and, for that reason, must be treated differently. It is important to encourage the patient to concentrate on the task at hand, particularly during the first several slides of this subtest, to ensure the best possible performance and to limit discouragement and resignation to failure.

The Booklet Category Test (BCT) (DeFilippis & McCampbell, 1979) has gained wide acceptance as an alternate, a less expensive, and a portable form of the Category Test, although there are limited data regarding the equivalence of the two tests. Jarvis, Hamlin and DeFilippis (in press) have identified a potential problem with its use, however. DeFilippis and McCampbell (1979) make it clear that the BCT is intended to be as precise a substitute for the original Category Test as possible so that normative data from the original test can be applied with the BCT. They stress the care taken to duplicate the characteristics of the test stimuli and even recommend that patients be prompted to point to the numbers on the card in front of them, instead of verbalizing them, to replicate the action of pressing the switches on the original version as closely as possible. Their instructions for administration are very similar to Reitan's (Reitan, 1959b, 1979; Reitan & Wolfson, 1985) original instructions, but they omit the additional prompts recommended for impaired subjects.

Recently, a computer version of the Category Test has become available (DeFilippis, 1993), but little is known yet about the equivalence of this version to the original. Reitan and Wolfson (1993) have expressed concerns about the effect of decreased examiner-patient interaction when a computer version of this test is used, and it seems advisable to have this version administered by an experienced examiner who can prompt the patient appropriately when indicated.

Patients who have little or no difficulty with this test may not need these additional "prompts," and their performance may not be much different if the BCT instructions (DeFilippis & McCampbell, 1979), which do not urge examiners to use them, are used as they are published. However, Jarvis, Hamlin, and DeFilippis (in press) have pointed out that some patients' performance suffers if they are not given. Therefore, it is strongly recommended that if the BCT test is used, the supplemental prompts be given as appropriate.

Although the Category Test is not timed, it is common practice to limit response time for each item to 15-20 seconds. The total number of errors is the score that contributes to the Halstead Impairment Index.

Tactual Performance Test

The Tactual Performance Test (TPT) is a test that utilizes an apparatus similar to the Seguin-Goddard form board. In the administration of this test, the patient is blindfolded and seated in front of a form board on a supporting rack. The patient is never allowed to see the board or the blocks. The 10 blocks, which fit on the board, are placed on the table immediately in front of the patient and below the board. The examiner quickly runs the patient's hand over the board and blocks to familiarize him/her with the nature of the task. The patient is then told to place the blocks, which are in front of him/her, in the correct slots on the board. This is a timed test and the patient is encouraged to perform the task as quickly as possible. The patient first performs the task with only the dominant hand. When this is completed, the blindfold is kept on and the blocks are removed from the board and replaced in front of the patient. The patient then performs this same task with the nondominant hand. The blindfold is kept on, the blocks are once again removed from the board, and the patient then performs the task with both hands. The three trials are timed with a maximum of 10 minutes per trial unless the patient is close to completion at the 10-minute mark with the dominant hand. In that case, each trial would be allowed to continue for a maximum of 15 minutes. Next, while the blindfold is kept on, the blocks and form board are removed and placed out of sight or covered up. The blindfold is then removed and the patient is given an 8½ x 11 sheet of white paper and a pencil and instructed to draw the outline of the form board with the blocks in the correct positions as nearly as he/she can remember them. Times and number of blocks placed correctly are recorded for the dominant hand, nondominant hand, and both hands. A total time is calculated and the number of blocks remembered and correctly located are recorded. This results, then, in a total of six scores—one each for the dominant hand, nondominant hand, both hands, total time, memory, and localization. These latter three— total time, memory, and localization—contribute to the Halstead Impairment Index.

In this complex test, the most obvious requirement for successful performance is the ability to sustain adequate strength and speed of movement. It also requires tactile perception and the ability to form a visual "map" of the board. Problem-solving ability is a major requirement, and new learning ability probably accounts for the usual improvement across trials. Since the patient is not told until after the third trial that he/she will be required to draw the board, there is an additional requirement for incidental memory.

There are a number of potential problems in the administration of this test. The first of these involves the adequacy of the blindfold. Since the test is completely useless if the patient ever sees the blocks or the board, this is a crucial requirement. The adequacy of the blindfold should be checked by making a movement of the examiner's hand toward the patient's eyes from below to see whether or not the patient can see this. It may be necessary to repeat this at times during the test. A number of different blindfolds have been suggested, but the best type appears to be one available from Lafayette Instruments, Inc., which is similar to a plastic ski goggle with an opaque lens. Since many patients find the blindfold uncomfortable, either physically or psychologically, they have a tendency to take it off as soon as they think the test is done. Consequently, it is important for the examiner to say "keep the blindfold on" at the end of each trial and to make certain that it is kept in place after the third trial until the form board and blocks are all out of sight.

Many patients will also have a tendency to use both hands on either one or both of the trials, which they are required to perform with one hand only. Similarly, they sometimes have a tendency to shift to the dominant hand when the nondominant hand is being tested. The examiner should be aware of these natural tendencies and stop the patient quickly if he/she attempts to do so. We have found that it is helpful to have the patient sit close to the edge of the table with the hand that is not being examined on his/her knee beneath the surface of the table, or even under their own knee. This makes it more difficult for the patient to shift hands inadvertently, as the hand that is not being examined will be stopped by the table if there is a tendency to utilize it.

Seashore Rhythm Test

The Seashore Rhythm Test was adapted from the Seashore Tests of Musical Ability. This test is administered by playing a tape recording that represents 30 pairs of rhythmic beats. The patient's task is to record on an answer sheet an S or a D indicating whether the second group of beeps in each pair was the same as, or different from, the first group of beeps in the pair. For example, the patient may hear a pair of beats that sounds like this:

    beep — beep beep beep — beep

    beep — beep beep beep — beep

The correct response to this stimulus is "S or Same." Alternately, the subject may hear a pair like this:

beep beep—beep beep beep—beep

beep beep—beep beep—beep beep

The correct response to this stimulus is "D or Different." The pace of this recording is quite rapid and no cues are given as to the number of the stimulus pair or the corresponding number on the answer sheet for the 10 pairs of beeps within any of the 3 subtests. The number of correct responses contributes to the Impairment Index.

The most obvious requirement for the successful performance of this test is the ability to discriminate between different patterns of nonverbal sounds. In addition, however, this test requires the ability to sustain attention and concentration without any cues as to where one should be on the response sheet. A significant degree of coordination among ear, eye, and hand is also necessary. A poor performance on this test, then, may have little to do with inability to discriminate auditory rhythmic patterns, but may indicate a severe impairment of attention or concentration.

Speech Sounds Perception Test

The Speech Sounds Perception Test is also administered with a tape recorder. On this test the patient has a response sheet with 60 groups of 4 "nonsense words," which all contain the "ee" sound. The patient's task is to listen to the tape and underline the correct nonsense word. For example, the first stimulus word is "theets" and the patient must choose the correct response on the answer sheet from the following words "theeks, zeeks, theets, and zeets." The patient then hears "the second word is weej." The patient's task is to underline the correct word from among weech, yeech, weej, and yeej. While this test is longer in duration than the Seashore Rhythm Test, having 60 stimuli as opposed to 30, the pace is much slower and the patient is cued prior to each stimulus regarding where on the answer sheet a response should be marked. The number of errors on this test contributes to the Impairment Index.

The most obvious way in which the Speech Sounds Perception Test differs from the Seashore Rhythm Test is that the stimuli are verbal ones as opposed to nonverbal rhythms. In addition, the pace is slower and the patient is given cues about where the responses should be marked on the answer sheet. The requirement for attention and concentration is more sustained, yet the task is somewhat simpler than that of the Rhythm Test since more cues are provided. The same requirements for ear, eye, hand coordination, and the same possibilities for interference with adequate performance are present on both tests. Some older patients may have difficulty with this test because high-frequency hearing loss impairs their discrimination of the sounds.

Finger Oscillation Test

The Finger Oscillation or Finger Tapping Test requires that the patient tap as rapidly as possible with the index finger on a small lever, which is attached to a mechanical counter. The patient is given five consecutive 10-second trials with the preferred hand and then five consecutive trials with the nonpreferred hand. The scores on this test are the average number of taps in a 10-second period for the dominant hand and a 10-second period for the nondominant hand. The score on the dominant hand contributes to the Halstead Impairment Index. This test is basically a test of simple motor speed, although some degree of coordination is required.

It is important in the administration of this test for the examiner to start the stopwatch or clock at the precise moment the patient taps the lever the first time. Similarly, it is important to note whether the patient continues to tap after the examiner says "stop" and, if so, to subtract the number of extra taps from the score. It is also important to make sure that the patient is using only the index finger in tapping and is not making extraneous movements of the entire hand or arm. This can generally be assured by making certain that the heel of the patient's hand remains flat on the table. Some patients will show a great deal of intertrial variability in speed, and it is important to get *five consecutive* trials that are within five taps of each other in terms of speed. It may be difficult to achieve this with some patients, and one may need to administer as many as 10 trials in cases of extreme variability. No more than 10 trials should be administered, and one may then drop the fastest and the slowest trials and take an average of the remaining eight trials as the score for that hand.

Halstead Impairment Index

The Halstead Impairment Index is computed from the seven scores derived from the above tests. The computation of this index is described in the section on scoring of the individual tests. Recently, Reitan has advocated the use of an additional summary measure, *The Neuropsychological Deficit Score* (NDS; Reitan & Wolfson, 1993). The NDS is a composite measure which takes into account certain aspects of the pattern of performance, right-left differences, and pathognomonic signs, as well as the level of performance on individual tests. It is not used in this volume because there is limited empirical research regarding its usefulness and there are as yet no demographically corrected normative data available.

Trail Making Test

Even though the Trail Making Test does not contribute to the Halstead Impairment Index, it is considered an integral part of the Halstead-Reitan Battery. The Trail Making Test is a timed paper-and-pencil test, which consists of Parts A and B. On each part the patient is given a sample page, which is used for practice to aid the patient in understanding the instructions. The examiner then gives the patient Part A, which is a white sheet of paper with 25 numbered circles distributed in a random pattern. The patient is required to connect the circles with lines in numerical order as quickly as possible. Part B, which is given after practice on a sample sheet, consists of 25 circles—some of which are numbered from 1 to 13 and the remainder lettered from A to L. The patient is required to connect the circles beginning with number 1, then going to A, and from A to 2, 2 to B, and so on, in an alternating sequence. The scores on this test are the total times in seconds for each part and the number of errors.

Part A requires that the patient be able to scan the page rapidly, finding the correct numbers and connecting them in numerical sequence. In addition to the perceptual and problem-solving requirements, it includes a significant requirement for motor speed and coordination. Part B has the same requirements but, in addition, the patient must be able to recognize the different significance of the two types of symbols within the circles, and to alternate from one set of symbols to the other appropriately and consistently. The patient must simultaneously maintain attention on two aspects of a stimulus situation.

The most common problem in the administration of this test is that of quickly correcting the patient's errors. If the patient makes an error, the clock is kept running and the examiner must rapidly and efficiently indicate that the move was an error and return the patient to the last correct point in the sequence with the instruction to continue. This requires that the examiner be constantly alert to the patient's performance and thoroughly familiar with the positions of the numbered and lettered circles on the page so that he/she can correct patient errors without unduly penalizing the patient in terms of the timed score.

Aphasia Screening Test

Most examiners using this battery follow Reitan's example by incorporating the Aphasia Screening Test, which was prepared by Reitan as a modification of the Halstead-Wepman Aphasia Screening Test. The stimuli for this test are incorporated into a small spiral bound notebook. The first stimulus is a picture of a square, which the patient is asked to draw on a sheet of paper without lifting the pencil from the paper. This procedure is often repeated to see if the drawing improves on a second trial. The patient is then asked to name the object and then to spell it.

The second and third stimuli are drawings of a Greek cross and a triangle. The patient is asked in sequence once again to draw them (twice), name them, and spell them. This is followed by a drawing of a baby, which the patient is asked to name.

The next stimulus is a picture of a clock. The patient is asked not to say anything about it, but just to write the name of the picture on the paper. A drawing of a fork is next and the patient is asked to name it.

The patient is asked to read out loud the next four stimulus cards, which have the following on them:

"7 six 2"

"MGW"

"See the black dog"

"He is a friendly animal, a famous winner of dog shows."

The following three items are presented verbally, and the patient is asked to repeat them after the examiner. These items are *triangle*, *Massachusetts*, and *Methodist Episcopal*." Next the patient is shown a card with the word SQUARE and asked not to say the word but to write it on the paper. Then the patient is shown a card with the word SEVEN on it and asked to read it out loud. Then he/she is asked to repeat the word seven after the examiner. Next, the patient is asked to repeat, "He shouted a warning" after the examiner and then to explain the meaning of that sentence. The patient is then asked to write the sentence on the paper.

The patient is then requested to write down the problem 85-27 on a piece of paper and to perform the calculation. The next item is also an arithmetic problem 17 x 3 which the patient is asked to do mentally and to write down only the answer. The patient is then shown a picture of a key and asked to name it. The examiner then says, "If you had one of these in your hand, show me how you would use it." Then the patient is asked to copy the picture of the key on paper.

A card is then shown to the patient which reads, "Place left hand to right ear." The examiner asks the patient to read the card and then to do what it says on the card. Finally, the examiner says, "Now I want you to put your left hand to your left elbow."

It is obvious that the Aphasia Screening Test taps a number of different areas of dysfunction. These include dysnomia, dyslexia, spelling dyspraxia, dyscalculia, dysgraphia, right-left confusion, dysarthria, and constructional dyspraxia. Patients may make a variety of errors on this test for many reasons that have nothing to do with brain dysfunction, and it is obvious that educational deficits can affect abilities such as reading, spelling, and calculation. Similarly, psychiatric disturbances, which include thought disorder, may result in a variety of errors. The most important consideration for the examiner is that all responses must be recorded verbatim, with the exception of absolutely correct responses, which are given without any hesitation or delay. Only in this way is it possible to interpret these responses and their relationship to etiologic factors. It is also important to recognize that this test does not constitute a complete examination for aphasia problems. It does not, for example, provide a clear determination of receptive versus expressive problems.

Sensory Perceptual Examination

The addition of the Reitan-Kløve Sensory Perceptual Examination (Reitan, 1984) to the battery augments the assessment of higher-order functions by including procedures that are common to most clinical neurological examinations. Administration of these procedures in a reliable manner requires a good deal of skill and practice by the examiner. They can only be learned by practicing under the guidance of an experienced examiner; therefore, only a brief description of these procedures will be given here. Tactile, auditory, and visual modalities are tested to make certain that the patient can perceive a very low intensity stimulus delivered unilaterally. Stimuli are then delivered bilaterally and simultaneously. Tactile stimuli are very light touches presented to the hands and face while the patient's eyes are closed. Auditory stimuli are presented from behind the patient by the examiner's rubbing the thumb and finger together gently next to the patient's ear. In the testing of visual perception the examiner sits in front of the patient and makes a slight movement of the fingers at the periphery of the patient's vision while the patient focuses on the bridge of the examiner's nose. Visual fields are checked by a gross direct confrontation method.

Further tests of tactile perception include a test of tactile finger recognition in which the patient is asked, with eyes closed, to identify the individual fingers that are touched by the examiner on each hand. In the fingertip number writing test, the patient is asked to identify numbers written with a stylus on the fingertips of his/her hand by the examiner while the patient's eyes are closed. Finally, the tactile coin recognition task requires the patient to identify, through touch alone, pennies, nickels, and dimes.

The Reitan-Kløve Tactile Form Recognition Test was developed separately from the rest of the Sensory Perceptual Examination, but is usually recorded on the same form. This procedure requires the patient to identify flat plastic shapes (cross, square, triangle, and circle), which are placed in the patient's hand after being inserted through a curtained opening in a vertical board. On the side of the board facing the patient is another set of the same stimulus figures (cross, square, triangle, and circle). The patient is instructed to point with the free hand to the figure that is being presented in the hand hidden by the board.

It is obvious that these procedures require adequate functioning in the tactile, auditory, and visual modalities. A comparison of the number of errors on the two sides of the body is, then, the critical data obtained from this portion of the battery. One of the more important kinds of information obtained is that concerning suppressions, or the failure to perceive a sensation on one side of the body when both sides are simultaneously stimulated.

The importance and significance of data about suppressions makes it imperative that the examiner determine initially that the patient is able to perceive unilateral stimulation. Sometimes, in the auditory modality, for example, a patient will have a higher threshold for perception on one side of the body than on the other. This may require the examiner to present simultaneous stimulation of unequal intensity in order to eliminate different threshold levels and purely test for cortical suppression. Another problem that many patients have is focusing steadily on the bridge of the examiner's nose during the visual portions of the examination. The examiner must be aware of any eye movement on the part of the patient and repeat instructions and procedures if necessary. It is also important to remember that this is essentially a physical examination—an assessment of tactile, auditory, and verbal perception—and is not an assessment of verbalization, memory, or attention. On the fingertip number writing test, for example, it is common to find patients who give responses other than the numbers included in the instructions and demonstration (3, 4, 5, 6). When numbers such as 2, 7, or 8 are given as responses, it is likely that the patient either has not understood or retained the instructions, or is not paying attention to the task. In this case, instructions may be repeated or Xs and Os substituted for the numbers to be drawn on the fingertips. In some cases it is useful to repeat all or parts of the Sensory Perceptual Examination. If visual suppressions are noted or if confrontation testing of visual fields suggests field defects, it is useful to examine visual fields with a perimeter examination.

Strength of Grip

A measure of Strength of Grip (Lezak, 1983) obtained with the Smedley hand dynamometer has also routinely been added to the battery by Reitan and others. This test is very simple and requires only a few minutes to administer. The instrument is adjusted to accommodate the size of the patient's hand, and the patient is instructed to stand, holding the instrument at his/her side, pointed toward the floor with the arm held straight at the elbow. The patient is simply instructed to squeeze the dynamometer as hard as he/she can. Alternating trials are given with the dominant and nondominant hands with a total of two trials for each hand.

This is a simple measure of motor strength with no other behavioral components required for adequate performance. There do not appear to be any common problems in administering the test. Unlike the finger oscillation test, it is quite easy to get fairly consistent measures on repeated trials, and a large number of trials is rarely required.

Additional Tests

Most neuropsychologists who use the HRB supplement it with additional tests. Reitan added the Wechsler Belvue Scale initially, and it was later replaced by the Wechsler Adult Intelligence Scale (WAIS; Wechsler, 1955). More recently, many neuropsychologists have replaced that with the WAIS-R (Wechsler, 1981). The Minnesota Multiphasic Personality Inventory (MMPI; Hathaway & McKinley, 1942) has also been a common addition to the battery. It provides an assessment of the patient's level of stress and coping style, which is essential in a comprehensive neuropsychological evaluation, and its use in forensic evaluations is particularly important. Since most readers of this volume should be familiar with these tests and their revisions, they will not be described further here.

Other additions to the battery vary widely both in terms of the specific tests and the number of tests added. A major constraint is the time required for testing, which can be a particular problem with severely impaired patients (Benton, 1992). This concern must be balanced against the need for an adequate assessment of the important functional areas.

An additional assessment of memory functioning is probably the need that is most often addressed. This is important both because memory is crucial for most types of adaptive functioning and it is frequently impaired by many types of brain injuries and diseases. Heaton et al. (1991) have described the Story Memory and Figure Memory Tests that are used by a number of neuropsychological laboratories and have provided demographically corrected normative data for them. The Russell Revision of the Wechsler Memory Scale (RRWMS; Russell, 1975) was also used fairly widely until the Wechsler Memory Scale-Revised (WMS-R; Wechsler, 1987) became available. This latter test yields Indices for Verbal Memory, Visual Memory, General Memory, Attention/Concentration, and Delayed Recall, each with a Mean of 100 and a Standard Deviation of 15. Either the RRWMS or the WMS-R was used in most of the cases discussed in this volume. Other additional tests were used in the cases discussed in this volume.

The Rey Auditory Verbal Learning Test (RAVLT; Lezak, 1983) consists of five presentations of a list of 15 words (List A), after each of which the patient is asked to recall as many words as possible. This is followed by a learning trial with a list of 15 different words (List B). Immediately after that, the patient is asked to recall as many words as possible from the original list, (List A). Finally, after a 30-minute delay, the patient's recognition of words from List A is tested. The test provides information about verbal learning abilities and interference tendencies.

The Grooved Pegboard Test (Kløve, 1963) requires patients to place 25 notched pegs in slotted holes, which are oriented in random directions on a board, as rapidly as they can. One trial is given with each hand, and the scores for each are the time, in seconds, required to place all 25 pegs. This test requires both motor speed and fine motor coordination (Lezak, 1983). Demographically corrected normative data for the test are available in Heaton et al. (1991).

On the Wisconsin Card Sorting Test (WCST; Berg, 1948; Grant & Berg, 1948; Heaton, 1981) four stimulus cards are displayed in front of the patient. One card has a red triangle on it, one has two green stars, one has three yellow crosses, and one has four blue circles on it. The subject is then given 128 response cards, each of which has a design on it similar to the ones of the stimulus cards. The patient is instructed to place each response card in front of the stimulus card which it "matches" and is told by the examiner whether the response is correct or not. The initial principle for the correct placement or sorting is *color*. After ten consecutive correct responses, the principle changes, without notice to the patient, to *form*, and then after ten consecutive correct responses, it changes to *number*. This sequence continues until the patient has completed six "categories" or until all 128 cards have been used. Several different scores may be calculated, but the one that is most sensitive to brain impairment, especially frontal lobe dysfunction, is the Perseverative Response score, and it is the only one for which demographically corrected normative data are available from Heaton et al. (1991). It is important to note, however, that the *T* score for perseverative responses can be misleading in certain cases. It is possible to obtain an acceptable *T* score for perseverative responses while completing only one or two categories, and that, of course, represents an impaired performance. One should always check to see how many categories were actually completed. There is also a computer version of the WCST available (Heaton, 1993), which simplifies administration and scoring and ensures reliability of them. A recently revised Manual for the WCST provides norms for all of the scores for ages 6.5 through 89 (Heaton, Chelune, Talley, Kay, & Curtiss, 1993). This test requires a flexibility in thinking in addition to the concept formation and problem-solving abilities similar to those required by the Category Test. It appears to be sensitive to frontal lesions, yet like the Category Test and Trail Making B, its scores are reflective of strengths and weaknesses throughout the brain.

The Thurstone Word Fluency Test (TWFT; Pendleton, Heaton, Lehman, & Hulihan, 1982) consists of two parts. On Part A, the patient has 5 minutes to write down as many words as he/she can that begin with the letter s. On Part B, the patient has 4 minutes to write down as many four-letter words beginning with the letter c as possible. The score, for which demographically corrected normative data are available from Heaton et al. (1991), is the total number of words from the two parts.

The Benton Judgment of Line Orientation Test (JOLO; Benton, Varney, & Hamsher, 1978) evaluates visual spatial perceptual abilities by requiring patients to identify the lines on a display that match the angle of separation of two line segments presented in each of 30 trials. Only a verbal response is required; no constructional, or practic, ability such as arranging blocks on the Block Design Subtest, is required. This aids in evaluating "pure" visual spatial perceptual abilities. The test is particularly sensitive to posterior parietal right-hemisphere lesions. Normative data are available for gender and age.

Scoring, Cutoff Scores, and Data Sheets

Scoring of tests on the battery ranges from simple, objective, and almost automatic procedures on some tests to complex, relatively subjective, and more time-consuming methods on others. The scoring of the Category Test is an example of the former, since the score is simply the total number of errors made by the patient in responding to the 208 stimulus slides. On this test, there is no ambiguity about the scoring since an error is indicated to the examiner by the sound of the buzzer. If, as unfortunately sometimes happens, the patient immediately corrects his/her response and gives a correct response, this is scored as an error, and every attempt is made to prevent the patient from giving more than one response to future items.

There are six scores that are recorded for the TPT. For the dominant hand, the time required to place all 10 blocks correctly is recorded. If the patient has not placed all 10 blocks correctly within 10 minutes, the time is recorded as 10 minutes and the number of blocks placed in 10 minutes is recorded in parentheses. The same procedure is followed for the nondominant hand and for both hands. If on the first trial the patient has nearly all of the blocks in at the end of 10 minutes, the examiner may permit the patient to continue working but should record the number of blocks placed after 10 minutes as well as the total time required to place all 10 blocks correctly. The total time is simply a sum of the times on the first three trials. The examiner should also indicate the number of blocks correctly placed for the total of the three trials. If the patient continued to work for more than 10 minutes on the first trial, the examiner should allow the patient the same amount of time on subsequent trials to provide consistency and aid in proper interpretation of right/left differences.

Although Reitan originally called for 15-minute trials with each hand, (Reitan & Wolfson, 1985) most users of the battery have found trials this long to be counterproductive with severely impaired patients and limit each trail to 10 minutes unless the patient is making progress with the task. The issue of comparable times is essentially resolved by calculating the time per block placed for each of the trials, and that is the measure that is used in calculating *T* scores in the Heaton et al. (1991) system.

Obtaining the memory score for the TPT is more difficult and somewhat subjective. The important thing to remember is that scoring for memory is very liberal. If a patient either draws a block correctly or names a drawing correctly, even though the drawing does not resemble the named block, credit is given for that drawing. This measure is not a test of verbal ability or drawing skill, but simply a measure of incidental memory. When the patient has completed the drawing of the board with whatever encouragement is needed (without specific hints to remember any missing pieces), the examiner should question the patient about the name of any ambiguously drawn block. Even if a drawing is not recognizable as any one of the blocks and if the patient gives it a name that corresponds (at least approximately) to the name of the shape of a block, credit is given for that figure.

Scoring of the localization component is also quite difficult at times. The easiest way to score for localization is to divide the outline of the board that the patient used and to position the blocks into nine equal sectors (see Reitan & Wolfson, 1993). The examiner should then give localization credit for any block, whose major portion falls within the proper sector of the drawing in relationship to similar sectors on the board itself.

Three of these six scores—total time, memory, and localization—are included in the Halstead Impairment Index. The other three scores—the times for dominant hand, nondominant hand, and both hands—are not included in the Impairment Index. They are examined using a different method of inference and have strong implications for lateralization of cerebral dysfunction.

The score on the Finger Oscillation Test is an objective one that is relatively easily obtained, although there may be difficulties during the administration of the test in obtaining consistency of performance for the required number of trials. The scores that are recorded are the average number of taps in 10 seconds with the dominant hand and the average number of taps in 10 seconds with the nondominant hand. The score with the dominant hand enters into the Halstead Impairment Index. As was indicated above for TPT, the comparison of the scores on the dominant and nondominant hand is considered from the perspective of a different method of inference and has strong implications for lateralization of cerebral dysfunction.

Cut-off Scores for Brain Damage

The cut-off scores which best separate groups of brain-damaged from nonbrain-damaged subjects as reported by Reitan (1959b) are shown in Table 1. The value of the Impairment Index obviously decreases as the number of test scores available declines and it is of little value when the number of scores available is less than five (see Table 2 for calculation of Impairment Index based upon 7, 6, or 5 tests).

The other tests that are commonly included in a standard battery do not have cut-off scores, and in some cases do not really lend themselves to calculating numerical scores. Instead, they are more often either evaluated from the perspective of the difference in performance on the two sides of the body or examined for evidence of pathognomonic signs. Strength of Grip is a measure that tends to fall into the former category. While one expects most adult female patients to have a strength of grip of at least 20 kilograms in the dominant hand and most adult male patients to have a strength of grip of at least 40 kilograms with the dominant hand, the more important consideration by far is the relationship of the two hands.

Until fairly recently, a 10% difference between the performance of the two hands on strength of grip, as well as on finger tapping speed and the time on the Grooved Pegboard, was considered to be normal, and deviations from that were considered to have implications for lateralization of a cerebral lesion. Thompson et al. (1987) have demonstrated that this is not always accurate. The relationships are not the same for all of those tests, and certain demographic variables have significant influences on some of them. The use of the Heaton et al. (1991) *T* scores will take these into account.

The Aphasia Screening Test is an example where pathognomonic signs may be the most useful data. While Russell et al. (1970) have developed a scoring system for the Aphasia Screening Test specifically for research purposes, quality of response is exceedingly important and may not lend itself to quantitative scoring. Certain types of clearly dysphasic errors must be considered to be pathognomonic signs, and one or two of them

Table 1
Halstead Cut-off Scores Suggesting Brain Damage*

Tests	Halstead Cut-off Scores
Category Test	51 or more errors
TPT Total Time	15.7 minutes or more
Memory	5 or less correct
Localization	4 or less correct
Seashore Rhythm	25 or less correct
Speech Sounds Perception	8 or more errors**
Finger Oscillation (Tapping) (Dominant hand)	50 or less taps in 10 seconds
Impairment Index	5 or above

	Normal	Mild	Moderate	Severe
	0.0-0.2	0.3-0.4	0.5-0.78	0.8-1.0

The following test, while not contributing to the Halstead Impairment Index, has established cut-off scores.

Trail Making	
Part A	40 seconds or more
Part B	91 seconds or more

*(From Reitan, 1955; 1959; and based upon Halstead, 1947)

To calculate the Halstead Impairment Index, one divides the number of scores from Table 1 which are in the impaired range, by the total number of tests given which contribute to the Halstead Impairment Index (maximum 7). This results in a decimal value between 0 and 1.0. If none of the scores were in the impaired range the Impairment Index would be 0.0, while if all of them were in the impaired range (7 divided by 7, or 6 divided by 6, etc.), the Impairment Index would be 1.0. Since it is traditional to round all the results of this to the nearest 1 decimal place, the number of tests in the impaired range and the resulting impairment indices are listed on the prorated schedule in Table 2.

**Reitan and Wolfson (1985) suggest a cut-off score of 11 or more errors on the Speech Sounds Perception Test based upon analysis of more recent data.

Table 2
Calculation of the Halstead Impairment Index Based on Number of Tests Used and Number of Test Scores Which Fall Within the Brain-Impaired Range

	Number of Halstead tests utilized		
	7 Tests	6 Tests	5 Tests
Number of tests in Impaired range	1 = 0.1	1 = 0.2	1 = 0.2
	2 = 0.3	2 = 0.3	2 = 0.4
	3 = 0.4	3 = 0.5	3 = 0.6
	4 = 0.6	4 = 0.7	4 = 0.8
	5 = 0.7	5 = 0.8	5 = 1.0
	6 = 0.9	6 = 1.0	
	7 = 1.0		

would have more significance in terms of interpretation than a greater number of more equivocal errors. This is further complicated by the fact that interpretation of responses to the Aphasia Screening Test must take into consideration features such as intelligence and education.

While interpretation of the Sensory Perceptual Examination is based more on inferences regarding differences in performance of the two sides of the body, there are also some pathognomonic signs that may be seen. Visual/field deficits such as those shown in the Neuroanatomical Illustrations (see Appendix C) are pathognomonic signs, and consistent, reliable suppressions on one side of the body in a single sensory modality should be considered to be pathognomonic signs since such suppressions are seldom found among neurologically intact patients.

Since administration of a standard battery such as this generates a large amount of raw data, it is helpful to use a form for recording a summary of the results. There is probably no special virtue in any single form and the major value of any summary form is to provide a consistent format for the organization and evaluation of results. Figure 1 offers an example of a basic summary data sheet which combines many of the positive aspects of several forms.

The scores that enter into the Halstead Impairment Index have asterisks on the far right-hand side of the page so that it is easy to calculate the Impairment Index from those seven scores. The Impairment Index, the score on the Category Test, the localization score on the TPT, and the score on Part B of the Trail Making Test are those scores that are the most sensitive to brain impairment; because we generally look first at those scores, they appear near the top of the list even though the Trail Making Test does not itself contribute to the Halstead Impairment Index.

DATA SUMMARY FORM
RESULTS OF NEUROPSYCHOLOGICAL EXAMINATION

Case Number: _____ Age: _____ Sex: _____ Education: _____ Handedness: _____

Name: _____ Employment: _____ Date of Testing: _____

WAIS or WAIS-R
VIQ
PIQ
FS IQ

Scaled Scores

Information
Comprehension
Digit Span
Arithmetic
Similarities
Vocabulary
Picture Arrangement
Picture Completion
Block Design
Object Assembly
Digit Symbol

**MINNESOTA MULTIPHASIC
PERSONALITY INVENTORY**

T Scores

?
L
F
K
Hs
D
Hy
Pd
Mf
Pa
Pt
Sc
Ma
Si

IMPAIRMENT INDEX   ☐ . ☐ *
CATEGORY TEST   *
TACTUAL PERFORMANCE TEST
                        Time _____ # of Blks. In
Dominant hand:
Nondomin. hand:
Both hands:
            Total Time: *
            Memory: *
            Localization: *

TRAIL MAKING TEST
Part A: seconds   errors
Part B: seconds   errors

SEASHORE RHYTHM TEST (correct)
Raw Score: *

SPEECH-SOUNDS PERCEPTION TEST
Errors: *

FINGER OSCILLATION TEST
Dominant hand: . ☐ *
Nondominant hand: . ☐

STRENGTH OF GRIP
Dominant hand: kilograms
Nondominant hand: kilograms

**REITAN-KLØVE TACTILE FORM
RECOGNITION TEST**

                        Errors   Seconds
Dominant hand: ☐
Nondominant hand: ☐

SENSORY SUPPRESSIONS
Dominant:
Nondominant:

APHASIA SIGNS:

Figure 1. Data Summary Form.

Chapter 3

Guide to Interpretation

The following chapters contain a number of hypotheses regarding the brain-behavior relationships demonstrated by the data obtained from the Halstead-Reitan Battery. This selection of hypotheses is by no means all-inclusive of those that have appeared in the neuropsychological research literature; rather, those that appear in these chapters were selected on the basis of their clinical utility in neuropsychological assessment. Many of these hypotheses have become common knowledge in the field and may not be associated with specific research or references. No attempt has been made to indicate the nature or extent of validational studies regarding the selected hypotheses, and readers interested in pursuing this subject are urged to study the original research literature. Reitan (1975), for example, gives a review of a number of important validation studies, and Hevern (1980) has reviewed others.

In performing a neuropsychological evaluation a number of questions should be considered. While there may at times be some variations, in general it is best to consider these questions in the sequence listed below:

1. **Is there cerebral impairment?** In asking this question we are essentially asking whether there is evidence of behavioral deficits (in the case of congenital damage), or behavioral changes (in the case of acquired lesions) that can be attributed to the presence of a brain lesion. In cases of acquired lesions, it is essential that one determine the premorbid level of functioning for comparison purposes (see chapter 10).

2. **What is the severity of the cerebral dysfunction?** Here two questions are implied. The first is whether the severity of the impairment is such that it is medically significant and requires medical and/or surgical intervention. Second, is whether the severity of the impairment is such that it will impair the person's ability to function in his/her daily activities.

3. **Is the lesion progressive or static?** This is obviously a matter of degree since there are some very slowly progressive, degenerative disorders and there are some very rapidly progressive, space occupying lesions, such as certain highly malignant neoplasms. Heaton, Grant, Anthony, and Lehman (1981) found that this is a very difficult question to answer solely on the basis of test scores. In addition to test data, information about the patient's history is critical in regard to this question in "real" clinical cases. The answer to this question has implications for whether a lesion is medically significant, as well as for prognosis.

4. **Is the lesion diffuse, lateralized, or are there multiple lesions?** Is the entire brain impaired, is one cerebral hemisphere primarily involved, or is there a "spotty"

impairment with pockets of damage along with relatively unimpaired areas of the brain? Similarly, we are asking whether all areas of functioning are impaired to the same extent or whether there are more isolated areas of impairment of functioning with concomitant sparing.

5. **Is the impairment in the anterior or posterior portions of the cerebral hemispheres, and can it be localized?** This is essentially a further refinement of question 4.

6. **What is the most likely pathological process, and what is the prognosis?** It is often helpful in answering this question to first ask whether, on the basis of the answers to prior questions, certain pathological processes can be ruled out. For example, if the answer to question 3 is that the lesion is a static one, then one can rule out certain major categories of pathology such as rapidly growing neoplasms. Here again, the patient's history is critical in real clinical cases.

7. **What are the individual's cognitive/behavioral strengths and weaknesses, and how do they relate to daily living skills, treatment, and rehabilitation?** Information about the patient's emotional status and coping style plays a very important role here as indicated in chapter 11.

It is important to answer certain questions in the previous sequence. One cannot ascertain which hemisphere is more impaired if one has not first answered the question about whether a lesion is lateralized or not. Similarly, one cannot answer the question about the nature of the pathological process without having answered questions about severity, velocity, and location. It is not critical that certain questions be answered in precisely the order listed above. One can, for example, decide whether a lesion is more likely to be diffuse or lateralized before deciding on the probable velocity of the lesion. In general, however, it is helpful to address these questions in the sequence indicated above.

Methods of Inference

In this chapter we will describe the use of the hypotheses presented in the following chapters in answering these seven questions. This approach is a multifaceted one that uses the four methods of inference suggested by Reitan (e.g., Reitan, 1967; Reitan & Wolfson, 1985). These are: (1) level of performance, (2) patterns of scores on different tests and subtests, (3) differences in functioning of the two sides of the body, and (4) presence of pathognomonic signs.

Before these methods of inference are discussed in detail, it is necessary to address the effects of certain demographic factors on test performance. The fact that performance on neuropsychological tests is influenced by factors other than impairment of brain functioning has long been known (e.g., Reitan, 1955b). Since then, others such as Long (Moehl & Long, 1989; Long & Klein, 1990) have identified the effect of age on a number of tests. The failure to take this into account in a systematic way has undoubtedly led to incorrect clinical inferences in some cases and has been used to discredit the testimony of neuropsychologists in forensic situations (Faust, Ziskin, & Hiers, 1991). Age, education, and in some cases gender, have been shown to have significant effects on the performance of various neuropsychological tests, in some cases accounting for more than 40% of the variance in performance (Heaton, Grant, & Matthews, 1986). Much less is known about the effect of ethnicity, although a review by Faust et al. (1991) of a number of relevant studies, suggests that this is an area requiring more study. Normative data for the effects of age, education, and sex are now available for the Halstead Reitan Battery and a number of other tests discussed in Heaton et al. (1991). The use of these norms allows one to apply the four methods of interference with a much higher degree of accuracy than was previously possible. The numbers of normal subjects on which these norms are based for each of the test are shown in Table 3.

Table 3
Number of Subjects for Tests in Normative Group

Test	Number
Halstead-Reitan Battery and WAIS	486
Aphasia Screening Test	352
Pegboard & Dynamometer	475
Wisconsin Card Sorting Test	195
Thurstone Word Fluency	202
Tonal Memory	196
Digit Vigilance Test	280
Story Memory Test	186
Figure Memory Test	166
Peabody Individual Achievement Test	135
Boston Naming Test	107
Boston Diagnostic Aphasia Exam (Complex Ideational Material)	186

Note. Reproduced by special permission from the Publisher, Psychological Assessment Resources, Inc., from *Comprehensive Norms for an Expanded Halstead-Reitan Battery: Demographic Corrections, Research Findings, and Clinical Applications* (p. 5) by R. K. Heaton, I. Grant, and C. G. Matthews, 1991, Odessa: Psychological Assessment Resources, Inc. Copyright 1991 by Psychological Assessment Resources, Inc. All rights reserved.

These subjects all "completed structured interviews in which they denied any history of learning disability, neurological disease, other illnesses that affect brain function, significant head trauma, serious psychiatric disorder (e.g., schizophrenia), or alcohol or other drug abuse" (Heaton et al., 1991, p. 5).

1. Assessment of *level of performance* is the most commonly used method of drawing inferences from test data. Most psychologists are familiar with this method of inference, having used it in evaluating data from intelligence tests and other types of assessment material. There is a long history, for example, in the psychological literature of tests such as the Benton Visual Retention Test (Benton, 1963), the Background Interference Procedures of Canter (1970), and the Memory for Designs Test (Graham & Kendall, 1960), which correlate the patient's overall level of performance with the presence or absence of brain impairment. We discussed in chapter 1 the problems inherent in the use of any single test for making inferences about this question. The sole reliance on the use of level of performance as a method of inference regarding brain damage is also subject to other frequent misunderstandings. The level of performance on any single measure is not in itself definitive evidence of the presence or absence of a brain lesion. "In fact, it is a serious mistake to assume that one or more test scores beyond the accepted cut-off scores always indicate the presence of an acquired cerebral disorder" (Heaton et al., 1991, p. 36). They point out that of 455 neurologically normal subjects from whom 40 test scores including the HRB and WAIS were available only 10% has no scores in the impaired range, and the group *median* was four scores in the impaired range.

Two additional factors should be considered in assessing the level of performance on the various test scores and indices of the battery. The first of these is that conditions other than identifiable brain damage can lower scores on many tests of the battery. Assessment of psychiatric patients particularly must be tempered with the fact that conditions such as depression and psychosis can lower these scores. Golden (1977), for example, has shown that the usual cut-off scores for the Halstead-Reitan Battery do not distinguish brain-damaged from neurologically intact patients in a psychiatric population as well as they do in a nonpsychiatric sample. There is, in fact, growing evidence for a neurochemical and/or metabolic basis for many psychiatric disturbances (e.g., Heaton & Crowley, 1981). The second factor that should be addressed is the fact that some patients with discrete localized brain lesions will perform in the nonimpaired range on many of the tests of the Battery. The implication of this is that the level of performance on tests of the Battery cannot by itself be taken as a definite indication of whether or not a patient has a brain impairing lesion.

2. Psychologists have also traditionally used the *pattern of performance* among different test scores as an indication of the presence or absence of brain impairment. Matarazzo (1972), for example, reviewed a number of studies in which Verbal IQ-Performance IQ differences were used to infer the presence or absence of brain damage. The Shipley Institute of Living Scale (Shipley, 1946) is one example of a number of other tests that have utilized comparisons of performance on different types of tasks as a means of inferring neurological disorder. Just as the sole reliance on level of performance as a method of inference will lead to many false conclusions, so will focusing only on interpretation of patterns of test scores.

In the following chapters the reader will find hypotheses regarding the implications of different patterns of test scores. These should be studied in such a way that the most common and most important of them will be obvious on inspection of test data. One of the relationships that illustrates the importance of answering the questions identified above in a logical sequence relates to the occasional effect of lateralized lesions on the difference between Verbal IQ and Performance IQ. One might mistakenly conclude that a patient has a right-cerebral hemisphere lesion because Performance IQ is considerably lower than Verbal IQ if one has not first arrived at a reasonable answer to the question of whether or not there is in fact sufficient evidence to conclude that the patient has brain damage.

Some of the other important hypotheses in subsequent chapters relate to interpretation of patterns on test scores (e.g., relationships between the scores on tests such as the

Seashore Rhythm Test and Speech Sounds Perception Test). The relationship between the scores on TPT, for example, and more purely motor tests have implications for anterior or posterior location of lesions. It is essential, however, to recognize the strength of the implications of each of these patterns, as well as any other patterns that one may consider.

3. While psychologists have historically tended to rely principally on the above two methods of inference, neurologists have focused more on differences in the sensory, motor, and reflex *functioning of the two sides of the body* to infer the presence and location of brain-impairing lesions. This method of inference results in the strongest implications for lateralization of the lesion. Data on the test battery that lead to this type of inference include the difference in performance of the two hands on the TPT, Finger Oscillation, Strength of Grip, Grooved Pegboard, and the Sensory Perceptual Examination. Discrepancies between the performance of the two sides of the body that exceed the normal expectations have very strong implications for lateralization and severity of a lesion.

4. Just as neurologists rely on differences in functioning of the two sides of the body, they also rely on the presence of *pathognomonic signs*, such as the Babinski reflex, in drawing conclusions about neurological disorders. The neuropsychologist also looks for such definitive signs of brain impairment, particularly on the Aphasia Screening Test and on the Sensory Perceptual Examination. When obvious aphasic signs are seen on the Aphasia Screening Test, or when consistent, reliable suppressions on one side of the body or visual field defects are found on the Sensory Perceptual Examination, these are pathognomonic signs of brain impairment, as well as indications of lateralization and sometimes localization.

Answers to the previously discussed critical questions should be attempted by the neuropsychologist using all four methods of inference. Reliance on only one or two of them may result in unfortunate false-positive or false-negative inferences. Use of level of performance alone, for example, may yield false-positive inferences because a number of other factors such as cultural deprivation, educational disadvantage, and various psychiatric conditions, may in turn lead to poor levels of performance on many tests. On the other hand, reliance only on the presence of pathognomonic signs, or differences in functioning of the two sides of the body, may lead to false-negative inferences, particularly when there are diffuse, generalized lesions. As Reitan (1967) and Reitan and Wolfson (1985) have suggested, the combination of these four methods of inference is the most powerful way of evaluating neuropsychological test data. When such data are considered from the perspectives of all four methods of inference, one is much less likely to make either false-negative or false-positive errors.

To summarize, these four methods of inference are complimentary and should be used in combination to interpret neuropsychological test data. In assessing the level of performance, the reader should refer to the section of the Guide on cut-off scores and consider the *T* scores for individual tests. Patterns of performance on different tests and subtests can be evaluated by referring to the individual test hypotheses. One should look for the presence of pathognomonic signs on the Aphasia Screening Test and the Sensory Perceptual Examination, while differential performance of the two sides of the body can be evaluated by comparing the results of the Sensory Perceptual Examination, Finger Oscillation Test, Strength of Grip, TPT, and Grooved Pegboard Test on the two sides of the body.

In analyzing neuropsychological test data from the Halstead-Reitan Battery, the use of this Guide should proceed through the following steps and questions.

First, transcribe the neuropsychological test data from the test records themselves onto a data summary sheet such as the one described in chapter 2 (Figure 1).

The next step for patients who are 20 years of age or older is to calculate T scores, which are corrected for age, education, and sex for the raw scores from the HRB tests, the WAIS, and certain other tests, using the norms provided by Heaton et al. (1991). The use of the norms is facilitated by entering data on the "Record Forms for Comprehensive Norms for an Expanded Halstead-Reitan Battery" in the following sequence:

1. Enter the age, education, and sex of the patient at the top of page 1. These will later be used to determine which T score table will be used.

2. Enter the raw scores for each measure under the proper column, being careful to use the correct unit of measure for each one: number of errors, number correct, time per block, and so forth.

3. Find the Scale Scores for each of the raw scores in Appendix C, and enter them in the correct column. The Scale Scores convert raw scores to a common metric, which has a Mean of 10 and a Standard Deviation of 3.

4. Find the correct table in Appendix D for the age, education, and sex of the patient and enter the T scores for each of the Scale Scores in the proper column. The T scores convert Scale Scores to a common metric, with a Mean of 50 and a Standard Deviation of 10, which are corrected for age, education, and sex.

5. Enter the T scores for each measure on pages 2 and 3 and plot them on the Profile.

Alternatively, one may use a computer program available from the same publisher. In that case, steps 1 and 2 are carried out by entering the same information into the computer, and the remaining steps are accomplished by the computer. Heaton et al. (1991, p. 21) note that the T scores generated by the computer program are "somewhat more precise," but that the differences between them and those derived from the printed manual are "fairly small." Use of the computer program also results in a significant saving of time and reduces the possibility of errors.

The computer program prints a # next to each T score that is below 40 to indicate that it is in the "impaired" range and prints an L next to each of the motor and sensory scores that has "possible lateralizing significance." In doing so it takes into consideration the effects of demographic variables identified by Thompson et al. (1987), rather than using the "traditional" rule of an expected 10% difference.

It is important to note that the WAIS (Wechsler, 1955), not the more recent WAIS-R (Wechsler, 1981), was used in the Heaton et al. (1991) study. Therefore, if one uses the WAIS-R, T scores should not be calculated from the tables in Heaton et al. (1991). Instead, Heaton (1992) should be consulted. This *Supplement* provides tables for determining T scores based on the WAIS-R (Wechsler, 1981) standardization sample. The computer program allows the use of either WAIS or WAIS-R scores.

Heaton et al. (1991, p. 16) have suggested a tentative classification of T scores for clinical interpretation. This is summarized in Table 4.

Table 4
Tentative Clinical Classification of *T* Scores

Classification	*T* score
Above Average	55+
Average	45-54
Below Average/Borderline	40-44
Mild Impairment	35-39
Mild-to-Moderate Impairment	30-34
Moderate Impairment	25-29
Moderate-to-Severe Impairment	20-24
Severe Impairment	1-19

Note. Adapted by special permission from the Publisher, Psychological Assessment Resources, Inc., from *Comprehensive Norms for an Expanded Halstead-Reitan Battery: Demographic Corrections, Research Findings, and Clinical Applications* (p. 16) by R. K. Heaton, I. Grant, and C. G. Matthews, 1991, Odessa: Psychological Assessment Resources, Inc. Copyright 1991 by Psychological Assessment Resources, Inc. All rights reserved.

It is important to note that these suggestions are more or less arbitrary and are based on clinical experience with a specific clinical population. With different populations, different cut-off scores for inferring brain impairment may be appropriate. Factors such as the acceptable false positive and false negative rates and the base rate for brain impairment in a population should be considered. Heaton et al. (1991, p. 16) have provided a detailed table for which the effect of changing the cut-off point for inferring impairment on the classification of their normal subjects can be determined. In a psychiatric population, for example, it may be appropriate to lower the cut-off score from 39 to 34, or even 29. A cut-off score of 39 will be used in the cases discussed in this volume.

There are certain situations in which raw scores or Scale Scores, rather than *T* scores, should be considered. On tests such as the Aphasia Screening Test (AST) and the Sensory Perceptual Examination (SPE), on which pathognomonic signs are sometimes seen, any errors are quite rare among normal subjects. Consequently, even a small number of errors will result in a lowered *T* score. When this occurs, it is important to examine the raw data to determine *how* and *why* the errors were made. When this is done, one may find, for example, that errors on the SPE were due to momentary lack of attention, or that spelling errors on the Aphasia Screening Test were due to lack of formal education.

Although the Adult version of the HRB is used with patients at least 15 years old, *T* scores can only be calculated for patients age 20 and older. Jarvis and Barth (1984) recommended the use of a profile which was an adaptation of the work of Russell et al. (1970). There were, however, only 26 neurologically normal subjects in the control group on which this profile was based. Furthermore, they were all male, and the mean age was 44.54 years, making this a clearly inappropriate group on which to base judgments about patients ages 15-19. At some point in the future, a truly equivalent normative group may become available for use with these younger "adult" patients. The mean age of the subjects in the Heaton et al. (1991) study was only slightly lower than those in the Russell et al. (1970) control group, but approximately 34% of them were females, and they were probably a more culturally diverse group, since the Russell et al. (1970) subjects were all patients in a Veterans Administration hospital. For these reasons, we recommend using a Profile of <u>Scale Scores</u> based on the Heaton et al. (1991) study. To do this, one should circle the raw score for each test on a Profile such as the one in Figure 2. It is important to recognize that these <u>Scale Scores</u> are *not* corrected for age, education, or gender.

The next step is to address each of the critical questions using the four methods of inference. The hypotheses used in this process are presented in chapters 4-7, and illustrations of the process are provided in chapter 11.

Questions to be Answered

1. *Is there cerebral impairment?*

Level of performance. T scores below 40 should be reviewed, with special attention paid to those tests most sensitive to cerebral impairment. The hypotheses in chapter 4 are most important here.

Pattern of performance. The relevant hypotheses in chapter 4 should be checked for relationships shown on the *T* score profile that are deviant from normal expectations. The hypotheses regarding the WAIS scores are particularly important here.

Right-left differences. The performance on the TPT, Finger Oscillation, and Strength of Grip Tests, and the difference in performance of the two sides of the body on the Sensory Perceptual Examination should all be checked for deviations from the expected performance. Such deviations have relevance for this question as well as the later one regarding lateralization.

Pathognomonic signs. Hypotheses regarding these signs will be found among those related to the Aphasia Screening Test and the Sensory Perceptual Examination. The presence of any such signs in the data is a strong argument for an affirmative answer to this question with regard to the presence or absence of brain impairment. As indicated earlier, it is important to examine the raw data in this regard.

2. *What is the severity of the cerebral dysfunction?*

Level of performance. The pattern of the *T* scores on the profile sheet should be examined in terms of the degree of impairment on each of the tests. Particular attention should be paid to those tests that are most sensitive to impairment and to those that represent functions most important to the patient being examined.

Pattern of performance. Here it is the magnitude of the deviation from expected patterns of performance that is most relevant regarding the question of severity. A particular relationship must be considered in the context of each individual patient. For example, a Verbal IQ 15 points below a Performance IQ has different implications for an attorney than for a mechanic.

Right-left differences. Once again the magnitude of the difference from expected performance is the key factor in assessing severity.

Pathognomonic signs. Generally, the presence of any pathognomonic sign indicates definite impairment, and, of course, a greater number of such signs suggests greater severity.

3. Is the lesion progressive or static?

Level of performance. The hypotheses regarding specific tests in chapter 4 should be checked for indications regarding velocity. One should note that it is often possible to state with more confidence that a lesion is relatively static than that it is progressive. For example, adequate performance on the Seashore Rhythm and Speech Sounds Perception Tests makes a progressive lesion less likely, but poor performance on these tests can result from factors other than a progressive lesion.

Pattern of performance. The hypotheses related to WAIS performance in chapter 4 are the most relevant ones regarding this question.

Right-left differences. This method of inference does not usually yield useful information regarding this question.

Pathognomonic signs. Certain pathognomonic signs are frequently seen in cases with rapidly progressive lesions, but one should note that they may still be present, if there has been actual tissue destruction, even after a lesion has become static and chronic.

4. Is the lesion diffuse or lateralized?

Level of performance. This method of inference does not yield information relevant to this question.

Pattern of performance. The hypotheses in chapter 4 should be checked against the data for lateralizing signs. One should note, however, that the lateralizing signs seen in patterns of performance are all relatively weak ones.

Right-left differences. This is the method of inference that is most useful in answering the question of diffuse versus lateralized lesions. Differences in the performance on the two sides of the body should be checked carefully on the TPT, Finger Oscillation, Strength of Grip, Grooved Pegboard Test, and Sensory Perceptual Examination. As indicated earlier, the use of the Heaton et al. (1991) computer program facilitates identification of potentially significant relationships.

Pathognomonic signs. Pathognomonic signs, which may be found on the Aphasia Screening Test and Sensory Perceptual Examination, are also among the most powerful indicators of lateralization.

5. Is the impairment in the anterior or posterior portion of the cerebral hemisphere?

Level of performance. This method of inference does not yield information relevant to this question.

Pattern of performance. The most useful patterns of performance to be considered are those described in the hypotheses relating performance on motor tasks compared to sensory tasks. Other hypotheses regarding patterns of WAIS subtest scores (e.g., BD-PA) and constructional dyspraxia should also be considered.

SCALED SCORE EQUIVALENTS OF TEST RAW SCORES

Scaled scores	HII	AIR	CAT ERROR	TRAIL A	TRAIL B	TPT TIME	TPT MEM	TPT LOC	SSHOR RHYM	SPCH PERC	APHAS SCRN	SPAT REL	SP TOTAL	Scaled scores
19	–	0.00-0.11	0-5	0-11	0-22	0-0.175	–	10	30	0	–	–	–	19
18	–	0.12-0.15	6	12	23-25	0.176-0.182	–	9	–	–	–	–	–	18
17	–	0.16-0.22	7-8	13	26-29	0.183-0.195	10	–	–	–	–	–	–	17
16	–	0.23-0.29	9-10	14	30-33	0.196-0.215	–	–	–	–	–	–	0	16
15	–	0.30-0.39	11-12	15-16	34-37	0.216-0.235	–	8	–	1	–	–	–	15
14	–	0.40-0.48	13-14	17	38-42	0.236-0.259	9	7	29	–	–	–	–	14
13	0.0	0.49-0.56	15-17	18-19	43-46	0.260-0.285	–	–	–	2	0	–	1.0	13
12	0.1	0.57-0.65	18-21	20-21	47-51	0.286-0.325	–	6	28	3	1	–	–	12
11	–	0.66-0.80	22-27	22-24	52-57	0.326-0.372	8	5	27	4	–	2	1.5-2.4	11
10	0.3	0.81-0.99	28-35	25-27	58-66	0.373-0.429	–	4	26	5	2-3	–	2.5-3.4	10
9	0.4	1.00-1.15	36-47	28-31	67-78	0.430-0.495	7	3	25	6	4	3	3.5-5.4	9
8	–	1.16-1.30	48-59	32-35	79-91	0.496-0.635	–	2	24	7	5-6	–	5.5-6.9	8
7	0.6	1.31-1.45	60-73	36-41	92-110	0.636-0.768	6	–	23	8-9	7-8	4	7.0-9.9	7
6	0.7	1.46-1.80	74-83	42-49	111-130	0.769-0.949	5	1	21-22	10-12	9-12	–	10.0-13.4	6
5	–	1.81-2.00	84-95	50-60	131-178	0.950-1.189	4	0	19-20	13-16	13-15	5	13.5-16.4	5
4	0.9	2.01-2.35	96-107	61-69	179-236	1.190-1.999	3	–	17-18	17-22	16-18	–	16.5-24.4	4
3	–	2.36-3.07	108-117	70-83	237-277	2.000-2.249	2	–	15-16	23-29	19-21	6	24.5-31.9	3
2	–	3.08-3.50	118-124	84-95	278-300	2.250-2.500	1	–	12-14	30-34	22-75	–	32.0-48.9	2
1	1.0	3.51-3.75	125-135	96+	301+	2.501-2.999	0	–	0-11	35-60	–	7-8	49.0+	1
0	–	3.76-5.00	136-208	–	–	3.000	–	–	–	–	–	9-12	–	0

Scaled scores	TAP DH	TAP NDH	GRIP DH	GRIP NDH	PEG DH	PEG NDH	TPT DH	TPT NDH	TPT BH	SP R	SP L	TFR R	TFR L	Scaled Scores
19	70.0+	66.1+	75.0+	70.0+	0-44	0-43	0-0.199	0-0.129	0-0.069	–	–	0-4.3	0-4.2	19
18	68.0-69.9	63.7-66.0	73.5-74.9	67.5-69.9	45	44-47	0.200-0.219	0.130-0.139	0.070-0.079	–	–	4.4-5.1	4.3-4.9	18
17	66.1-67.9	59.2-63.6	70.0-73.4	65.5-67.4	46	48-50	0.220-0.239	0.140-0.149	0.080-0.089	–	–	5.2-5.5	5.0-5.3	17
16	63.1-66.0	57.1-59.1	66.1-69.9	62.0-65.4	47-48	51	0.240-0.269	0.150-0.179	0.090-0.099	0	–	5.6-6.3	5.4-5.7	16
15	60.5-63.0	55.3-57.0	62.5-66.0	58.0-61.9	49-50	52-54	0.270-0.299	0.180-0.209	0.100-0.119	–	–	6.4-6.9	5.8-6.5	15
14	57.8-60.4	53.4-55.2	58.5-62.4	55.0-57.9	51-53	55-56	0.300-0.339	0.210-0.239	0.120-0.139	–	–	7.0-7.9	6.6-7.0	14
13	55.9-57.7	51.2-53.3	54.5-58.4	51.0-54.9	54-55	57-59	0.340-0.389	0.240-0.269	0.140-0.159	–	–	8.0-8.5	7.1-7.9	13
12	54.0-55.8	49.0-51.1	51.0-54.4	46.5-50.9	56-59	60-62	0.390-0.429	0.270-0.319	0.160-0.189	1.0	–	8.6-9.5	8.0-8.4	12
11	52.0-53.9	46.6-48.9	46.5-50.9	43.0-46.4	60-62	63-66	0.430-0.489	0.320-0.379	0.190-0.219	–	0.0-0.4	9.6-10.5	8.5-9.4	11
10	49.5-51.9	44.4-46.5	40.0-46.4	37.5-42.9	63-66	67-70	0.490-0.569	0.380-0.439	0.220-0.259	1.5-2.4	0.5-1.4	10.6-12.0	9.5-11.1	10
9	46.3-49.4	42.0-44.3	34.0-39.9	30.5-37.4	67-70	71-75	0.570-0.669	0.440-0.539	0.260-0.319	2.5-3.4	1.5-1.9	12.1-14.4	11.2-13.2	9
8	43.2-46.2	38.8-41.9	29.5-33.9	26.0-30.4	71-74	76-80	0.670-0.779	0.540-0.669	0.320-0.399	3.5-4.4	2.0-2.9	14.5-16.9	13.3-15.2	8
7	41.0-43.1	36.0-38.7	26.0-29.4	23.0-25.9	75-82	81-86	0.780-0.939	0.670-0.869	0.400-0.539	4.5-5.4	3.0-3.9	17.0-19.0	15.3-17.4	7
6	37.7-40.9	34.0-35.9	24.0-25.9	21.0-22.9	83-89	87-97	0.940-1.299	0.870-1.109	0.540-0.689	5.5-7.4	4.0-5.4	19.1-22.0	17.5-19.4	6
5	34.0-37.6	31.3-33.9	21.5-23.9	19.0-20.9	90-101	98-110	1.300-1.749	1.110-1.559	0.690-0.899	7.5-10.9	5.5-6.9	22.1-24.4	19.5-23.4	5
4	31.0-33.9	28.8-31.2	18.0-21.4	16.0-18.9	102-119	111-122	1.750-2.339	1.560-2.699	0.900-1.599	11.0-13.4	7.0-10.9	24.5-27.9	23.5-25.9	4
3	27.1-30.9	26.4-28.7	14.1-17.9	14.0-15.9	120-149	123-169	2.340-2.779	2.700-3.799	1.600-2.999	13.5-17.9	11.0-19.0	28.0-29.9	26.0-28.4	3
2	23.1-27.0	25.8-26.3	9.6-14.0	9.6-13.9	150-165	170-178	2.780-10.00	3.800-4.499	3.000-6.999	18.0-24.9	19.5+	30.0-32.9	28.5-31.9	2
1	19.9-23.0	19.9-25.7	5.0-9.5	5.0-9.5	166-200	179-200	10.01+	4.500-6.999	7.000+	25.0+	–	33.0-99.9+	32.0-99.9+	1
0	0-19.8	0-19.8	0-4.9	0-4.9	201-300	201-300	–	7.000+	–	–	–	–	–	0

Figure 2. Profile of scale scores.

Note. Reproduced by special permission from the Publisher, Psychological Assessment Resources, Inc., from *Comprehensive Norms for an Expanded Halstead-Reitan Battery: Demographic Corrections, Research Findings, and Clinical Applications* (pp. 46-47) by R. K. Heaton, I. Grant, and C. G. Matthews, 1991, Odessa: Psychological Assessment Resources, Inc. Copyright 1991 by Psychological Assessment Resources, Inc. All rights reserved.

Scaled scores	WORD FLUEN	BOST NAME	BDAE COMP	WCST PSVR	SSHOR TONAL	DIGIT TIME	DIGIT ERROR	STORY LEARN	STORY LOSS	FIGUR LEARN	FIGUR LOSS	PIAT RECOG	PIAT COMP	PIAT SPELL	Scaled scores
19	–	–	–	–	–	–	–	–	–	–	–	–	–	–	19
18	104+	85	–	–	–	0-242	–	25.01+	–	21.5+	–	–	–	–	18
17	102-103	84	–	0-4	30+	243-263	–	24.01-25.00	–	20.00-21.40	–	95+	95+	99	17
16	89-101	–	–	–	–	264-270	–	23.01-24.00	–	19.10-19.90	–	91-94	93-94	–	16
15	85-88	83	–	–	–	271-279	–	21.51-23.00	–	18.80-19.00	–	86-90	91-92	–	15
14	76-84	82	–	5	29	280-293	0	21.01-21.50	–	17.81-18.70	–	81-85	90	98	14
13	66-75	81	–	–	28	294-318	–	18.51-21.00	0-2.5	17.31-17.80	–	74-80	89	95-97	13
12	58-65	79-80	12	6	27	319-339	1	17.51-18.50	2.6-6.5	15.71-17.30	0.0-5.0	67-73	88	89-94	12
11	54-57	77-78	–	7-9	25-26	340-362	2	15.01-17.50	6.6-9.5	15.01-15.70	5.1-5.6	55-66	84-87	77-88	11
10	47-53	76	–	10-14	22-24	363-388	3-4	10.76-15.00	9.6-11.5	14.01-15.00	5.7-10.5	44-54	80-83	66-76	10
9	42-46	73-75	11	15-21	20-21	389-408	5-7	9.81-10.75	11.6-15.5	8.01-14.00	10.6-15.7	36-43	65-79	42-65	9
8	35-41	67-72	–	22-28	17-19	409-460	8-10	8.60-9.80	15.6-19.2	5.81-8.00	15.8-22.5	27-35	47-64	27-41	8
7	29-34	62-66	10	29-38	14-16	461-511	11-15	7.55-8.59	19.3-22.0	4.50-5.80	22.6-30.0	19-26	32-46	9-26	7
6	25-28	56-61	–	39-45	11-13	512-554	16-21	6.31-7.54	22.1-27.5	2.80-4.49	30.1-37.5	8-18	22-31	5-8	6
5	21-24	52-55	9	46-53	8-10	555-598	22-27	4.91-6.30	27.6-32.4	2.21-2.79	37.6-43.8	6-7	5-21	2-4	5
4	16-20	42-51	–	54-78	0-7	599-601	28-35	4.01-4.90	32.5-40.6	1.96-2.20	43.9-52.9	4-5	3-4	1	4
3	10-15	35-41	8	79-90	–	–	36-47	2.71-4.00	40.7-43.2	1.20-1.95	53.0-73.3	2-3	1-2	–	3
2	0-9	18-34	4-7	91-100	–	–	48-59	0-2.70	43.3-50.4	0-1.19	73.4-100.0	1	–	–	2
1	–	0-17	0-3	101-110	–	60-69	–	–	50.5-70.0	–	–	–	–	–	1
0	–	–	–	111-127	–	70+	–	–	70.1-100.0	–	–	0	0	0	0

Scaled scores	VIQ	PIQ	FSIQ	INFO	DIGIT SPAN	VOCAB	ARITH	COMP	SIMIL	PICT COMP	PICT ARR	BLOCK DESGN	OBJ ASSMB	DIGIT SYM	Scaled scores
19	–	–	–	–	–	–	–	–	–	–	–	–	–	–	19
18	142+	140+	141+	–	19	–	–	–	–	–	18	–	–	19	18
17	139-141	137-139	139-140	19	–	19	–	–	19	18	17	–	18	18	17
16	138	134-136	135-138	18	–	18	–	19	18	–	16	17	17	17	16
15	134-137	130-133	132-134	17	16	17	17	18	17	16	15	16	16	16	15
14	130-133	125-129	129-131	16	15	16	16	17	16	–	14	15	15	15	14
13	126-129	121-124	124-128	15	14	15	15	16	15	14	13	14	14	14	13
12	122-125	117-120	121-123	14	–	14	14	15	14	13	12	13	13	13	12
11	118-121	114-116	117-120	13	12	13	13	14	13	12	11	12	12	12	11
10	111-117	109-113	111-116	12	11	12	12	13	12	11	10	11	11	11	10
9	105-110	106-108	106-110	11	10	11	11	12	11	10	9	10	10	10	9
8	100-104	102-105	103-105	10	9	10	10	11	10	9	8	9	9	9	8
7	96-99	99-101	99-102	9	–	9	9	10	9	8	7	8	8	8	7
6	93-95	95-98	94-98	8	7	8	8	9	8	7	6	7	7	7	6
5	88-92	90-94	90-93	7	6	7	7	8	7	6	5	6	6	6	5
4	84-87	86-89	85-89	6	–	6	6	7	6	5	4	5	5	5	4
3	82-83	82-85	83-84	5	4	5	5	6	5	4	3	4	4	4	3
2	76-81	76-81	76-82	4	–	4	4	5	4	3	2	3	3	3	2
1	70-75	70-75	70-75	3	2	3	3	4	3	2	1	2	2	2	1
0	<70	<70	<70	0-2	0-1	0-2	0-2	0-3	0-2	0-1	0	0-1	0-1	0-1	0

Figure 2. Profile of scale scores (continued).

Right-left difference. This method of inference does not yield information relevant to this question.

Pathognomonic signs. Some pathognomonic signs may have very specific implications for localization, and the hypotheses related to any such signs should be checked carefully. Visual field defects are a prime example of this.

6.   *What is the most likely neuropathological process?*

The answer to this question is based first on a review of the answers to the preceding five questions. On this basis one can first determine which broad neuropathological category must be considered. For example, if a diffuse, slowly progressive lesion is involved, the focus must be on the degenerative or infectious processes. On the other hand, if a highly lateralized, acute, or progressive picture is presented, the destructive neoplastic and vascular conditions should be considered. Once such a general process category has been identified, it is necessary to review the specific hypotheses related to all of the individual possibilities within that category described in chapter 7. In this way, fairly accurate answers can frequently be formulated to this question. This can be a very intriguing result. It is important to remember, however, that this is not the most important function of the neuropsychologist. It is, of course, essential to consider the patient's history in real clinical cases.

7.   *What are the implications for daily functioning and treatment?*

The patient's performance on the tests in the battery provides the neuropsychologist with a sample of the abilities required for everyday activities. In order to generalize from this sample or to predict functioning in other activities, the requirements for performance of the tests described in chapter 2 must be considered. It is also important to evaluate both the strengths and weaknesses shown by the patient and consider them in relationship to the hypotheses on functional implications in chapter 8 and the suggestions for rehabilitation in chapter 11. As those chapters indicate, the data supporting inferences in these areas are less well established than those in some other areas, and appropriate caution should be observed. These are the areas of clinical neuropsychology in which the most important developments should be expected in the next few years.

CAVEAT

Although significant new developments, which should improve the accuracy of interpretation, are described in this volume the caveat offered earlier by Jarvis and Barth (1984) remains pertinent:

> While it is hoped that this Guide will be an aid, particularly for psychologists in mental health settings, to the better understanding of and cautious interpretation of neuropsychological test data on adult patients, it must be emphasized that users not overextend the limits of this Guide and their formal training. Some of the developments in the field of clinical neuropsychology have been dramatic, and one may be tempted to

> make highly specific diagnoses or predictions about the location and nature of brain lesions. To do so, however, without a high level of accuracy, will not only decrease the credibility of the individual practitioner and the entire profession, but more importantly, will do grave disservice to many patients. It is to these concerns that this caveat is addressed. (p. 36)

By now many psychologists have been exposed to the extremely detailed and usually accurate interpretation that experts such as Reitan can make from standardized test battery data. Furthermore, Goldstein, Daysack, and Kleinknecht (1973) have demonstrated that psychology interns can be trained in a relatively short period of time to make valid identifications of the presence of brain impairment using the Halstead-Reitan Battery. One must remember, however, that the predictions made by the subjects in the Goldstein et al. (1973) study were not as detailed as the predictions made by many of the experts in the field. It is also important for the clinical psychologist working in the typical mental health setting to remember that Reitan and his associates have worked primarily in neurosurgical departments of medical schools. In these settings they were dealing with very different populations than those with which most psychologists in the typical clinical settings are faced. Also, it is important to remember that they had exposure to thousands of cases with demonstrated cerebral pathology. This Guide is in no way intended to substitute for this type of vast experience.

There are other problems in making highly refined diagnoses and specific statements regarding localizations of lesions that some psychologists may have overlooked. The first of these is that many of our anatomical descriptions are quite general. Meyer (1955), quoting Bailey, states, "It must be realized that the various regions of the brain do not constitute functional subdivisions in any sense. The lobes were originally named after the cranial bones under which they lie and as such represent a crude anatomical classification" (1961, p. 555).

A further complication of this general "map" of the cortex stems from the nature and effect of pathological lesions with which we are dealing. Any lesion, whether due to atrophy, tumor, trauma, or other pathology may not affect a clearly limited area of the brain and the functions mediated by that area. Instead, it may exert effects through disruption of blood supply, pressure effects on other parts of the brain, and disruptions of connections between various areas of the cerebral hemispheres. Surgical intervention can have similar effects, although in many of these cases there remains considerable uncertainty as to the extent of pathology in portions of the brain that were not directly exposed during surgery. Another factor limiting even the work of Reitan and others who have been involved in his tradition with neurosurgical patients is that it is frequently not possible to obtain definite information about either the premorbid condition of the brain or the premorbid functioning of the patient. This factor is certainly more significant to psychologists working in a mental health setting where this evidence is even more difficult to obtain in a way that would permit detailed comparison with current performance on a complex neuropsychological test battery.

As a final word in this admonitory section, it must be stressed again that the psychologist in most mental health settings seldom sees the "clean" cases on which the Halstead-Reitan Battery research was developed. Instead, one is more likely to see a 60-year-old chronic alcoholic patient who has incurred multiple head injuries while intoxicated, suffers from malnutrition, and has been institutionalized for a long period of time either in a traditional institution or in one of our newer community settings. There is frequently little reliable medical or social history available and there are few cues from the fragmentary vocational background as to the patient's premorbid or optimal level of functioning in almost any area. If this is not complicated enough, the patient may be psychotic at times and the referral question may be "Please differentiate organicity from schizophrenia or other psychosis." While this case is extreme, it is not uncommon for referrals to present several of the above complications. This illustrates the difficulties and dangers of extrapolating from clean neurosurgical case to the complex realities of life of many practicing clinical psychologists.

The reader should also note that this Guide addresses only the neuropsychological evaluation of adult patients. While there is a growing body of literature in the field of clinical neuropsychology of children, results are not generally as clear-cut and one should not attempt to extrapolate totally from the hypotheses or inferences included here to the assessment of children.

It is hoped that these cautionary statements will prompt the reader not to overdiagnose or make unwarranted statements about the presence or absence of brain damage and not to formulate rash predictions concerning the location and nature of brain pathology. It is instead hoped that this Guide will be a useful tool in understanding and interpreting neuropsychological test data, and that it will aid in formulating more useful treatment plans for patients.

Chapter 4

Test Hypotheses

Impairment Index

As indicated earlier, the Halstead Impairment Index is a composite measure of the level of performance on the tests of the Halstead-Reitan Battery. It simply indicates the proportion of those test scores that are in the range characteristic of brain-impaired patients; therefore, all of the considerations regarding interpretation of level of performance indicators identified in chapter 2 should be observed in evaluating the Impairment Index. One should also note that this Index is correlated with age and education and that the significance of an elevated Impairment Index decreases with increasing age or low education as indicated below. Taking these factors into consideration, however, the Impairment Index is still the most sensitive indicator of brain impairment (Wheeler, Burke, & Reitan, 1963).

While the level of the Impairment Index is often interpreted as an indicator of the severity of brain damage, one needs to recognize that it is possible to have an Impairment Index of 1.0 (all of the tests in the battery in the impaired range) with only a mild degree of impairment. For example, if a patient has 52 errors on the Category Test; scores on the TPT of 16 minutes total time, memory-5 and location-4; 24 items correct on the Seashore Rhythm Test; 14 errors on the Speech Sounds Perception Test; and a Finger Tapping score of 50 with the dominant hand, he/she would have an Impairment Index of 1.0. Since each of these scores is just barely in the impaired range, however, it should be clear that the overall impairment is mild even though all of the scores fall beyond the cut-off points.

(4-1) The most sensitive general indicators of brain impairment (level of performance scores) are: 1) Impairment Index, 2) Category, 3) TPT Localization, and 4) Trails B, in that order of significance (Reitan, 1959a).

(4-2) The significance of an elevated Impairment Index decreases with age, particularly after age 40. This is corrected for by the use of T Scores (Heaton et al., 1991).

(4-3) Prognosis for recovery of language functions is relatively good even with clear-cut indications of left-cerebral hemisphere damage if the Impairment Index is relatively low and certain other scores such as Category, Speech Sounds Perception and Seashore Rhythm are adequate (Reitan, 1959a).

(4-4) Patients with Parkinson's disease often perform poorly on the Category Test, tend to have relatively high impairment indices, and perform poorly on Trail Making; their IQs may be in the average range (Reitan & Boll, 1971).

(4-5) The Impairment Index tends to be higher in cases with tissue destruction such as intracerebral neoplasms, cerebrovascular accidents (CVAs), and penetrating head injuries, and may be lower in cases of extracerebral neoplasms and some mild-to-moderate closed head injuries (Golden, 1978).

WAIS or WAIS-R

The Full Scale IQ on the Wechsler Adult Intelligence Scale, when viewed from the perspective of level of performance, is primarily useful when it is compared to other data. Previous performance on this same test is the best comparative data to determine whether or not there is an overall deterioration in intellectual functioning. Many times previous testing is not available, however, and one must use estimates of previous level of intellectual functioning such as educational and vocational background. A person with a college degree and a vocational history consistent with his/her education, for example, who achieves a Full Scale IQ of only 80 is demonstrating a significant level of impairment whether this is due to identifiable brain damage or a psychiatric condition.

The data from the WAIS, however, should also be considered in terms of the pattern of scores on the Verbal IQ (VIQ), Performance IQ (PIQ), and the individual subtests. The hypotheses in this section indicate a number of important relationships among scores. The pattern of subtest scores often yields valuable information about strengths and weaknesses that may be useful in planning rehabilitation programs.

(4-6) IQ tends to be negatively correlated with Category scores (Cullum, Steiner, & Begler, 1984).

(4-7) If there is a strong indication of cerebral impairment, yet IQ scores are relatively unimpaired, a static lesion is suggested and possibly a more anterior lesion (Golden et al., 1981).

(4-8) Patients with Parkinson's disease often perform poorly on the Category Test, tend to have relatively high impairment indices, and perform poorly on Trail Making; their IQs may be in the average range (Reitan & Boll, 1971).

(4-9) Closed head injuries can produce mild and often diffuse damage, which may not significantly affect Full Scale IQ or create a difference between VIQ and PIQ. With this type of pathology one may see mixed signs or different levels of impairment because of the contrecoup and shear strain effects (Binder, 1986).

VIQ-PIQ Differences

(4-10) When PIQ is 20 or more points lower than VIQ on the WAIS, this suggests the possibility of right-cerebral hemisphere impairment. When the reverse is true, left-cerebral hemisphere impairment is suspected. One must temper this finding with the fact that the PIQ is more likely to be affected by a cerebral lesion than is VIQ due to the fact that the Performance subtests involve new and unique learning; while Verbal subtests measure accumulated knowledge, which is the least affected by brain impairment (Reitan, 1955a, 1959a).

(4-11) Extracerebral tumors rarely result in significant VIQ-PIQ differences (Reitan, 1972; Reitan & Wolfson, 1993).

(4-12) Localizing or lateralizing signs in the *absence* of depressed FSIQ and with little PIQ/VIQ difference suggest the absence of intracerebral tumor or vascular disorder (Golden et al., 1981; Reitan, 1959a).

(4-13) No significant difference between VIQ and PIQ suggests either diffuse impairment and/or a static (or slowly progressive) lesion (Reitan, 1959a).

(4-14) When there are definite indications of left-cerebral hemisphere damage such as dysphasia and lowered VIQ but no indication of left-cerebral hemisphere signs on TPT and Tapping, this suggests a focal lesion located at some distance from the motor strip (Reitan, 1959a).

(4-15) The greatest VIQ/PIQ differences are often seen with intrinsic neoplasms (Reitan & Wolfson, 1993).

(4-16) Extrinsic neoplasms frequently do not show any differences between VIQ and PIQ (Reitan & Wolfson, 1993).

Similarities

(4-15) A very low score on Similarities suggests left temporal lobe impairment. A normal score on Similarities, however, does not suggest the absence of left temporal lobe impairment (Reitan, 1959a), but this is a weak indicator of a focal lesion.

Block Design and Picture Arrangement

(4-16) A Block Design score significantly lower than the Picture Arrangement score suggests a right parietal-occipital lesion, while a Picture Arrangement score lower than the Block Design score suggests a right anterior temporal lobe lesion (Reitan, 1959a).

(4-17) If Picture Arrangement and Block Design scores are both depressed, a right temporal-parietal lesion is suggested (Reitan, 1959a).

(4-18) Although low Picture Arrangement scores are most often associated with right anterior temporal lobe lesions, they are more often associated with right frontal lobe lesions when several of the pictures are left in the original, but incorrect, order (McFie & Thompson, 1972).

Digit Symbol

(4-19) One of the most sensitive general indicators of cerebral impairment is Digit Symbol, provided there are other signs of impairment on the Halstead-Reitan Battery (Golden, 1978).

Digit Span

(4-20) Although Digit Span may be affected by neurological impairment, it is also affected by many other factors. Therefore, a low score on this subtest is not a good indication of brain damage (Reitan & Wolfson, 1993).

Information and Vocabulary

(4-21) Mortenson, Gade, and Reinisch (1991) have cast doubt on the notion that Information and Vocabulary are less susceptible to the effects of brain impairment than other subtests, and for this reason, other indications of pre-morbid cognitive functioning should be sought.

Picture Completion

(4-22) Picture Completion is not particularly sensitive to neurological impairment, and low scores on this subtest have no special significance (Reitan & Wolfson, 1993).

Category Test

As indicated, the Category Test is the single test most sensitive to damage to any area of the brain. Occasionally, however, one will see a patient with demonstrable neurological impairment who performs quite well on this test. One young man, for example, who had suffered a severe closed head injury, performed very well on the Category Test, making only 14 errors. This is a very good score on this test (*T* score = 63) for a person with his education (12 years) and IQ (Full Scale IQ 114). This level of performance obviously has major implications for the rehabilitation of this man who has severe motor and sensory impairments due to his injury.

(4-23) The most sensitive general indicators of brain impairment (level of performance scores) are: (a) Impairment Index, (b) Category, (c) TPT Localization, and (d) Trails B, in that order of significance (Reitan, 1959a).

(4-24) IQ, particularly PIQ, tends to be negatively correlated with Category scores (Logue & Allen, 1971; Cullum et al., 1984).

(4-25) If scores on both Category and Part B of Trail Making are poor, while other tests are near normal, a focal and static lesion of one or both anterior frontal lobes may be suggested (Reitan, 1959a).

(4-26) Adequate performance on the Category Test and the Seashore Rhythm Test, even in the presence of a high Impairment Index and poor performance on other tests, does not appear consistent with either intracerebral tumors or massive CVAs (Reitan, 1972; Reitan & Wolfson, 1993).

(4-27) Prognosis for recovery of language functions is relatively good even with clear-cut indications of left-cerebral hemisphere damage if the Impairment Index is relatively low and certain other scores such as Category, Speech Sounds Perception, and Seashore Rhythm are good (Reitan, 1959a).

(4-28) Patients with Parkinson's disease often perform poorly on the Category Test, Trail Making and motor tests and tend to have relatively high impairment indices; their IQs may be in the average range (Reitan & Boll, 1971).

(4-29) Alcoholics may perform very poorly on the Category Test and memory tests and show impaired performance on other tests of the HRB, but have intact IQs (Grant, 1987).

(4-30) Patients with MS often perform well on the Category Test, but poorly on the TPT (Reitan & Wolfson, 1993).

Trail Making Test

The Trail Making Test, particularly Part B, is one of the more sensitive general indicators of neurological impairment. The score on Part B may also have implications for certain aspects of the patient's daily functioning. For example, a particularly poor score on Part B indicates that the patient has difficulty in following complex patterns of visual stimuli involving alternation between two sets of symbols.

One of the hypotheses in this section indicates that the difference between the scores on Part A and Part B on the Trail Making Test may have some implications for lateralization to one cerebral hemisphere or the other. It should be noted, however, that the implication of this difference for lateralization is not a strong one, and inferences about lateralization of a lesion should never be based on this relationship alone.

(4-31) The most sensitive general indicators of level of brain impairment (performance scores) are: (a) Impairment Index, (b) Category, (c) TPT Localization, and (d) Trails B, in that order of significance (Reitan, 1959a).

(4-32) A score on Trails B that is substantially poorer than the score on Trails A suggests left-hemisphere impairment, while a lower score on Part A suggests right-cerebral hemisphere impairment. This is a weak hypothesis unless substantiated by other data (Reitan & Tarshes, 1959).

(4-33) If scores on both Category and Part B of Trail Making are poor while other tests are near normal, a focal and static lesion of one or both anterior frontal lobes may be suggested (Reitan, 1959a). This is a weak hypothesis since neither test is sensitive only to frontal pathology.

(4-34) Patients with Parkinson's disease often perform poorly on the Category Test, tend to have relatively high impairment indices, and perform poorly on Trail Making; their IQs may be in the average range (Reitan & Boll, 1971).

Tactual Performance Test

While the localization score on the TPT is one of the more sensitive general indicators of neurological impairment, the most valuable information derived from the scores on this test is the difference in performance between the dominant and nondominant hands. As indicated in the following hypotheses, this has strong implications for lateralization of lesions.

Since the TPT is a test with very complex requirements for satisfactory performance, having both motor and sensory components, it is important to compare the scores on this test with those on other tests that have some (but not all) of the same requirements that the TPT does. For example, it is often useful to compare performance on the TPT with test results from Finger Oscillation, which has only simple motor speed requirements. This, of course, has implications for location of the lesion more anteriorly or posteriorly, depending on which test score is more impaired. If one were to use only the Halstead-Reitan cut-off scores, such a comparison would be difficult. The use of the Heaton et al. (1991) profile simplifies such comparisons.

It has traditionally been assumed that there is a consistent relationship between the times required to perform the TPT on the first and second trials, with the preferred and nonpreferred hands, respectively, among neurologically normal subjects, with the non-preferred hand performing 30-40% faster than the preferred hand because of learning and interhemispheric transfer to information (e.g., Golden, 1978). Deviations from this expected relationship have been interpreted as an indication of cerebral impairment and lateralization of a lesion. More recently, however, research has shown that this relationship is more complex and is influenced significantly by other variables. An important study by Thompson et al. (1987) examined the effects of age, education, sex, and lateral preference (handedness) on the "intermanual difference scores" on the TPT, finger tapping, strength of grip, and Grooved Pegboard tests with 426 neurologically normal subjects.

This study identified lower percent differences between the two hands than those that had previously been considered normal and disclosed significant effects of age and education on the TPT. This leads to the following hypotheses regarding the TPT:

(4-35) If the nonpreferred hand does not perform 20% faster than the preferred hand on the TPT, a lesion in the hemisphere contralateral to the nonpreferred hand is possible *for patients age 40 or below who have more than 9 years of education* (Thompson et al., 1987).

(4-36) If the nonpreferred hand performs more than 30% faster than the preferred hand on the TPT, a lesion in the hemisphere contralateral to the preferred hand is possible *for patients age 40 or below who have more than 9 years of education* (Thompson et al., 1987).

(4-37) For patients above age 40, reversals of the relationships in (4-35) and (4-36) do not necessarily have any clinical significance (Thompson et al., 1987).

(4-38) For patients with less than 9 years of education, reversals of the relationships in (4-35) and (4-36) do not necessarily have any clinical significance (Thompson et al., 1987).

(4-39) A single discrepancy from the expected right/left relationship among the TPT, finger tapping, strength of grip, and Grooved Pegboard tests does not necessarily have any clinical significance since 57% of normal subjects show at least one such discrepancy. On the other hand, the presence of three or more such discrepancies (of more than one standard deviation from the mean), *in a consistent direction*, is very rare among normal subjects and should be considered to suggest cerebral impairment and the possibility of a lateralized lesion. The presence of two or more discrepancies greater than two standard deviations from the mean is equally rare, and when two or more such discrepancies in a consistent direction are found, this should also be considered to suggest cerebral impairment and the possibility of a lateralized lesion (Thompson et al., 1987).

Regardless of which of the first two trials was better, one should consider the time on the third trial (with both hands). The time on this trial should be less than the time on the faster of the first two trials. When it is not, or when the difference does not reach the expected degree of improvement, this suggests that the more impaired hand may be interfering with the performance of the other hand when both are used. This is an indication of severe impairment, which is often seen in patients with significant tissue-destroying lesions such as intracerebral neoplasms. An example of this would be a patient who only placed 7 blocks correctly in 10 minutes with the dominant hand, placed all 10 blocks correctly with the nondominant hand in 5 minutes and placed all ten blocks correctly with both hands in 4.5 minutes. This results in Scale Scores of 5 for the dominant hand, 9 for the nondominant hand, and 7 for both hands (Heaton et al., 1991, p. 46); thus the dominant right hand (left-cerebral hemisphere) interference effect is obvious.

Finally, one may sometimes encounter cases in which the performance gets steadily slower as the trials progress. In such cases, particularly if the number of blocks placed correctly also decreases with each succeeding trial, fatigue may be a factor. If this is the case, there should be supporting data seen on other motor tests and in general observations of the patient's performance.

Another hypothesis that may need to be considered, particularly in psychiatric populations, is that the patient is becoming more resistant, less motivated, or depressed over perceived failures as testing progresses. Evaluation of these hypotheses is aided by careful observation and recording of the patient's cooperation, effort, and general approach to the testing situation.

(4-40) The most sensitive general indicators of brain impairment (performance scores) are: (a) Impairment Index, (b) Category, (c) TPT Localization, and (d) Trails B, in that order of significance (Reitan, 1959a).

(4-41) If TPT performance is more impaired than Finger Tapping performance with the same hand, a posterior lesion is suggested, that is, at some distance from the motor strip. If Finger Tapping is more impaired than TPT with the same hand, a lesion in the anterior part of the contralateral hemisphere is suggested (Reitan, 1959a).

(4-42) When there are definite indications of left-cerebral hemisphere impairment such as dysphasia and lowered Verbal IQ, but no indication of left-cerebral hemisphere signs on TPT and Tapping, this suggests a focal lesion located at some distance from the motor strip (Reitan, 1959a).

(4-43) The Memory and Localization scores on the TPT do not have any lateralizing significance (Reitan & Wolfson, 1993).

Seashore Rhythm Test

As indicated in chapter 2, the Seashore Rhythm Test is not simply a test of auditory discrimination of different patterns of rhythms; instead, it has complex attention and concentration requirements for satisfactory performance. It is important to determine which of these requirements the patient was not able to meet satisfactorily in order to interpret the score on the Seashore Rhythm Test most accurately. Precise information about how the patient performed or failed to perform adequately on this test is important and a second trial on the test with modified requirements for performance may supply additional information (see chapter 1 for further suggestions about modifications that may be useful.)

One should note that the indication of possible lateralization of a lesion derived from the relationship between the score on this test and the score on the Speech Sounds Perception Test is at best a weak one and should not by itself be taken as a valid indication of lateralization of a lesion (Golden et al., 1981; Long & Hunter, 1981). More recent literature (Reitan & Wolfson, 1989, 1993) does not support such a relationship.

(4-44) Intact scores on the Speech Sounds Perception Test and the Seashore Rhythm Test indicate that there probably is *not* a rapidly progressive lesion. These scores are also good measures of recovery following a CVA or trauma (Reitan, 1959a, 1972; Reitan & Wolfson, 1993).

(4-45) Very poor Seashore Rhythm and Speech Sounds Perception scores may suggest general destruction of brain tissue (Golden, 1978).

(4-46) If aphasic signs are present and Speech Sounds Perception is depressed, a left temporal lesion may be suspected (Reitan & Wolfson, 1993).

(4-47) A very low score on Speech Sounds Perception compared to Seashore Rhythm may suggest a left-hemisphere lesion, while the reverse may suggest a right-hemisphere lesion (Golden et al., 1981; Long & Hunter, 1981), although Reitan and Wolfson (1989, 1993) have indicated that Seashore Rhythm does not have lateralizing significance. Therefore, this hypothesis should be considered cautiously.

Speech Sounds Perception Test

The comments in the preceding section on the Seashore Rhythm Test generally apply to interpretations of the Speech Sounds Perception Test and will not be repeated here.

Finger Oscillation Test

The level of performance on this test is a relatively weak indicator of brain damage since there is a wide range of scores achieved by both brain-damaged and intact patients. On the other hand, a difference in the performances of the dominant and nondominant hands may have implications for lateralization of lesion. As indicated above, it is often useful to compare performance on this test with performance on other tests, such as the TPT, in drawing inferences about anterior versus posterior location of a lesion.

Traditionally, a 10% difference in tapping speed between the two hands, with the preferred hand being faster, has been considered normal. Deviations from this expected relationship have been interpreted as an indication of cerebral impairment and lateralization of a lesion. The results of the Thompson et al. (1987) study require certain modifications in this.

(4-48) For *right-handed* patients, the finger tapping speed should be approximately 10% faster with the preferred hand than with the nonpreferred hand. A deviation from this expected relationship may contribute to a suspicion of impairment of the functioning of the hemisphere which is contralateral to the less adequately functioning hand. For left-handed subjects, this relationship does not hold up: The mean difference between the two hands is less, and reversals are fairly common in a group of normal left-handed subjects. One should note that even though the mean difference between the two hands on finger tapping for right-handed subjects in the Thompson et al. (1987) study is approximately 10%, the standard deviation is 9.4; therefore, deviations from the 10% expectation are not at all uncommon. This makes the following hypothesis extremely important.

(4-49) A single discrepancy from the expected right/left relationship among the TPT, finger tapping, strength of grip, and Grooved Pegboard tests does not necessarily have any clinical significance since 57% of normal subjects show at least one such discrepancy. On the other hand, the presence of three or more such discrepancies (of more than one standard deviation from the mean), *in a consistent direction*, is very rare among normal subjects and should be considered to suggest cerebral impairment and the possibility of a lateralized lesion. The presence of two or more discrepancies greater than two standard deviations from the mean is equally rare, and when two or more such discrepancies, in a consistent direction, are found, this should also be considered to suggest cerebral impairment and the possibility of a lateralized lesion (Thompson et al., 1987).

(4-50) Retention of simple motor function (tapping speed) in the presence of other severe deficits is sometimes seen in cases of extracerebral neoplasms.

(4-51) If TPT performance is more impaired than Finger Oscillation with the same hand, a posterior lesion in the contralateral hemisphere is suggested, specifically at some distance from the motor strip. If Finger Oscillation is more impaired than TPT with the same hand, a lesion in the anterior part of the contralateral hemisphere is suspected (Reitan, 1959a).

(4-52) When there are definite indications of left-cerebral hemisphere impairment such as dysphasia and lowered VIQ, but no indication of left-cerebral hemisphere signs on TPT and Tapping, this suggests a focal lesion located at some distance from the motor strip (Reitan, 1959a).

(4-53) If motor functions such as tapping and strength of grip are depressed, one would expect a lesion in the anterior part of the brain near the motor strip (Reitan, 1959a).

(4-54) If Finger Oscillation scores are vastly different, a CVA should be considered (Reitan & Wolfson, 1993).

(4-55) If TPT scores are depressed and Finger Tapping is within normal limits, this suggests sensory strip involvement (Reitan, 1959a).

Strength of Grip (Hand Dynamometer)

Scores on the Strength of Grip may have implications for lateralization of cerebral lesions. In interpreting Hand Dynamometer scores, one needs to take into consideration not only sex differences, but also age, physical activity, and occupation. A low score, for example, would be more significant in a young male patient who had engaged previously in heavy manual labor than it would be in an older patient who had engaged only in relatively sedentary occupations and little other physical activity requiring the use of his hands.

In general, the hypotheses regarding finger tapping also apply to strength of grip, with the additional caution that the mean difference between the two hands on strength of grip for normal subjects is only 7.7% and variability in the difference between the two hands is even greater for strength of grip. Reversals from the expected relationship are, consequently, even more common than for finger tapping (Thompson et al., 1987).

Grooved Pegboard

In general, the hypotheses for strength of grip hold true for the Grooved Pegboard Test, with the following additional considerations: Both the mean differences between the two hands and the standard deviations of the differences are generally greater for the Grooved Pegboard Test, resulting in even more frequent deviations from expectations. Furthermore, females show greater variability than males on the Grooved Pegboard Test. Consequently, any suggestions of lateralization of a lesion based on this test should be very conservative (Thompson et al., 1987).

Aphasia Screening Test

The Reitan Indiana Aphasia Screening Test, which is part of the Halstead-Reitan Battery, does not contribute to the Halstead Impairment Index and is a general screening examination rather than a thorough assessment of all possible aphasic disorders. Nevertheless, pathognomonic signs elicited by this examination are quite significant.

It is important in administering the Aphasia Screening Test to make a verbatim recording of everything that the patient says in response to the questions and instructions. This may help later in distinguishing between true aphasic signs and indications of thought disorder or limited education. A verbatim recording will also assist in detecting mild dysphasic signs that would otherwise go unnoticed if the examiner simply records the correct responses, which may be given following several false starts. A common example of this is the patient who responds to the stimulus picture of a fork in a halting manner with "sp sp sp fork," or the patient who responds to the stimulus picture of a Greek cross by saying, "ah ah ah red red cross ahhh cross." Such false starts in identifying the stimulus may represent mild dysphasic signs resulting from certain left-cerebral hemisphere lesions.

It is important to distinguish between educational deficits and dysphasic signs. The use of this aphasia screening test assumes at least a fourth grade reading level with the significance of dysphasic signs increasing as educational level increases. For example, if a patient spells SQUARE as "SQUAR," (particularly if he/she has a limited education), this may reflect an educational deficit, while spelling it "SQU" may be a dysphasic error. Similarly, the spelling of CROSS as "CROSSSS" is a dysphasic error, especially if it is done by a patient with a twelfth grade education. When one can assume an adequate education, the presence of two or more definite dysphasic errors strongly suggests brain impairment.

(4-56) Aphasia signs are among the strongest indicators of left-cerebral hemisphere impairment (Reitan, 1959a; Reitan & Wolfson, 1993).

(4-57) Dysnomia, dyslexia, dysgraphia, spelling dyspraxia, and dyscalculia, in that order of significance suggest left-hemisphere impairment. Constructional dyspraxia usually suggests right-hemisphere impairment; it is important to recognize, however, that 15-20% of subjects who show constructional dyspraxia have left-cerebral hemisphere impairment only. This is therefore a relatively weak lateralizing sign (Reitan, 1959a).

(4-58) Expressive aphasic signs, dysnomia, spelling apraxia, and dysgraphia suggest left-anterior impairment (Reitan, 1959a).

(4-59) Receptive aphasic signs, visual form agnosia, visual letter agnosia, dyslexia, auditory verbal agnosia, and auditory number agnosia suggest left posterior impairment. It should be noted that determination of whether certain dysphasic problems are expressive or receptive in nature may require a more thorough aphasia examination than the brief one that is typically part of the battery (Reitan, 1959a).

(4-60) If constructional dyspraxia is evident and Block Design is much lower than Picture Arrangement, a right-parietal lobe lesion is suggested (Golden, 1978).

There are certain other relatively infrequent deviant responses on this test that should be noted. These include the following:

(4-61) An attempt to draw the clock instead of writing the word for it as instructed may be a sign of left-hemisphere impairment (Reitan & Wolfson, 1993).

(4-62) Central dysarthria, which is indicated by addition, omission, or substitution of syllables, as opposed to slurring of speech, suggests a left-hemisphere lesion (Reitan & Wolfson, 1993).

(4-63) If a patient with an adequate education adds 85 and 27 instead of subtracting, this may indicate impairment to the left-cerebral hemisphere and is considered a dyscalculia (Reitan, 1975).

(4-64) Some patients may be unable to demonstrate the use of the key without actually having a key in their hand. This is called *ideokinetic dyspraxia* and suggests the presence of neurological impairment.

(4-65) Most patients read the stimulus 7 SIX 2 as "7-6-2." When a patient reads it as "7-S-I-X-2," this suggests left-hemisphere impairment (Reitan, 1972).

(4-66) Ignoring the left side of a stimulus, as in responding "6-2" to the stimulus 7 SIX 2, suggests a right-parietal lobe lesion (Golden, 1978).

(4-67) Rotation of the key drawing has no significance for brain damage since controls rotate as often as brain-damaged patients (Reitan, 1975; Reitan & Wolfson, 1993).

Sensory Perceptual Examination

The most useful data from the Sensory Perceptual Examination is that which shows the differential functioning of the right and left sides of the body. Major differences in performance of the two sides of the body are among the stronger indicators of lateralized lesions.

Special note should be made of the performance of some severely impaired patients on the fingertip number writing task. Some people, whether their impairment in functioning is due to a brain lesion or to a psychiatric disturbance, may show many errors on both hands. These multiple errors on both hands are often due to confusion or difficulty in understanding the instructions, particularly when the patient reports numbers that were not included in the instructions. Such errors may have little to do with impaired tactile sensation, particularly when there are no similar errors on other related tasks such as Finger Agnosia, Tactile Coin Recognition, and Tactile Form Recognition. (Tactile Coin Recognition is no longer considered a standard part of the test battery.) Readministration of this part of the examination using Xs and Os instead of numbers may be indicated.

(**4-68**) Visual suppressions suggest impairment in the contralateral cerebral hemisphere (Golden, 1978; Golden et al., 1981).

(**4-69**) Visual field defects suggest parietal or temporal lobe impairment, often from an intracerebral neoplasm or CVA (Reitan & Wolfson, 1993) (see Appendix C).

(**4-70**) Loss of sight in one eye suggests damage anterior to the optic chiasm, often from an extracerebral neoplasm or from a peripheral lesion affecting the eye itself (see Appendix C).

(**4-71**) A lesion near the optic chiasm may result in one blind eye and one eye with half field loss. This is sometimes seen in cases with pituitary tumors (Reitan, 1972).

(**4-72**) Suppressions seldom occur in nonimpaired populations (Golden, 1978; Heaton et al., 1991).

(**4-73**) The absence of any suppression suggests the absence of an acutely destructive, space-occupying lesion in the posterior part of the cerebral hemisphere (Reitan, 1959a).

(**4-74**) Auditory suppressions suggest a lesion in the contralateral temporal lobe (Reitan, 1959a).

(**4-75**) Tactile perception is related primarily to parietal lobe functioning; poor scores on Fingertip Number Writing, Finger Agnosia, Tactile Coin Recognition, and Tactual Form Recognition suggest parietal lobe lesions (Golden et al., 1981).

(**4-76**) Misidentification of the circle on the Tactile Form Recognition test is the most serious error on that test.

(4-77) Patients with multiple sclerosis will often show both weakness and transient or spotty sensory perceptual deficits (Golden et al., 1981).

(4-78) Severe motor and sensory perceptual loss on one side may be associated with either a rapidly progressive intracerebral neoplasm or more likely an acute cerebrovascular disorder (Reitan, 1959a, 1972).

(4-79) Sensory suppressions and visual field deficits are associated with tissue destroying lesions (Reitan & Wolfson, 1993).

Chapter 5

Lateralization and Localization Hypotheses

Diffuse Impairment

Diffuse impairment most often results from degenerative processes such as senile dementia of the Alzheimer's type, cerebral arterial sclerosis, or infectious diseases such as meningitis. Closed head injuries will often show diffuse impairment but may also exhibit focal signs in the area of greatest trauma. Cases with diffuse impairment must be distinguished from those with multiple localizing signs. With diffuse impairment, if there are motor or sensory deficits on one side of the body, usually there will be similar deficits shown on the other side of the body. In cases of diffuse impairment usually there will be deficits in many functional areas with relatively few areas of cognitive/behavioral functioning remaining intact. In cases with multiple localizing signs, on the other hand, the test battery profile is more varied. If there are motor or sensory deficits on one side of the body, for example, functioning on the other side may be relatively well preserved. Similarly, while many functions may be impaired, others may remain relatively intact. Implications for the most likely pathological process are quite different for these two profiles. It may be difficult to distinguish between diffuse and bilateral impairment in some cases.

(5-1) The absence of lateralizing signs suggests diffuse impairment (Golden, 1978).

(5-2) No significant difference between VIQ and PIQ suggests either diffuse impairment or a static (or slowly progressive) lesion (Reitan, 1959a).

(5-3) Clear, sharp focal deficits and mild-to-severe generalized impairment are sometimes seen with penetrating head injuries (Golden, 1978).

(5-4) Very poor Seashore Rhythm and Speech Sounds Perception scores may suggest general destruction of brain tissue (Golden, 1978).

(5-5) Closed head injuries often produce mild diffuse damage, which may demonstrate no gross or severe signs with no effect on Full Scale IQ or the differences between VIQ and PIQ. With this type of pathology one may also see mixed signs or different levels of impairment because of the contrecoup and shear/strain effect (Binder, 1986).

(5-6) Infections, general cerebral arteriosclerosis, and degenerative processes that result in atrophy yield generalized deficits (Golden, 1978).

(5-7) Chronic alcoholics often show diffuse impairment with some prominent focal signs in areas such as memory (Golden, 1978) depending on the stage of the disease.

Lateralizing Signs

The most powerful signs of lateralized lesions are generally those that indicate discrepancies in performance on the two sides of the body and aphasia symptoms. The former are seen on the Sensory Perceptual Examination and on the various tests of motor performance while the latter are found on the Aphasia Screening Test. Other possible indicators of lateralization, such as the difference between Verbal IQ and Performance IQ, the difference between scores on the Seashore Rhythm Test and the Speech Sounds Perception Test, and the difference between scores on Parts A and B on the Trail Making Test, are weak indicators of lateralization and should be interpreted much more cautiously (only when confirming data is established on the sensory and motor tests). One also needs to recognize that certain pathognomonic signs such as visual field defects have priority in terms of interpretation. They are not only definite indications of lesions, but they define the locations of the lesions.

(5-8) When PIQ is at least 20 points lower than VIQ on the WAIS, this suggests possible right-cerebral hemisphere impairment. When the reverse is true, left-cerebral hemisphere impairment is suspected (Reitan, 1955a). One must temper this finding with the fact that the PIQ is more likely to be affected by a cerebral lesion than is VIQ due to the fact that the Performance subtests involve new and unique learning, while Verbal subtests measure accumulated knowledge, which is the least affected by brain impairment (Reitan, 1955a, 1959a).

(5-9) A score on Trails B that is substantially poorer than the score on Trails A suggests left-hemisphere impairment, while a lower score on Part A suggests right-cerebral hemisphere impairment (Reitan & Tarshes, 1959). This is a weak hypothesis unless substantiated by other data.

(5-10) Reversal of TPT relationship becomes more common and, therefore, less significant with age above 40 and education below 9 years because transfer of information across the corpus callosum deteriorates and fatigue becomes a more important factor (Thompson et al., 1987).

(5-11) Differences between the two hands on Finger Oscillation speed and Strength of Grip that exceed the expectations described in chapter 2 are strong lateralizing signs (Ross et al., 1990).

(5-12) A very low score on Speech Sounds Perception compared to Seashore Rhythm may suggest a left-hemisphere lesion, while the reverse may suggest a right-hemisphere lesion (Golden et al., 1981; Long & Hunter, 1981), although Reitan and Wolfson (1989, 1993) have indicated that Seashore

Rhythm does not have lateralizing significance. Therefore, this hypothesis should be considered cautiously.

(5-13) Dysnomia, dyslexia, dysgraphia, spelling dyspraxia, dyscalculia, and right-left confusion, in that order of significance, suggest left-hemisphere impairment (Reitan, 1959a). Constructional dyspraxia usually suggests right-hemisphere impairment. It is important to recognize, however, that 15-20% of patients who show constructional dyspraxia have left-cerebral hemisphere impairment only, and this is, therefore, a relatively weak lateralizing sign (Golden, 1978).

(5-14) Auditory suppressions suggest a lesion in the contralateral temporal lobe (Reitan, 1959a).

(5-15) Extracerebral tumors rarely result in significant VIQ-PIQ differences (Reitan, 1972).

(5-16) Localizing or lateralizing signs in the absence of depressed FSIQ and with little PIQ-VIQ difference suggest the absence of intracerebral tumor or vascular disorder (Golden et al., 1981).

(5-17) Tumors and CVAs generally result in clear-cut lateralizing signs, although the latter will sometimes be superimposed on a more diffuse picture.

(5-18) A lack of lateralizing signs in the records of patients who have schizophrenia may sometimes aid in differentiating them from some brain-damaged patients (Golden, 1978).

Right Hemisphere

In addition to indications of lateralization to the right-cerebral hemisphere mentioned in the immediately preceding section, the following hypotheses refer specifically to the right hemisphere:

(5-19) Visual memory that is less adequate than verbal memory suggests a right-hemisphere lesion (Russell, 1975).

(5-20) A Block Design score significantly lower than the Picture Arrangement score suggests a right parietal-occipital lesion, while a Picture Arrangement score lower than the Block Design score suggests a right-anterior temporal lobe lesion (Reitan, 1959a).

(5-21) If Picture Arrangement and Block Design scores are both depressed, a right temporal-parietal lesion is suggested (Reitan, 1959a).

(5-22) If constructional dyspraxia is evident and Block Design is much lower than Picture Arrangement, a right-parietal lobe lesion is suggested (Golden et al., 1981).

(5-23) Ignoring the left side of a stimulus, as in responding "6-2" to the stimulus 7 SIX 2 suggests a right-parietal lobe lesion (Golden, 1978).

(5-24) Poor performance on the JOLO suggests a posterior right-hemisphere lesion (Benton et al., 1978).

Left Hemisphere

Left-hemisphere lesions may be more obvious than right-hemisphere lesions on testing because of the importance of the left hemisphere for language functions. The following hypotheses refer specifically to the left hemisphere:

(5-25) Verbal memory that is less adequate than visual memory suggests a left-hemisphere lesion (Russell, 1975).

(5-26) A very low score on Similarities suggests left-temporal lobe impairment. An intact Similarities score, however, does not suggest the absence of left-temporal lobe impairment (Reitan, 1959a).

(5-27) If aphasic signs are present and Speech Sounds Perception score is depressed, a left-temporal lobe lesion may be suspected (Long & Hunter, 1981).

(5-28) Aphasic signs are among the strongest indicators of left-cerebral hemisphere impairment (Reitan, 1959a).

(5-29) An attempt to draw the clock instead of writing the word for it as instructed may be a sign of left-hemisphere impairment (Reitan & Wolfson, 1993).

(5-30) If a patient with an adequate education adds 85 and 27 instead of subtracting, this may indicate impairment to the left-cerebral hemisphere (Reitan & Wolfson, 1993).

(5-31) Most patients read the stimulus 7 SIX 2 as "7-6-2". When a patient reads it as "7-S-I-X-2," this suggests left-hemisphere impairment (Reitan & Wolfson, 1993).

Localizing Signs

In attempting to localize a lesion, it is common to consider first whether the lesion is located more anteriorly or more posteriorly. Since the motor strip is anterior to the fissure of Rolando and the sensory strip is posterior to it, the relative degree of impairment of motor and sensory functions has implications for anterior or posterior location of a lesion. The following hypotheses are relevant to this question:

(5-32) If motor performance such as on Finger Tapping and Strength of Grip is depressed, one would expect a lesion in the anterior part of the brain near the motor strip (Reitan, 1959a).

(5-33) If TPT performance is more impaired than Finger Oscillation performance with the same hand, a posterior lesion is suggested (i.e., at some distance from the motor strip). If Finger Oscillation is more impaired than TPT with the same hand, a lesion in the anterior part of the contralateral hemisphere is suspected (Reitan, 1959a).

(5-34) If TPT scores are depressed and Finger Oscillation is within normal limits, sensory strip involvement is suggested (Reitan, 1959a).

One should next examine the data to see whether or not still more specific localization to one of the lobes of the cerebral hemisphere is indicated.

Frontal Lobes

Lesions of the frontal lobes, especially if they are at some distance anterior to the motor strip, in the prefrontal area, are among the most difficult to identify with the Halstead-Reitan Battery. Emotional reactions are common, and impairment of higher level functions such as those seen on the Category Test are often seen; however, one must recognize that the Category Test is sensitive to damage to any part of the brain. Right frontal lobe lesions may be particularly "silent" on the results of the Halstead-Reitan Battery. One patient was seen with a verified right frontal lobe lesion whose only demonstrable deficit on the Battery was an exceptionally low score on the Picture Arrangement subtest of the WAIS. Lezak (1983) has also reported a similar case.

(5-35) If scores on both Category and Part B of Trail Making are low, while other tests are near normal, a focal and static lesion of one or both anterior frontal lobes may be suggested (Reitan, 1959a).

(5-36) Expressive aphasic signs, dysnomia, spelling apraxia, and dysgraphia suggest left-anterior impairment (Reitan, 1959a).

(5-37) The WCST is sensitive to frontal lesions (Heaton, 1980; Pendleton & Heaton, 1982); however, like the Category Test and Trail Making B, its scores are reflective of strengths and weaknesses throughout the brain.

(5-38) Although low Picture Arrangement scores are most often associated with right anterior temporal lobe lesions, they are more often associated with right frontal lesions when several of the pictures are left in the original, but incorrect, order (McFie & Thompson, 1972).

Temporal Lobes

Temporal lobe lesions may show a number of complex patterns of deficit. Auditory deficits of various kinds are common. If dysphasic signs are seen on the Aphasia Screening Test, it may be useful to examine these further to determine whether the deficits are primarily receptive or expressive. Receptive deficits are more common with temporal lobe involvement. Visual field defects may also result from some temporal lobe lesions and if the medial temporal region is involved, memory impairment may be present. In order to assess memory deficits we recommend that a more thorough evaluation of memory should be added to the battery, such as the one suggested by Russell (1975) or the Wechsler Memory Scale-Revised (Wechsler, 1987).

(5-39) A very low score on Similarities suggests left-temporal lobe impairment. A normal Similarities score, however, does not suggest the absence of left-temporal lobe impairment (Reitan, 1959a).

(5-40) A Block Design score significantly lower than the Picture Arrangement score suggests (right) parietal-occipital lesions, while a Picture Arrangement score lower than the Block Design score suggests (right) anterior temporal lesions (Reitan, 1959a).

(5-41) If Picture Arrangement and Block Design scores are both depressed, a right temporal-parietal lesion is suggested (Reitan, 1959a).

(5-42) If aphasic signs are present and Speech Sounds Perception is depressed, a left temporal lesion may be suspected (Long & Hunter, 1981).

(5-43) Receptive aphasic signs, visual form agnosia, visual letter agnosia, dyslexia, auditory verbal agnosia, and auditory number agnosia suggest left-posterior temporal lobe impairment (Reitan, 1959a).

(5-44) Visual field defects suggest parietal or temporal lobe damage, often from an intracerebral neoplasm or CVA (Reitan & Wolfson, 1993) (see Appendix C).

(5-45) Auditory suppressions suggest a lesion in the contralateral temporal lobe (Reitan, 1959a).

(5-46) Fingertip Number Writing errors are sometimes seen with temporal lobe lesions (Long & Hunter, 1981).

Parietal Lobes

Parietal lobe lesions are most commonly reflected in tactile perceptual deficits. They may also affect motor performance on tasks in which effective sensory feedback is necessary for completion of the task. Right parietal lobe lesions may be reflected by difficulty in design copying tasks (constructional dyspraxia), although such deficits are sometimes seen with lesions in the left hemisphere as well. Lack of response to the left half of a stimulus figure is one of the stronger indications of right parietal lobe impairment.

(5-47) A Block Design score significantly lower than the Picture Arrangement score suggests (right) parietal-occipital lesions; a Picture Arrangement score lower than the Block Design score suggests (right) anterior temporal lesions (Reitan, 1959a).

(5-48) If Picture Arrangement and Block Design scores are both depressed, a right temporal-parietal lesion is suggested (Reitan, 1959a).

(5-49) Although low Picture Arrangement scores are most often associated with right anterior temporal lobe lesions, they are more often associated with right frontal lesions when several of the pictures are left in the original, but incorrect, order (McFie & Thompson, 1972).

(5-50) If constructional dyspraxia is evident and Block Design is much lower than Picture Arrangement, a right parietal lesion is suggested (Reitan, 1959a).

(5-51) Ignoring the left side of a stimulus, as in responding "6-2" to the stimulus 7 SIX 2 suggests a right parietal lesion (Golden, 1978).

(5-52) Visual field defects suggest parietal or temporal lobe damage, often from an intracerebral neoplasm or CVA (Reitan & Wolfson, 1993) (see Appendix C).

(5-53) Tactile perception is related primarily to parietal lobe functioning; poor scores on Fingertip Number Writing, Finger Agnosia, Tactile Coin Recognition, and Tactual Form Recognition suggest parietal lobe lesions.

(5-54) Poor performance on the JOLO suggests posterior right parietal lobe impairment (Benton et al., 1978).

Occipital Lobes

(5-55) A Block Design score significantly lower than the Picture Arrangement score suggests (right) parietal-occipital lesions, while a Picture Arrangement score lower than the Block Design score suggests (right) anterior temporal lesions (Reitan, 1959a).

(5-56) Visual suppressions suggest impairment in the contralateral cerebral hemisphere posterior to the optic chiasm (Golden, 1978).

Chapter 6

Process Hypotheses

This chapter includes hypotheses regarding severity, velocity (whether a lesion is static or progressive), prognosis for recovery, and the effects of hospitalization on performance. Although severity can be determined fairly easily, as Heaton et al. (1981) have shown, it is very difficult to answer questions about factors such as the velocity of a lesion solely on the basis of test data. Consequently, the hypotheses related to acuity and progression of lesions should be considered cautiously, and additional sources of information are essential in real clinical cases.

Severity

In determining the degree of severity, one should consider the general level of performance indicated by the Impairment Index and the T scores for individual tests. These judgments must, however, be tempered by certain other factors, which are indicated in the following hypotheses:

(6-1) The significance of an elevated Impairment Index decreases with age beginning with age 45-50. Age corrected T scores take this into consideration (Heaton et al., 1991).

(6-2) IQ tends to be negatively correlated with Category scores (Cullum et al., 1984).

(6-3) Mortenson et al. (1991) have cast doubt on the notion that information and vocabulary are less susceptible to the effects of brain impairment than other subtests, and for that reason other indications of premorbid cognitive functioning should be sought.

(6-4) For patients above age 40, reversals of the relationships in (4-35) and (4-36) do not necessarily have any clinical significance (Thompson et al., 1987).

(6-5) Misidentification of the circle on the Tactile Form Recognition Test is the most serious error on that test.

(6-6) Sensory suppressions and visual field defects are associated with tissue destroying lesions (Reitan & Wolfson, 1993).

If the patient under consideration has been hospitalized for a significant time, the hypotheses in the section on Effects of Hospitalization should also be considered in judging severity.

Velocity

In determining whether a lesion is static or progressive, and, if progressive, how rapidly, the following hypotheses should be considered:

(6-7) If there is a strong indication of cerebral impairment yet IQ scores are relatively unimpaired, this suggests a static lesion (Reitan, 1959a).

(6-8) No significant difference between Verbal and Performance IQ suggests diffuse impairment and/or a static (or slowly progressive) lesion (Reitan, 1959a).

(6-9) If scores on both Category and Part B of Trail Making are poor while other tests are near normal, a focal and static lesion of one or both anterior frontal lobes may be suggested (Reitan, 1959a).

(6-10) Adequate performance on tests such as Category, Trails B, and Speech Sounds Perception are rarely seen in cases with acute, destructive lesions (Reitan & Wolfson, 1993).

(6-11) Intact scores on the Speech Sounds Perception Test and the Seashore Rhythm Test indicate that there probably is *not* a rapidly progressive lesion. These scores are good measures of recovery following a CVA or trauma (Reitan, 1959a, 1972; Reitan & Wolfson, 1993).

This last hypothesis appears to be a particularly important one since patients with rapidly progressive, destructive lesions almost always have severe impairment of attention and concentration, which makes adequate performance on these two tests unlikely. It should be noted, though, that the converse of this hypothesis is not necessarily true. That is, a very poor performance on these tests does not always imply a rapidly progressive lesion, since many factors may impair performance on these tests, which, as indicated in chapter 2, have complex requirements for successful performance. Careful observation of the precise nature of the patient's performance should aid in identifying the type of deficit that causes the impairment in individual cases.

Recovery and Prognosis

Knowledge of the nature and time of occurrence of a lesion provides certain implications for recovery and prognosis. For example, there is a commonly seen recovery curve following head injuries that shows a gradual improvement of functioning that may take up to 2 years post coma to reach maximum spontaneous recovery. The time interval between the injury and the testing, then, has implications for prognosis. The following hypothesis regarding test data also has implications for recovery and prognosis:

(6-12) Intact scores on the Speech Sounds Perception Test and the Seashore Rhythm Test indicate that there probably is *not* a rapidly progressive lesion. These are also a good measure of recovery following a CVA or trauma (Reitan, 1959a, 1972; Reitan & Wolfson, 1993).

Effects of Hospitalization

The overall level of performance of schizophrenics on the battery is generally more impaired than that of nonschizophrenics. At least part of this impairment can probably be attributed to the general effects of hospitalization or institutionalization, and one should expect to see a relatively lower level of performance by most patients who have been hospitalized for a significant period at the time of testing, regardless of the reason for hospitalization. For example, many hospitalized patients show a low score on Digit Span; therefore, this is one of the poorest predictors of brain impairment (Reitan, 1972; Reitan & Wolfson, 1993).

Strength of Grip and Finger Oscillation speed usually also decline significantly during lengthy hospitalization, but should do so bilaterally, with no indication of lateralization.

Effect of Psychiatric Disorders

Severe psychiatric disorders such as the schizophrenic and major affective disorders frequently have an adverse effect on performance on neuropsychological tests. There are several factors that may be involved: Motivation is often less than adequate; intrusive thoughts, hallucinations, or delusions may interfere with attention and concentration; and the memory impairment, psychomotor slowing, and slowed thinking associated with depression result in inadequate performance on some tests.

(6-13) When a patient has a major psychiatric disorder, one cannot rely solely on the level of performance to determine the presence of brain injury or disease. The use of multiple methods of inference and a detailed history are critical in such cases (Golden et al., 1981).

(6-14) A diagnosis of dementia, as differentiated from depression, should never be made solely on the basis of memory deficits, since they are commonly seen with severe depression (American Psychiatric Association, 1987).

(6-15) Constructional dyspraxia in copying drawings and evidence of dyspraxia noted on tests such as Object Assembly and Block Design are frequently seen in patients with dementia.

(6-16) It is important to distinguish the unusual use of language of some patients who have a schizophrenic disorder from aphasia. In some cases, the assistance of a speech and language pathologist may be needed to accomplish this (Golden et al., 1981).

(6-17) The behavior of patients who have a major psychiatric disorder should be observed closely during testing to determine whether they are responding to internal stimuli at times. If this occurs, it may not be possible to interpret test results validly (Golden et al., 1981).

(6-18) It is advisable to defer testing of patients who are receiving neuroleptic or antidepressant medications until the dosage of their medications has been stabilized to minimize the effects of the medications on test performance (Heaton & Crowley, 1981).

Chapter 7

Neuropathological Condition Hypotheses

This chapter lists the hypotheses regarding the implications of test data for various neuropathological conditions or lesions. It also includes comments about the epidemiology of various lesions and the expected severity, velocity, and prognosis. The list of neuropathological conditions is not exhaustive, but it includes those most frequently encountered by neuropsychologists as well as a number of others that are important either because of the risk of confusing them with more common disorders or because of the importance of identifying infrequently encountered but potentially treatable ones.

Trauma

Two types of brain trauma are generally recognized: closed head injuries and penetrating head injuries. The former are most often caused by motor vehicle accidents, and the latter are exemplified by gunshot wounds.

In their discussion of the pathophysiology of closed head injuries, Teasdale and Mendelow (1984) distinguish between primary causes of brain damage, that is, those due to immediate impact, and secondary causes. The primary causes are cerebral contusions with hemorrhages, which are most common in the frontal/temporal regions and diffuse axonal injuries. It is these latter injuries in the brain stem area, caused by a shearing mechanism (stretching or breaking of axons and dendrites) or rotational forces, that are largely responsible for the coma that frequently results from closed head injuries. The secondary causes of brain damage are factors such as intracranial hematomas, cerebral edema, infection, subarachnoid hemorrhage, and hydrocephalus, as well as hypoxia and hypotension (Teasdale & Mendelow, 1984, p. 9).

Penetrating head injuries, while common in military combat, are much less common than closed head injuries among noncombatants. Fifty percent of all penetrating head injuries are fatal. The primary effects resulting from penetrating head injuries are the tissue destroyed in the path of the penetrating missile and bleeding. The secondary factors described for closed head injury can also complicate the picture.

This leads to several hypotheses regarding performance on neuropsychological test batteries:

(7-1) Static velocity is consistent with a closed head injury, particularly when the injury occurred some time prior to testing.

(7-2) Closed head injuries may produce mild diffuse damage, which may reveal no gross or severe signs and often does not affect Full Scale IQ or differences between VIQ and PIQ. With this type of pathology one may see mixed signs or different levels of impairment because of contusions in different regions and shear/strain effects (Binder, 1986).

(7-3) The Impairment Index tends to be higher in causes of tissue destruction such as intracerebral neoplasms, CVAs, and penetrating head injuries and may be lower in cases of extracerebral neoplasms and some mild-to-moderate closed head injuries (Golden, 1978).

(7-4) If Finger Oscillation scores are vastly different, a CVA or penetrating head injury should be considered (Reitan & Wolfson, 1993).

If a patient has recently suffered a significant head injury, this information will usually be available and the referral question will often be one regarding cognitive and behavioral strengths and weaknesses, prognosis, and implications for rehabilitation rather than diagnosis. In cases of more remote trauma, this information may not be available and diagnostic questions may be more important. In these cases, epidemiological factors may be helpful. It is clear that people of any age, sex, or position in society may suffer head injuries, but the incidence among some groups is considerably higher. Adolescents and young adults are at particularly high risk as are substance abusers.

(7-5) Young adults who engage in hazardous occupations show a pattern of impulsive, reckless behavior, and/or substance abusers frequently experience closed head injuries.

(7-6) A history of repeated, relatively mild closed head injuries may result in significant evidence of impairment (Boll, 1986; Saunders & Harbough, 1984; School Health and Sports Medicine Committee, 1990).

The severity of impairment following head trauma can vary from mild to extremely severe. Although approximately 50% of all patients with gunshot wounds to the head die, some may exhibit very mild impairment on the Halstead-Reitan Battery. On the other hand, it is not uncommon to see patients who have suffered closed head injuries in automobile accidents that did not result in any penetration of the skull, but who evidence severe cognitive and behavioral impairment on these tests. The reverse may also be true, of course, since there are people who demonstrate severe impairment following penetrating head injuries and some who exhibit only mild impairment following closed head injuries.

There may be progressive deterioration immediately following traumatic head injury if there is significant uncontrolled bleeding, edema, or other secondary factors. In addition to shear-strain itself, some of the subsequent damage that occurs following head injury involves the effects of excitation of neurotransmitters and eventual breakdown of cell membranes due to increased lactic acid and resultant acidosis (Dixon, Taft, and Hayes, 1993; Hayes, Jenkins, and Lyeth, 1992; and Povlishock, 1992). If the patient survives moderate-to-severe head trauma, there is an expected course of spontaneous recovery of some function over the following 18-24 months. For the most part, only minor spontaneous improvement takes place after this period, although further recovery is certainly possible over many years, particularly if neuropsychological and family-oriented rehabilitation efforts continue (see chapter 11).

The prognosis following head injury is determined largely by the severity of the trauma and to some extent by the location of the lesion and the resulting deficits in functioning. Severity of trauma is perhaps best indicated by depth of coma as measured on the Glasgow Coma Scale (which assesses eye opening, verbal responses, and motor responses) (Brooks, 1984) and length or duration of coma. In terms of location of lesion and resulting specific deficits, a person with a relatively mild trauma that results in a circumscribed lesion may have a very poor prognosis for returning to his/her former activities if functions that were critical for the performance of those activities are impaired.

A discussion of traumatic brain injury would not be complete without reference to mild head injury. In 1981 Rimel, Giordani, Barth, Boll, and Jane defined mild head injury in three ways: (1) Glasgow Coma Scale of 13-15; (2) loss of consciousness of less than 20 minutes; and (3) hospitalization under 48 hours. In an epidemiological study of over 1,200 head-injured patients who were brought to emergency rooms across central and western Virginia, they found that over 50% fit the criteria for mild head injury. Of the mild head-injured patients followed up at 3 months post trauma (over 400 patients), approximately one-third had not returned to work, most of whom also demonstrated significant neuropsychological deficits. This study, among others, began the modern debate over the neurocognitive effects and recovery curves in mild head injury.

Much has been written in this areas over the ensuing 12 years, including an excellent review by Binder in 1986 entitled "Persisting symptoms after mild head injury: A review of the postconcussive syndrome." His review of the literature suggests that mild acceleration-deceleration (nonimpact) and impacts to the head can cause brain injury and resultant postconcussion symptoms such as headaches, dizziness, memory dysfunction, attention deficits, fatigue, irritability, anxiety, depression, sleep disturbance, and other neuropsychological deficits.

The majority of the recent literature suggests that most mild head injured patients either experience no significant cognitive/emotional sequelae or make a rapid and full recovery over the first few weeks or months following their injuries (see Barth, Ryan, Schear, & Puente, 1992). Yet as Binder (1986) points out, "despite some methodological problems and negative results, the preponderance of literature supports the notion that persisting cerebral dysfunction <u>sometimes</u> can result from seemingly mild head injury even in the absence of gross neurological complications" (p. 341). It is in these complicated mild head injury cases (particularly those that end up in the forensic arena) that the neuropsychologist must be particularly careful to utilize the available age and education-based norms provided by Heaton et al. (1991), carry out exhaustive medical record and psychosocial history review, and be well acquainted with the scientific literature when discussing diagnosis, recovery, treatment, and functional outcome.

Neoplasms

Cerebral neoplasms or brain tumors received a great deal of study and attention by neuropsychologists in the early stages of development of the Halstead-Reitan Battery (e.g., Reitan, 1959a) in spite of their relative infrequency of occurrence. Kaufman (1981), for example, estimates that they occur less than 5% as often as CVAs. Most neuropsychologists will examine few, if any, patients with neoplasms of the brain, and those cases they do see will usually have already been diagnosed prior to neuropsychological evaluation. The very fact of this low incidence, along with the serious medical implications of the diagnosis, makes it important for every neuropsychologist to be familiar with the type of neuropsychological data resulting from them.

Fundamental understanding of neoplastic disease requires knowledge of five diagnostic subcategories: (1) malignancy, (2) velocity or grade, (3) location, (4) capsulation, and (5) histology or type. Malignancy refers to determining whether a tumor is benign or malignant, or whether it is growing. Speed of growth is termed *velocity* and designated as grades from I to IV (I being slow growing and IV referring to fast growing tumors). Location, in its broadest sense is associated with discovering whether the neoplastic lesion is inside the brain tissue (intracerebral or intrinsic) or outside the cerebrum (extracerebral or extrinsic). This latter distinction typically has implications for overall severity since intracerebral tumors infiltrate and directly destroy more tissue than extracerebral ones, which exert pressure on the brain but may not cause lasting damage if treated or removed. Tumors are also categorized as encapsulated versus unencapsulated depending upon whether they have a hard layer of cells surrounding the neoplasm or are more free-form and infiltrating. Finally, tumors are identified by the cell types from which they arise. For example, neoplasms which arise from the connective tissue in the brain or glioblast cells are referred to as *glioblastomas* (or *glioblastoma multiforma*) and are intracerebral in nature. The other most common tumor types are *astrocytomas* (which grow from connective tissues like the gliomas), *meningioma* (which arise from the meninges and are typically extracerebral) and *oligodendrogliomas*, which are often slow growing and intracerebral. An additional type of tumor merits special mention. Although metastatic tumors are typically intracerebral, they are secondary tumors that have metastasized from a primary cancer elsewhere in the body, most often from the breasts or lungs. This typically results in multiple tumors within diverse parts of the brain, and the resulting picture on the Halstead-Reitan Battery is one of severe, rapidly progressive, "spotty" impairment.

The following additional hypotheses relate test data to neoplasms:

(**7-7**) The absence of any suppression on the Sensory Perceptual Examination suggests the absence of an acute destructive lesion in the posterior part of the cerebral hemisphere (Reitan, 1959a).

(**7-8**) Extracerebral tumors rarely result in significant VIQ-PIQ differences (Reitan, 1972).

(**7-9**) Extreme sparing of some functions suggests the possibility of an extracerebral neoplasm rather than an intracerebral neoplasm. An example of this is retention of simple motor speed (tapping) in the presence of other severe deficits (Reitan & Wolfson, 1993).

(7-10) The Impairment Index tends to be higher in cases with tissue destruction such as intracerebral neoplasms, CVAs, and penetrating head injuries, and may be lower in cases of extracerebral neoplasms and some mild-to-moderate closed head injuries (Golden, 1978).

(7-11) Localizing or lateralizing signs in the absence of depressed FSIQ and with little PIQ-VIQ difference suggest the absence of intracerebral tumor or massive CVA because such disorders cause more global damage and generally lower PIQ (Golden et al., 1981; Reitan, 1959a).

(7-12) Adequate performance on the Category Test and the Seashore Rhythm Test, even in the presence of a high Impairment Index and poor performance on other tests does not appear consistent with either intracerebral tumors or massive CVAs, since damage of this type usually impairs abstraction ability, regardless of the location of the lesion (Reitan, 1972; Reitan & Wolfson, 1993).

(7-13) Severe motor and sensory perceptual loss on one side may be associated with either a rapidly progressive intracerebral neoplasm or more likely an acute cerebrovascular disorder (Reitan, 1959a, 1972).

(7-14) If Finger Oscillation scores are vastly different, a CVA should be considered (Reitan & Wolfson, 1993).

(7-15) Ignoring the left side of a stimulus, as in responding "6-2" to the stimulus 7 SIX 2, suggests a right-parietal lobe lesion (Golden, 1978).

(7-16) A lesion near the optic chiasm may result in one blind eye and one eye with a half field loss. This is sometimes seen in cases with pituitary tumors (Reitan, 1959a, 1972).

(7-17) Metastatic carcinomas generally show multiple focal signs plus very poor overall performance. For example, if the nonpreferred hand is much poorer than the preferred hand on TPT, time with both hands should be low also. That is, the poor functioning of the nonpreferred hand should interfere with the functioning of the preferred hand. If it does not, the absence of an intracerebral neoplasm, particularly metastatic carcinoma, is suggested (Golden, 1978).

Cerebrovascular Disorders

There is a wide variety of cerebrovascular disorders, ranging from congenital arteriovenous malformations to general arteriosclerotic conditions, internal bleeding within the brain (hemorrhages and hematomas), and infarcts resulting from thrombi and emboli. Congenital malformations are frequently asymptomatic, and a general arteriosclerotic condition will produce a picture of diffuse impairment on the HRB with severity depending on the stage of the disease. Strokes, or CVAs characterized by bleeding or occlusion, may show highly focal, severe impairment when they occur in a major artery or may show less severe, multifocal or spotty pictures when there have been several "minor" incidents, such as in transient ischemic attacks (TIAs).

(7-18) Localizing or lateralizing signs in the absence of depressed FSIQ and with little PIQ-VIQ difference suggest the absence of intracerebral tumor or massive CVA, because such disorders cause more global damage and generally lower PIQs (Golden et al., 1981; Reitan, 1959a).

(7-19) Adequate performance on the Category Test and the Seashore Rhythm Test, even in the presence of a high Impairment Index and poor performance on other tests, does not appear consistent with either intracerebral tumors or massive CVAs since damage of this type usually impairs abstraction ability regardless of the location of the lesion (Reitan, 1972; Reitan & Wolfson, 1993).

(7-20) Severe motor and sensory perceptual loss on one side may be associated with either a rapidly progressive intracerebral neoplasm or more likely an acute cerebrovascular disorder (Reitan, 1959a, 1972).

(7-21) If Finger Oscillation scores are vastly different, a CVA should be considered (Reitan & Wolfson, 1993).

(7-22) Ignoring the left side of a stimulus, as in responding "6-2" to the stimulus 7 SIX 2, suggests a right-parietal lobe lesion (Golden, 1978).

(7-23) Even though CVAs generally occur in older people, if one sees a picture consistent with a stroke in a young adult female, injury should be made about use of oral contraceptives, since they increase the risk of strokes (Burns, 1984).

[handwritten margin note: inquiry]

Infections

Infections of the brain may be generalized or focal; they may invade the meninges or brain tissue itself, and may be caused by bacterial, viral, or fungal agents. Consequently, the picture seen on neuropsychological testing will vary greatly. The type most commonly seen by neuropsychologists is meningitis, which is usually an arrested and generalized infection in which the question is one of identifying the residual damage and remaining intact functions. This can produce diffuse, static impairment, and it is important to ascertain the strengths and weaknesses that should be the focus of rehabilitation efforts.

(7-24) Infections, general cerebral arteriosclerosis, and degenerative processes that result in atrophy yield generalized deficits (Golden, 1978).

Abscesses of the brain are focal infections that may result from infections of the mastoid or nasal sinuses or from penetration of the skull. They may be of virtually any size and distribution, sometimes several occurring at quite different locations. They may occur at any age, but are most common in childhood and early adulthood (Berg, 1984). Consequently, this possibility should be considered when a focal or multifocal, spotty picture of impairment, which is quite severe, is seen in a young person. Once the infection has been treated, the neuropsychological picture should appear static and less severe, but still can produce evidence of focal deficits due to the local tissue destruction. Delineation of the pattern of strengths and weaknesses is important in planning rehabilitation at this point.

One rare, but dramatic, viral infection, Creutzfeldt-Jacob's disease, deserves special note because of its grim prognosis. It occurs in middle age, or even earlier, and is characterized by a rapidly progressive dementia, highly variable movement disorders, and abnormal behavior, all without the usual signs of infection such as fever; it progresses to death in a few years (Jubelt & Harter, 1984). On neuropsychological examination patients should show a diffuse, fairly rapidly progressive dementing picture. The features that should alert one to this rare possibility in contrast to the more common dementing disorders are the early age of onset, the more rapid progression, the unusual combination of dementia with varied movement disorders, and psychiatric symptoms, which might sometimes be the earliest cause for concern. When this latter is the case, the psychiatric picture will probably be a puzzling one that does not fit the pattern of any common psychiatric disorder.

Degenerative Diseases

The disorders discussed here all result from a gradual deterioration of tissue in one or more parts of the brain. While some of them have several features in common, the striking differences require that they be considered separately.

Primary Degenerative Dementia

Primary degenerative dementia or Alzheimer's disease, often referred to as senile dementia Alzheimer's type (SDAT) is widely recognized today as the most common of the degenerative dementing diseases (e.g., Katzman, 1984; Barth & Macciocchi, 1986). The process usually begins in the 50s or 60s with changes occurring in both cortical and subcortical levels. There is cortical atrophy, ventricular dilatation, and cell loss with dendritic spine degeneration, as well as changes at the histological level including development of neurofibrillary tangles, neuritic plaques, and granulovacuolar bodies.

Behaviorally the disease is characterized by general cognitive decline. Memory problems are often among the first seen, particularly recent memory with remote memory remaining relatively intact. New learning ability and mental flexibility become impaired fairly early, and various dysphasic, dyspraxic, and visual-spatial disorders are often seen. Apathy or depression are frequent, and this complicates the differential diagnosis from psychiatric disorders.

The severity of impairment at any point in time ranges from mild to very severe. Most cases seen for neuropsychological assessment will evidence at least moderate severity, and the most severely impaired patients will be virtually untestable with many of the assessment procedures in the HRB. This results from their extreme impairment of concentration and attention and their inability to follow complex instructions, as well as confusion and disorientation.

This disorder is progressive and the rate of progression may range from relatively slow to fairly rapid. Definite evidence of deterioration can usually be seen on retesting after a year, which can assist in diagnosis. Definitive diagnosis is only possible through brain tissue biopsy. Since there is no effective treatment, prognosis must always be considered poor. The most important questions for the neuropsychologist are usually the ones related to how much self-care these people are capable of, and how structured and protected their living situation needs to be at any point in time. Most of them will eventually require skilled nursing care, but through identification of strengths and weaknesses, one may be able to avoid premature institutionalization. This is important since overly protective and restrictive environments will almost always result in regression and more rapid deterioration of functioning. The identification by the neuropsychologist of strengths and weaknesses and their implications for daily functioning is important to help other clinicians and family members understand the optimal amount of care that these patients need at any point in time.

Although SDAT is the most common of the dementing disorders, there are many other medical diseases and the affective psychiatric disorders that may be mistaken for it. Because a number of these other conditions are reversible, it is essentially that they be eliminated before the diagnosis of SDAT is made. Diagnosis and treatment of conditions such as kidney, liver, and lung disease; hormonal disorders; toxic conditions; and infectious disorders are obviously not within the purview of the neuropsychologist, but one should not support a diagnosis of SDAT unless one is certain that reasonable medical steps have been taken to rule them out.

There are two areas of this differential diagnostic dilemma, however, of which the neuropsychologist should be particularly aware. The first of these is the frequent toxic effect of many medications on older people. A detailed listing of *all* medications (both prescription and over-the-counter drugs) being taken should be obtained and verified by an independent source. Of particular concern are drugs with sedating effects, those with anticholinergic effects, and most psychotropic drugs, even at dosages that would be well within the therapeutic range for younger people. This last point is important because older people frequently have more extreme reactions to such medications at the doses that are "usual" for younger people. At times, the patient's physician may not be aware of the combination of drugs being taken, having relied solely on the patient's unreliable report; any suspicions of problems resulting from this should be passed on to the physician. A more difficult problem may arise when there is a suspicion that sedative or psychotropic medications prescribed by the physician may be creating a problem. In such cases the best course may be to recommend consultation with a psychiatrist who is a specialist in gerontology. In any event, if the dementia seen on testing was caused by medications, retesting after the problematic drugs have been withdrawn should provide confirmation.

The second area that should be of particular concern to the neuropsychologist is depression. As noted, depression is sometimes a part of the picture in SDAT, but the affective disorders often present similar pictures. This can pose one of the most difficult diagnostic problems in this area. First, one should look for all the elements of dementia in the neuropsychological data; the more that features such as dysphasia, dyspraxia, and visual-spatial deficits are present in addition to a general "mental slowing," the better the case is for dementia as opposed to depression. In testing the patient, one should not readily accept "I don't know" answers, but should push for maximum effort, which may reveal abilities hidden by depression. The patient's history should be studied carefully for evidence of past depressive episodes as well as possible recent precipitants of depression such as the loss of a spouse. (It is important to remember, however, that such a loss may represent the loss of structure and support, which kept an existing dementia from being recognized until it was withdrawn.) Retesting after a year or more may be necessary in some cases. With SDAT one should see evidence of further deterioration while with a primary affective disorder one should see little change, or even improvement. Whenever there remains any unresolved question, appropriate treatment for an affective disorder with psychotherapy, medication, or even electroconvulsive therapy should be recommended with repeat neuropsychological evaluation to assess the outcome.

Finally, multi-infarct dementia (MID) must also be considered as part of a differential diagnosis. MID is characterized by a stepwise decline of cognitive functions due to multiple, focal, vascular insufficiencies.

(7-25) Diffuse impairment, with no significant signs of lateralization or focal lesions, is seen in SDAT (Barth & Macciocchi, 1986).

(7-26) Impairment of recent memory, with remote memory relatively intact, is seen in the early stages of SDAT (Barth & Macciocchi, 1986).

(7-27) In early stages of SDAT, PIQ is often more impaired than VIQ.

(7-28) Confusion manifested by difficulty in understanding test instructions is common in SDAT.

(7-29) A variety of aphasic signs is often seen in SDAT (American Psychiatric Association, 1987).

(7-30) Visuospatial problems manifested in constructional dyspraxia, poor performance on the JOLO, and difficulty finding the way around in unfamiliar surroundings may be shown by patients with SDAT.

(7-31) Dyspraxias may be shown on the Object Assembly subtest of the WAIS when the patient with SDAT recognizes what the object to be assembled is but is unable to put the parts together correctly. (When this type of test performance is noted, the patient's abilities to perform a variety of essential "real life" tasks such as dressing, operating familiar appliances, and so on should be evaluated because similar dyspraxias may exist in these areas, and they have major implications for treatment if they do.)

(7-32) SDAT may be distinguished from MID by the presence of focal signs of impairment and a stepwise course of decline in the latter disorder in contrast to more diffuse impairment and a more steady course of decline in the former (Katzman, 1984).

Hydrocephalus

Prockop (1984) has described in detail several different types of hydrocephalus. Of these, the one most likely to be seen by adult neuropsychologists is normal pressure hydrocephalus, the cause of which is not well understood. It presents with a classic triad of symptoms, dementia, urinary incontinence, and ataxic gait (with ventricular dilatation and normal intracranial pressure), and it may be either progressive or static. Unlike SDAT, for which it may be mistaken, it is potentially treatable with a shunt (even though it represents a degenerative condition); therefore the differential diagnosis is critical.

The pattern of performance on neuropsychological tests will not differ significantly between patients with SDAT and NPH, and the hypotheses regarding SDAT apply as well to NPH. In addition, the following hypotheses should be considered:

(7-33) A patient with test results characteristic of SDAT, but with a more rapid onset and progression than would ordinarily be expected in SDAT, should be suspected of having NPH, and appropriate medical tests should be recommended (Golden, 1978).

(7-34) A patient with test results characteristic of SDAT who also has urinary incontinence and an ataxic gait may be suspected of having NPH, and appropriate medical tests should be recommended (Prockop, 1984).

NPH is diagnosed readily with CT scan, MRI, and lumbar puncture. Furthermore, surgical shunting to drain excess CSF from the brain may produce improvement in as many as 60% of patients (Prockop, 1984). If shunting is performed, serial neuropsychological evaluations may be performed to document improvement following surgery and to monitor cognitive functioning on an ongoing basis. This latter may be important since sudden cognitive decline may be one of the first signs that the shunt is not functioning properly.

Huntington's Disease

Huntington's disease (HD), sometimes referred to as *Huntington's Chorea*, is a progressive degenerative, hereditary neurological disorder in which symptoms usually first appear between the ages of 35 and 40, although they have been reported as early as age 5 and as late as 70 years. Eventually there are symptoms of dramatic, disabling movement disorder, personality changes, and progressive dementia. The hereditary pattern of transmission is one that results in a 50% chance of each child of an effected parent acquiring the disease (Fahn, 1984). Medical tests now exist to diagnose this condition before symptoms develop.

A wide range of neuropsychological deficits on the HRB associated with HD has been identified by Boll, Heaton, and Reitan (1974). This study does not, however, demonstrate a single pattern of performance that one can use to suggest a diagnosis of HD, partly because of the wide range of stages of the disease at the time their subjects were tested.

When signs of dementia are noted in patients of younger ages than those at which the major dementing disorders such as SDAT and MID are usually seen, accompanied by personality changes and otherwise unexplainable movement disorders, one must consider the genetic characteristics of HD. A genetic profile or genealogy should be constructed, obtaining as complete a family history for as many earlier generations as possible. This is important because a number of factors may "hide" the presence of HD in the family, including the deaths of some people who actually had the disease before it became clinically apparent, failure to acknowledge the disease because of its stigma, and simple misdiagnosis. Oltman and Friedman (1961) identified a surprisingly wide range of other diagnostic labels that have been mistakenly assigned to people with HD, and it is reasonable to assume that this may have been even more common in earlier years.

In those cases in which one is asked to evaluate a patient who is known to be at risk for HD, the studies by Lyle and Gottesman (1977) and Butters, Sax, Montgomery, and Tarlow (1978) may be of some help. These studies suggest that signs of "mental decline," particularly in memory functioning, may be seen on testing those people at risk who later develop the disease. Unfortunately neither study uses a truly comprehensive neuropsychological test battery. Consequently, serial testing with the HRB over a period of several years appears to be the most prudent approach. If this is done, one would expect to see a decline in most areas of functioning tapped by the HRB preceding the appearance of choreiform movements and frank dementia in those people who eventually develop the disease, and this may be of value in helping the patient and family cope with this devastating disease.

Parkinson's Disease

Parkinson's disease is a disorder of the basal ganglia resulting in a dopamine deficiency state. The most commonly reported initial symptoms in order of their frequency are tremor, stiffness and slowness of movement, loss of dexterity and/or handwriting disturbance, and gait disturbance. Cognitive losses occur in some, but not all, patients, and this may reflect underlying difference in the pathology present in these two subgroups (Yahr, 1984).

This is a progressive disorder, with variable rates of decline, which most often occurs first between the ages of 50 and 65. Medical treatment may be helpful, and surgery is indicated in some cases. Neuropsychological evaluation is often indicated to assess the existence and extent of cognitive loss and aid in planning psychological aspects of treatment in view of the variability of this aspect of the disorder.

(7-35) Micrographia is sometimes seen in patients with Parkinson's disease and may be noted when the person is required to write various words and sentences on the Aphasia Screening Test. Tremor may be evident in drawings (Reitan, 1959a).

(7-36) Patients with Parkinson's disease often perform poorly on the Category Test and Trail Making and motor tests, and tend to have relatively high impairment indices; their IQs may be in the average range (Reitan & Boll, 1971).

Multiple Sclerosis

Multiple Sclerosis (MS) is a demyelinating disease of the central nervous system in which widely disseminated plaques occur in the white matter of both the brain and spinal cord. Its cause is unknown, but current theories implicate both viral and immunological factors. It first appears most often between the ages of 20 and 40 and is slightly more common in women than in men. A wide range of symptoms may be seen with muscle weakness, ocular dysfunction, urinary disturbances, gait ataxia, paresthesias, dysarthria or scanning speech, and mental disturbances among them in that order of frequency. The course is highly variable, ranging from some cases with early symptoms that go into complete remission to cases that show a chronic, progressive course. Many cases fall in between these extremes, showing a pattern of relapses and remissions of some symptoms and gradual progression of others. This pattern, and particularly the fact that some symptoms such as visual disturbances may appear bizarre and last for only a few days, understandably lead to misdiagnosis of "hysteria" in some cases. There are no absolute pathognomonic tests, and a neurological diagnosis generally required demonstration of a characteristic course, onset at the typical age, evidence of multiple lesions of the white matter of the brain and/or cord, and no better neurologic explanation for these findings (Poser, Alter, Sibley, & Scheinberg, 1984). Recently, however, MRI scans and CSF analyses have made more definitive diagnoses possible at earlier stages in the disease.

A review of neuropsychological studies of MS by Peyser and Poser (1986) reveals changes in impressions regarding the cognitive effects of the disease in recent years, due to improvements in sampling procedures and research design. A study by Heaton, Nelson, Thompson, Burks, and Franklin (1985) demonstrates that deficits on the HRB are more common among patients with a "chronic-progressive" course than among those with a "relapsing-remitting" course. In spite of the fact that they report reliability in classification of patients into these two categories, this appears to be an over-simplification of the highly variable forms in which this disease presents and is of doubtful value in examining individual cases. It is clear, however, that neuropsychological impairment does occur in many cases and that it is not limited to sensory and motor deficits and not related to the extent of physical disability.

Because of the highly variable pattern of symptoms and the unpredictable course of the disease, as well as the fact that there are no pathognomonic neurologic tests for MS, neuropsychological assessment may aid in diagnosis. More importantly, it may aid in planning psychological aspects of treatment. It is often important to identify the neurological/neuropsychological bases for some of the complaints of patients and identify the interaction of them with emotional and social factors. Only if this is done can psychotherapy be directed appropriately toward those emotional factors that may be amenable to change and only then can patients and families be helped to deal with those deficits that have a "real" physical basis.

In evaluating individuals, the following hypotheses may be useful:

(7-37) Motor and sensory perceptual problems are common (Golden et al., 1981).

(7-38) A spotty pattern of impairment may be seen, reflecting multiple, widely dispersed lesions (Golden et al., 1981).

(7-39) Patients with MS often perform adequately on the Category Test, but show significant deficits in performance on the TPT (Reitan & Wolfson, 1993).

(7-40) Patients with MS often have adequate IQs but have low scores on the Digit Symbol and Picture Arrangement subtests (Reitan & Wolfson, 1993).

(7-41) When a suspicion of MS exists, one should obtain a *thorough* medical history, looking for any of the wide range of symptoms described in the beginning of this section, even of very brief duration (Scheinberg & Smith, 1987).

Alcohol and Drug Abuse

Alcohol

As Parsons and Farr (1981) and Parsons, Butters, and Nathan (1987) pointed out in their reviews of research on the effects of alcohol and drug use on neuropsychological performance, this is an extremely complex area for clinical assessment. There is no doubt that chronic severe abuse of alcohol has detrimental effects, but the precise relationship between it and a number of other factors such as age, length of time, and quantity of alcohol use, period of abstinence at the time of testing, nutritional status, other medical problems, and history of head trauma is much less clear. Nevertheless, these factors must all be considered in each individual case, and data regarding them should always be validated from independent sources since alcoholics are often unreliable informants. The following hypotheses are relevant in evaluating alcoholics:

(7-42) Alcoholics generally perform poorly on the Halstead-Reitan Battery, especially on the Category Test, TPT total time and location, and Trails B, and on the Digit Symbol and Block Design subtests of the WAIS, but may perform normally on Seashore Rhythm and the Vocabulary, Information, and Digit Span subtests of the WAIS (Grant, 1987; Parsons & Farr, 1981; Wilkinson, 1987).

(7-43) Memory deficits are commonly seen in chronic alcoholics (Parsons, 1987). Even when performance on the Wechsler Memory Scale is adequate, significant deficits may be demonstrated by using the 30-minute delayed recall procedure designed by Russell (1975). When this procedure is used, the stories, which may have been repeated fairly accurately on the initial trial often become woefully distorted on the delayed recall. These distortions can show indications of confabulation, with frequent personal references, even in patients who do not demonstrate clinical evidence of a fully developed Korsakoff's Syndrome.

This type of memory deficit may have definite implications for the ability to function independently. Sometimes such patients appear to be capable of independent functioning on the basis of observations of their behavior in an institutional setting, but their impairment of short-term memory may cause serious problems if they are living in an independent environment.

Prescription Drugs

The prescription drugs most likely to be abused are those with sedative/hypnotic or antianxiety effects. Even in therapeutic doses these can have adverse effects on neuropsychological performance for at least several hours, and in some cases, for up to 24-48 hours after ingestion (Heaton & Crowley, 1981). There is less clear evidence regarding the long-term effects of chronic use of most prescription drugs. At a minimum, however, one should make an effort to test patients in a drug-free condition, or when they are well stabilized on regular doses of their medications, but certainly not when they are undergoing withdrawal.

Other Drugs and Environmental Toxins

If the research of the effects of alcohol on neuropsychological performance results in a murky picture from the clinician's viewpoint, the prospects for understanding the effects of the so-called recreational or street drugs based on the research are even dimmer. A major complicating factor in this is the fact that most users of these drugs are polydrug users, making studies attempting to understand the effects of individual drugs futile. Furthermore, if alcoholics are often unreliable informants regarding their consumption, street drug users are even more so because of the fear of the consequences of revealing illegal activities. It is also more difficult to be certain that any such patient is actually detoxified than is the case with alcoholics.

> **(7-44)** Polydrug abusers may show depressed performance on the Finger Tapping, Seashore Rhythm, Category, and Trails B tests (Parsons & Farr, 1981).

> **(7-45)** At a more speculative level it seems likely that when polydrug abuse has included the use of PCP, the effects are more severe, longer lasting, and adversely affect all areas of functioning tapped by the Halstead-Reitan Battery, particularly attention and concentration.

In addition to the voluntary use of various drugs, there is a potential for exposure to thousands of other chemicals that have associated toxic risks (Hartman, 1988). These range from substances such as lead and mercury whose effects have long been known and are relatively well understood, to exotic, newly synthesized substances the effects of which are, in many cases, uncertain. When such exposure is suspected, a resource such as Hartman (1988) should be consulted.

Anoxia

Anoxia may result from a variety of causes, with accidents and suicide attempts being common ones. Carbon monoxide poisoning has similar results. In any case, the result of neuropsychological examination is a picture of static, diffuse impairment with memory deficits often being among the most prominent. Occasionally one may see a strikingly lateralized picture of impairment when the causal event was an attempted hanging in which the person's body fell in such a way that the carotid artery on one side was severely occluded.

A less well known phenomenon is the one in which an interval of relatively normal functioning for several days to a month or more after apparent recovery from coma is followed by a rapid and severe deterioration of neurologic and psychiatric functioning. This has been demonstrated with both carbon monoxide poisoning (Vicente, 1980) and a variety of other forms of anoxia (Plum & Posner, 1962). Consequently, patients who have suffered anoxia should not only be tested shortly after initial recovery, but should be followed for several months and retested if there are signs of further deterioration.

It also appears that the effects of repeated or chronic hypoxia, much like those of repeated mild head injuries, are cumulative. Prigatano, Parsons, Wright, Levin, and Hawryluk (1983) demonstrated that patients with chronic obstructive pulmonary disease show significant, but mild, impairment on the HRB, with deficits in abstract reasoning, memory, and speed of performance being seen consistently. This should alert one to the possibility of chronic hypoxia as a causal factor when such a pattern of deficits, which is otherwise unexplainable, is found. This is important because medical treatment may prevent further deterioration, although it will not necessarily reverse existing impairment.

Seizures

"Seizures are paroxysmal events of cerebral origin that have a wide variety of manifestations" (Dodrill, 1981, p. 366). The older terms *grand mal*, *petit mal*, and *psychomotor* seizures have been replaced with a more detailed classification system of seizures under the broad categories of *generalized* and *partial* seizures. In any event, seizures are symptoms of a wide range of neuropathology, and, as such, will not show any single characteristic pattern of performance on neuropsychological tests.

In addition to tonic-clonic (grand mal) seizures, there are two types of seizures which the alert neuropsychologist may aid in identifying. The first is the absence seizure, formerly called petit mal. This is characterized by a brief period of unresponsiveness to the environment, without loss of consciousness. It may be manifested to the observant examiner as periods of inattention or periodic "blank staring" during testing and may be suspected on examination of data when performance within a single test is characterized by variability suggestive of lapses of awareness.

The second type, complex partial seizures, formerly called psychomotor seizures, will rarely be observed during testing, but evidence of the underlying causal lesion may be seen on examination of test data, which shows a very focal deficit in an otherwise quite intact profile. If either of these two types of seizures is suspected, referral for medical diagnosis and treatment is indicated since both may respond favorably to appropriate anticonvulsant medications. Regardless of the type of seizure disorder, patients frequently have numerous adjustment problems, including emotional, interpersonal, vocational, and medication compliance problems. Dodrill (1986) has discussed these in detail, and the neuropsychologist working with such patients should be prepared to identify them and treat both patients and their families in this regard.

Chapter 8

Functional Implication Hypotheses

In recent years there have been major advances in medical treatment of the acute effects of brain injuries and disease, resulting in increased survival rates. Chapter 11 describes the role of neuropsychology in providing rehabilitation services for these survivors. Regardless of whether or not patients receive such neuropsychological rehabilitation services, there are frequently questions regarding their abilities to care for themselves, live independently, manage their own affairs, and return to work or school. These are often the most pressing questions involved in resolving claims for compensation. Partly because of the complex interaction of sensory, motor, cognitive, personality, and environmental factors (Jarvis & Barth, 1979; Jarvis & Vollman, 1983; Mooney, 1988), there are few definitive answers to these questions. Hart and Hayden indicate that, "there are very few empirical data supporting such predictions" (Hart & Hayden, 1986, p. 22); however, there are a number of hypotheses with varying degrees of empirical support that will assist in making predictions in individual cases. These are the hypotheses presented in this chapter.

Self-Care

In the area of self-care, the basic everyday activities of feeding, dressing, and hygiene, often called Activities of Daily Living (ADL), are considered. On the surface, it may appear that little sophistication is required to assess these abilities, but there is a trap here for the too narrowly focused neuropsychologist. Consider the case of the patient who arrives for a neuropsychological evaluation appearing well nourished, neatly dressed, and well groomed. Findings of significant motor or sensory deficits might arouse suspicions about the ability to function independently in this area, and an absence of them might lead one to conclude that the patient is capable of self-care. The trap is the assumption that because the patient is neatly dressed and groomed, for example, he/she actually performs the activities in an independent fashion leading to this appearance. This may not always be the case.

Patients with deficits in executive functions resulting from frontal lobe impairment may possess the skills required to perform the functions of ADLs but may not actually carry them out independently. They may require coaching or prompting to initiate the activities and, sometimes, to proceed through each of the steps in the required sequences. For example, a patient with a frontal meningioma, when asked to count backward from 10 required prompting after each number. (Patient, "10..."; Examiner, "What comes next?"; Patient, "9…"; Examiner, "What comes next?"; and so on…) Shortly after successful surgical removal of the tumor she was able to perform this task without prompting.

Another patient was evaluated about a year after he suffered a severe closed head injury. At the time of the evaluation he was neatly dressed and groomed. After interviewing his wife, however, it was determined that it was she who was responsible for the patient's favorable appearance. Left to his own devices, the patient would *never* bathe or change his clothes. In fact, he typically went to bed with all of his clothes on, including his boots.

(8-1) Interviews with family members or others who are familiar with the daily activities of the patient are critical and should always be conducted. These should focus on what the patient actually does independently and how much coaching or prompting is required.

(8-2) Patients whose performance is severely impaired on tests sensitive to frontal lobe impairment (among other neurological deficits), such as the Category Test, Part B of the Trail Making Test, and the Wisconsin Card Sorting Test, may have deficits in executive functions involving the initiation, inhibition, sequencing, and monitoring of behavior. Consequently, they may not care for themselves adequately without supervision, coaching, or prompting even though they possess the requisite skills to do so.

(8-3) Observations of the *quality* of patients' performance on tests may reveal features such as difficulty in initiating behavior (failure to start a task promptly when told to do so, even when the instructions are clearly understood); inhibiting behavior, or impulsiveness (attempting to start a task before being told to do so, or failure to wait until all of the instructions have been given); or failure to shift behavior appropriately (continuing to repeat digits instead of shifting to reversing them when told to do so). These may be related to deficits in executive functions resulting from frontal lobe impairment, which can lead to difficulty in caring for one's self independently (Lezak, 1983).

(8-4) Severe deficits in delayed recall on memory testing associated with temporal lobe impairment may result in self-care deficits when a person forgets to perform important ADL tasks. Simple prompts, reminders, or prominently posted schedules of activities may be effective in cases where there are not accompanying major deficits in executive functions.

(8-5) Evidence of constructional dyspraxia on tests such as those requiring design copying, Block Design, or Object Assembly suggests that a person may have difficulty dressing himself/herself properly and efficiently (Baum & Hall, 1981). Acker (1984) reviewed several additional studies that show relationships between constructional dyspraxia as well as impaired visual perception and scores on the Block Design and Object Assembly subtests and dressing dyspraxia.

Management of One's Own Affairs

In this area the management of finances is generally the most important issue, and environmental factors play a crucial role. The skills required to manage small amounts of money for personal purchases in an environment where one's housing and meals are provided are obviously less demanding than those required to pay rent, utility, and food bills when living in an apartment. Additional skills are, of course, required to manage a business or investment income.

(8-6) Performance in the mentally deficient range on the Arithmetic Subtest of the WAIS-R and achievement tests such as the WRAT-R suggests that a person will have trouble handling even routine, small personal purchases competently. When this level of test performance is observed, it is advisable to assess the person's ability further with exercises simulating making purchases and getting the correct change.

(8-7) Performance in the low average range or above on the Arithmetic subtest of the WAIS-R appears necessary to manage routine payments for things such as food, rent, and utilities. In marginal cases, exercises simulating activities such as writing checks to pay bills appear indicated.

(8-8) Moderately to severely impaired performance on tests requiring adequate new problem-solving abilities, such as the Category Test, suggests that a person may have trouble making competent decisions about major, nonroutine purchases or investment decisions (Heaton & Pendleton, 1981).

Independent Living

The question of how independently a person is capable of living is a complex one. Severe motor and sensory deficits obviously impose limitations, but a neuropsychological evaluation is usually not required to identify problems of this magnitude. At least minimally adequate self-care skills are required, and either the ability to manage one's own financial affairs or the availability of appropriate assistance with this, and willingness of the person to accept it, are necessary. Beyond these factors, several other considerations are relevant.

(8-9) The more severe a brain injury, as indicated, for example, by such measures as the length of coma and posttraumatic amnesia, the score on the Glasgow Coma Scale, and CT or MRI scans, the less satisfactory the outcome is likely to be in terms of independent living and productivity. However, it is important to keep in mind that there are exceptions to this, both severely injured people with good outcomes and mildly injured people with poor outcomes (Vogenthaler, Smith, & Goldfader, 1989).

(8-10) Deficits in visuospatial abilities and nonverbal memory are more likely to be associated with deficient independent living skills in people with senile dementia of the Alzhiemer's type (SDAT) than are deficits in verbal memory (Mahurin, DeBettingies, & Pirozzolo, 1991).

(8-11) Severely impaired performance on tasks requiring divided attention, such as Part B of the Trail Making Test, may be associated with deficits in attending to certain aspects of the environment such as fire hazards. Therefore, people who show this type of impaired performance should have their functioning monitored in an environment similar to the independent one where they want to live before being recommended for independent living.

(8-12) Severe memory impairment, particularly for delayed recall, may lead to dangerous situations such as fire resulting from leaving a stove on or flooding caused by leaving water running.

(8-13) Significant impairment of right-hemisphere functioning, particularly visual spatial perceptual deficits and nonverbal memory impairments may result in a person getting lost easily (Jarvis & Hamlin, 1991).

Return to Work or School

Determination of the ability to return to work or school involves questions regarding the nature of work or study and the related cognitive demands; the match between the person's remaining cognitive abilities and those demands; and, particularly in cases of mild brain injury, the timing of the attempt to return to work or study.

(8-14) Significant problems with attention, memory, and slowed information processing are the most commonly cited cognitive problems causing employment failure following brain injury (Wehman, Kreutzer, Sale, West, Morton, & Diambra, 1989).

(8-15) Scores on tests that tap retention of previously learned knowledge, such as the Information and Comprehension Subtests of the WAIS-R, which are significantly lower than the estimated premorbid scores on the same tests suggest that a patient may not retain enough job-related knowledge to return successfully to a previously held job. Supplemental testing of job-specific knowledge can be used to make finer discriminations.

(8-16) Severely impaired performance on tests that require new learning ability, such as the Category Test, the TPT, and the Digit Symbol Subtest of the WAIS-R, suggest that a patient may have difficulty returning to a job or field of study that requires adaptation to rapidly changing demands. Such people may also have difficulty learning the tasks required by new, unfamiliar jobs. They may learn new information and tasks more slowly than usual and will probably do best on jobs that limit demands to the repetitious performance of routine tasks. Additional tests of learning ability such as the Rey Auditory Verbal Learning Test (RAVLT) or the California Verbal Learning Test (CVLT) may provide additional relevant information in such an evaluation.

(8-17) Intact left-hemisphere functioning may allow adequate performance of language-related tasks such as mail sorting or filing, even in the presence of right-hemisphere deficits. Intact right-hemisphere functioning, on the other hand, may allow performance of tasks requiring visual-spatial functioning such as assembly work (Goldstein, 1987).

(8-18) Significantly more impairment on Part B of the Trail Making Test than on Part A of the same test suggests that, even if attention skills are generally adequate, there will be problems when "divided attention" is required. Patients who show this pattern of performance may be able to perform adequately when they do not have to attend to more than one thing at a time or when there are no distracting stimuli present in the environment, but their performance may deteriorate significantly in the presence of such distractions. This may have implications for structuring the patient's work environment in a way that will facilitate optimal performance (Lezak, 1987).

(8-19) Attention deficits may result in feelings of being "overloaded" and fatigue in work environments that are busy and include competing stimuli (Bennett, 1988). This may be a particularly common problem when people return to work too soon after a brain injury. Returning to work on a part-time basis or modifying the work environment may be helpful (Reitan, 1975; Reitan & Wolfson, 1993).

(8-20) People with only mild deficits on the Aphasia Screening Test can usually perform adequately on nonverbally oriented jobs, but will show impaired performance on jobs that require more verbal facility such as sales, teaching, counseling, and the law (Bennett, 1988).

(8-21) Significantly impaired performance on the Category Test and the Wisconsin Card Sorting Test reflect difficulty with concept formation, problem solving, and flexibility of thinking. People with these problems are not likely to perform well on supervisory, managerial, or most professional jobs (Bennett, 1988; Heaton & Pendleton, 1981).

(8-22) Impaired social interaction skills will generally hinder a person's ability to perform successfully at work or in school. On some types of jobs, such as management or sales, they may make performance impossible. Marsh and Knight (1991) found that impaired performance in an *in vivo* social interaction situation was highly correlated with impaired verbal fluency.

(8-23) The more pervasive the impairment (Impairment Index above .5) and the more severe the impairment, the less likely it is that a patient will be employed (Heaton et al., 1978).

(8-24) The greater the severity of psychological disturbance shown on the MMPI, the less likely it is that a brain-injured person will be employed (Heaton et al., 1978).

General

There are several other significant activities that, although they may not fit neatly into any one of the preceding categories, should be considered in a comprehensive neuropsychological evaluation.

(8-25) The presence of a seizure disorder requires medical evaluation to determine whether or not a person can drive a motor vehicle safely.

(8-26) Heaton and Pendleton (1981) list a number of areas of deficits including attention, right-left discrimination, nonverbal memory, visuoconstructional ability, and concept formation, which should be considered in evaluating driving ability. Acker (1986) also suggests that low test scores on the Picture Completion and Picture Arrangement subtests are related to impaired driving ability, and Chelune and Moehle (1986) suggest seven additional tests that may be relevant. Since driving safely is such a complex activity, it is clear that deficits in any of a variety of motor, perceptual, and cognitive skills can impair this activity. This is also an area that involves significant legal issues, and laws vary from one state to another. Although there are many people who have deficits in some of these skills but are driving every day, it is wise to recommend an evaluation of actual driving ability by a trained driving evaluator whenever significant deficits in any of these skills are found on neuropsychological evaluation. Sophisticated, computerized driving simulators may also be used in such assessments.

(8-27) Severe memory deficits suggest that Antabuse (disulfram) should be used with caution for treatment of alcoholism. The problem is that the patient may either forget that he/she has taken the Antabuse or forget what the consequences of drinking are after taking it. This may result in life-threatening behavior.

(8-28) A significant discrepancy between a patient's own assessment of abilities and the level of functioning shown on neuropsychological evaluation may result in problems in everyday functioning. If the patient's assessment is that his/her abilities are more impaired than formal evaluation indicates, the patient may resist return to the level of functioning that is predicted by the evaluation. Appropriate psychotherapy is indicated in such cases. Patients who underestimate or deny the severity of their disability may set themselves up for repeated failures in a variety of activities and a further reduction in self esteem (Heaton & Pendleton, 1981).

(8-29) The discrepancy between actual memory functioning and self-assessment of memory functioning may be estimated by comparing the results of formal memory testing to a patient's self-report on an instrument such as the Memory Functioning Questionnaire (Gilewski & Zelinski, 1988).

(8-30) Patients with significant deficits on tests which are sensitive to frontal lobe functioning may be particularly prone to inaccurate self-assessment of their own functional abilities (Taylor, 1990). Therefore, it is important to take this into consideration when making arrangements for the daily living situations, care, and supervision of such patients.

(8-31) Those people who show the greatest loss of intellectual functioning (difference between premorbid and postinjury IQs) have the greatest difficulty adjusting because they tend to compare their postinjury abilities to their premorbid expectations (Mayes, Pelco, & Campbell, 1989).

In 1981 Heaton and Pendleton stated, "Clearly, more research is needed to demonstrate that specific neuropsychological tests measure abilities that are required in specific aspects of patients' everyday functioning" (Heaton & Pendleton, 1981, p. 815). Nearly a decade later Heinrichs (1990) claimed that the "ecological validity" of neuropsychological tests had yet to be demonstrated. In view of the limited progress in this area, caution is indicated in drawing inferences about everyday functioning from neuropsychological test data in individual cases.

In some cases, interview data, ratings on behavioral rating scales, and/or the use of specific task-related simulations may improve predictions. Lawton (1988) reviewed a number of potentially useful rating scales. In addition, the Memory Functioning Questionnaire (Gilewski & Zelinski, 1988) and the Structured Assessment of Independent Living Skills (SAILS) (Mahurin, DeBettingies, & Pirozzolo, 1991) appear to have promise for quantifying patients' functional status.

Chapter 9

Illustrative Cases

Raw score transformations for the tests of the Halstead-Reitan Battery, the WAIS-R, and certain other tests are provided in the form of a printout from the Heaton et al. (1991) computer program, and T Scores are generally used in interpretation. When additional tests were administered, interpretation of scores is based on the best normative data available for each test. Each of the seven questions listed in chapter 3 is addressed from the perspectives of the four methods of inference: Level of Performance, Pattern of Performance, Right/Left Differences, and Pathognomonic Signs. Some interpretive statements are followed by numbers, which refer to the hypotheses presented in earlier chapters. For example, (x-y) would refer to Hypothesis y in chapter x.

The cases are all drawn from the hospital and outpatient practices of the authors. In some cases, information from imaging studies or other medical tests was actually available prior to the neuropsychological testing, but the interpretations of the neuropsychological test data are presented "blind" to such additional information to illustrate the methods of interpretation. In other cases, the medical tests were not performed until the neuropsychological evaluation had been completed. Finally, there are some cases for which a definitive neurological diagnosis was never established.

Most of the interpretations are provided blind to the patients' histories. This method has been widely used in validation studies, and it is used here for teaching purposes. It illustrates the value of the hypotheses presented in chapters 4 through 8 and the method of applying them to interpretation of test data. It also demonstrates some of the limitations of blind interpretation, which should never be the basis for actual clinical evaluations. The material presented in chapter 10 is essential in all real clinical applications.

Case 1

This is a 63-year-old, white, married, right-handed male accountant with 18 years of education. His work as a CPA had become increasingly erratic over the past several years. His employment was finally terminated after he had failed to file income tax returns for several of his firm's clients.

He had a great deal of difficulty understanding instructions for several of the tests and was completely unable to comprehend some of them. He could not, for example, perform either the TPT or the Category Test. He was very pleasant and polite and related to the female examiner in a rather childlike manner. Because of the level of his impairment, testing required several relatively short sessions. He was neatly and formally dressed,

```
                         HRB NORMS PROGRAM
                      Raw Score Transformations


Name:        Case1                      Sex:         M
Age:         63               Years of Educ:         18
Date:        02/26/93             File Name:         CASE1
Handedness: Right


                                             Raw    Scaled      T
Measure                          Abbreviation Scores  Scores  Scores


HALSTEAD REITAN
BATTERY SCORES

Halstead Impairment Index        HII
Average Impairment Rating        AIR
Category Test                    CAT ERROR
Trail Making Test-A (secs)       TRAIL A       124      1      17#
Trail Making Test-B (secs)       TRAIL B       264      3      24#
Tact Perf Test-Time (min/blk)    TPT TIME
Tact Perf Test-Memory (correct)  TPT MEM
Tact Perf Test-Location (correct) TPT LOC
Seashore Rhythm (correct)        SSHOR RHYM     15      3      28#
Speech Perception (errors)       SPCH PERC      18      4      26#
Aphasia Screening (errors)       APHAS SCRN     13      5      28#
Spatial Relations (rating)       SPAT REL        2     11      55
Sensory-Perceptual Total (errors) SP TOTAL

LATERALIZED SENSORIMOTOR/
PSYCHOMOTOR INDICES

Finger Tapping-Dom (taps)        TAP DH
Finger Tapping-Non-dom (taps)    TAP NDH
Hand Dynamometer-Dom (kgs)       GRIP DH      40.3     10      45
Hand Dynamometer-Non-dom (kgs)   GRIP NDH     37.3      9      41
Grooved Pegboard-Dom (secs)      PEG DH        106      4      31#
Grooved Pegboard-Non-dom (secs)  PEG NDH       133      3      32#L
Tact Perf Test-Dom (min/blk)     TPT DH
Tact Perf Test-Non-dom (min/blk) TPT NDH
Tact Perf Test-Both Hands (min/blk) TPT BOTH
Sensory-Perceptual-Right (errors) SP R
Sensory-Perceptual-Left (errors) SP L
Tactile Form Recog-Right (secs)  TFR R           9     12      52
Tactile Form Recog-Left (secs)   TFR L           9     11      49


# = Impaired
L = Right-left difference, with possible lateralizing significance
```

Figure 3. Case 1.

Note. Cases 1-15 are reproduced by special permission from the Publisher, Psychological Assessment Resources, Inc., from *HRB Norms Program* by R. K. Heaton and PAR Staff, 1991, Odessa: Psychological Assessment Resources, Inc. Copyright 1991 by Psychological Assessment Resources, Inc. All rights reserved.

```
                      HRB NORMS PROGRAM
                   Raw Score Transformations

                          Page 2

Name:        Case1                    Sex:        M
Age:         63              Years of Educ:       18
Date:        02/26/93           File Name:        CASE1
Handedness:  Right
```

Measure	Abbreviation	Raw Scores	Scaled Scores	T Scores
WAIS-R SCORES				
Verbal IQ (VIQ)	VIQ	80	6	15#
Performance IQ (PIQ)	PIQ	85	7	27#
Full Scale IQ (FSIQ)	FSIQ	81	6	17#
Information	INFO	2	2	2#
Digit Span	DIGIT SPAN	8	10	42
Vocabulary	VOCAB	4	4	12#
Arithmetic	ARITH	10	10	39#
Comprehension	COMP	6	6	24#
Similarities	SIMIL	4	4	21#
Picture Completion	PICT COMP	5	5	30#
Picture Arrangement	PICT ARR	4	4	28#
Block Design	BLOCK DESGN	9	9	48
Object Assembly	OBJ ASSMB	6	6	37#
Digit Symbol	DIGIT SYMB	3	3	30#

```
# = Impaired
```

Figure 3. Case 1 (continued).

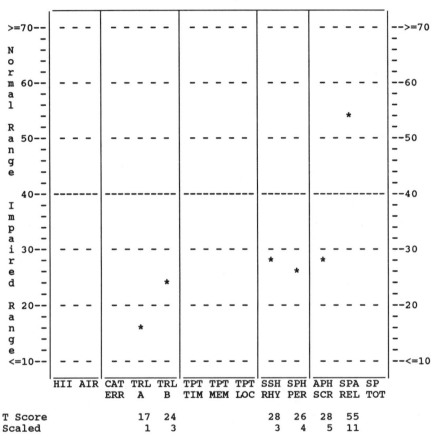

Figure 3. Case 1 (continued).

Page 4

Name: Case1   Sex: M
Age: 63   Yrs of Educ: 18
Date: 02/26/93   File Name: CASE1
Handedness: Right

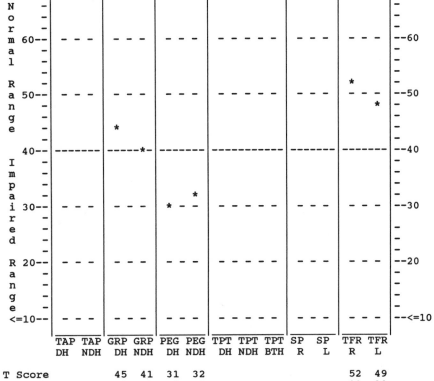

Lateralized Sensorimotor/Psychomotor T Score Profile

	TAP DH	TAP NDH	GRP DH	GRP NDH	PEG DH	PEG NDH	TPT DH	TPT NDH	TPT BTH	SP R	SP L	TFR R	TFR L
T Score			45	41	31	32						52	49
Scaled			10	9	4	3						12	11

Figure 3. Case 1 (continued).

Page 5

Name: Case1   Sex: M
Age: 63   Yrs of Educ: 18
Date: 02/26/93   File Name: CASE1
Handedness: Right

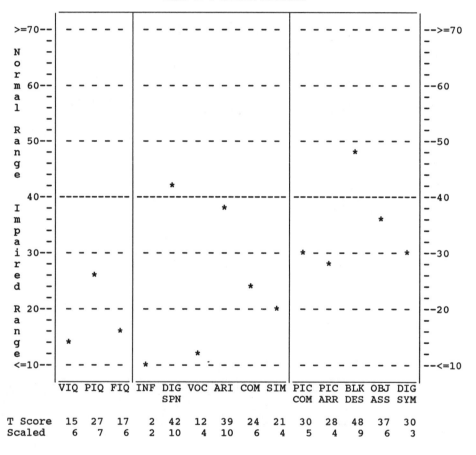

T Score   15 27 17   2 42 12 39 24 21   30 28 48 37 30
Scaled   6   7   6   2 10   4 10   6   4   5   4   9   6   3

Figure 3. Case 1 (continued).

SENSORY—PERCEPTUAL EXAMINATION Case 1

Indicate Instance in which stimulus is not perceived or is incorrectly perceived.

Error Totals

Tactile:

E wrote instructions
S: "you touched my R with your left" etc.

Right Hand/Left Hand — RH [| | |] LH [| | |] Both: RH [X|X|X] LH [| | |] RH __0__ LH __3__

Right Hand/Left Face — RH [| | |] LF [| | |] Both: RH [| | |] LF [| | |] RH _____ LF _____

E could not get S to understand

Left Hand/Right Face — LH [| | |] RF [| | |] Both: LH [| | |] RF [| | |] RF __—__ LH __—__

Auditory:

This ear (R) has been dead for 61 years, you know. My L ear

Right Ear/Left Ear — RE [| | |] LE [| | |] Both: RE [| | |] LE [| | |] RE __—__ LE __—__

Works real well, you know (Q) when I was 2½ yrs old
I was real sick + my (R) ear died, you know.

Visual:

Above eye level
Eye level   { RV [grid] LV [grid] Both: RV [grid] LV [grid]   RV _____ LV _____
Below eye level

↑
Could not understand instructions
↓

Finger Agnosia:

Right: 1 [grid] 2 [grid] 3 [grid] 4 [grid] 5 [grid] R __/__
Left: 1 [grid] 2 [grid] 3 [grid] 4 [grid] 5 [grid] L __/__

Could not understand instructions

Finger-tip Number Writing Perception:

Right: [4|6|3|5] [3|5|4|6] [6|5|4|3] [5|4|6|3] [6|3|5|4] R __/__
Left: L __/__

Astereognosis:

Right: [P|N|D]   Left: [D|N|P / D]   Both: Right: [N|P|D / D] R __1__
                                              Left: [D|D]   L __3__

Tactile Form Recognition:

"Wheel"

Errors: RH [○|□|△|✚] LH [△|✚|○|□] RH [✚|○|□|△] LH [□|△|✚|○] R __0__
Response Time: [1|1|1|1]   [1|1|1|1]   [2|1|1|1]   [1|2|1|1]   L __0__

Total Time: R _9"_ L _9"_

Visual Fields: Left   Right

[circle diagram]   [circle diagram]

Figure 3. Case 1 (continued).

APHASIA SCREENING TEST   **Case 1**

Form for Adults and Older Children

Name: _____ Age: **63**   Date: **1/31/83**   Examiner: _____

1. Copy SQUARE *(Pt. insisted on making a double line and shading figure outline although instructed otherwise. He also printed in center.)*	17. Repeat TRIANGLE *SAY TRIANGLE*
2. Name SQUARE *THAT'S JUST A SQUARE.*	18. Repeat MASSACHUSETTS *WHAT?! (Then ok)*
3. Spell SQUARE *(Printed. Would not spell aloud. May not have understood instr.)*	19. Repeat METHODIST EPISCOPAL *MASSODIS EPISCOPAL*
4. Copy CROSS *(See note for #1.)*	20. Write SQUARE *THAT'S A SQUARE UP THERE.* *(Indicated his drawing of a square and wrote "square" next to the word he'd printed when he made the drawing.)*
5. Name CROSS *(pause) LIKE A PLUS, YOU KNOW. (pause) SIMILAR TO ONE OF THESE (DREW "+.")*	21. Read SEVEN *(OK. then wrote "seven 7")*
6. Spell CROSS *C - R - O - S - S - S*	22. Repeat SEVEN *OK.*
7. Copy TRIANGLE *(See #1 and #4)*	23. Repeat/Explain HE SHOUTED THE WARNING. *WHAT?! - SHOUTED THE WARNING. WHO DID? (Q) HE TALKED TOO LOUD, YOU KNOW. (Q) I DON'T KNOW.*
8. Name TRIANGLE	24. Write HE SHOUTED THE WARNING. *WHAT?! (See his response) CAN I PLAY WITH THE CALCULATOR A LITTLE? (Referred to E's desk calculator)*
9. Spell TRIANGLE *(pause) (Insisted upon writing. Wrote, "T-R-I-A-A-N-G-L-E")*	25. Compute 85 − 27 = *85. 85. (Pause, then ok.) THE DIFFERENCE IS 58.*
10. Name BABY *(Tilted his head)* *THAT'S A BABY.*	26. Compute 17 X 3 = *57. (E: 15 X 3?) (Very long pause, then ok)*
11. Write CLOCK *A CLOCK, YOU KNOW.* *(Printed, then printed "next ." Then wrote when asked to do so.)*	27. Name KEY *THAT'S A - UH - KEY, YOU KNOW. KIND OF LIKE I HAVE IN MY HOME, YOU KNOW.*
12. Name FORK *A FORK, YOU KNOW.* *(Printed, then wrote)*	28. Demonstrate use of KEY *(Uses pencil as a "prop" to demonstrate) YOU PUT IT IN THE HOLE IN THE DOOR AND TURN IT.*
13. Read 7 SIX 2 *OK*	29. Draw KEY *(See drawing)*
14. Read M G W *OK*	30. Read PLACE LEFT HAND TO RIGHT EAR. *(Read haltingly)*
15. Reading I *SEE THE BLACK DOG, YOU KNOW . (Printed the sentence and (A WORD))*	31. Place LEFT HAND TO RIGHT EAR *HERE'S MY LEFT HAND AND HERE'S MY RIGHT EAR. (didn't do task)*
16. Reading II *SHE IS - HE IS A FAMILY - HE IS A FRIENDLY ANIMAL, A FAMOUS (pronounced făm ous) WINNER OF DOG SHOWS. I DON'T EXACTLY KNOW WHAT THAT MEANS, THOUGH.*	32. Place LEFT HAND TO LEFT ELBOW *HERE'S MY LEFT ELBOW. I JUST CAN'T PLACE IT TOO MANY PLACES on MY BODY, YOU KNOW. (Made various attempts) CAN I PLAY WITH THAT (calculator)? (Pt. was unable to figure out how to turn it on. E showed him.) I DIDN'T NOTICE THAT, THIS IS NOT LIKE MINE. (Cont.)*

32. Cont. LET ME SHOW YOU SOMETHING. MINE IS NICER. TAKE ME HOME TO GET IT SO I CAN SHOW YOU. (Pt. was unable to operate E's calculator.)

Figure 3. Case 1 (continued).

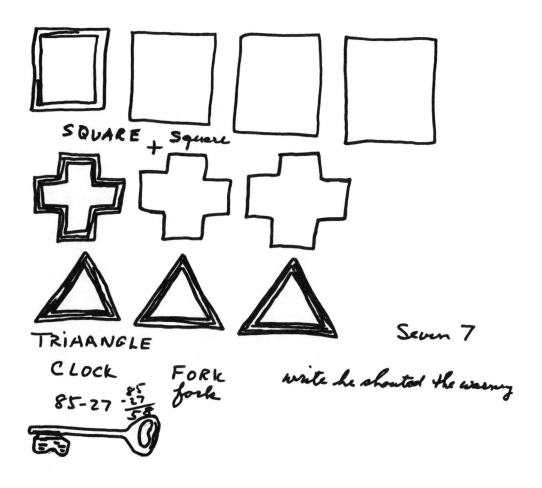

Figure 3. Case 1 (continued).

wearing a suit and tie, and treated the walk on the hospital grounds from his ward to the Neuropsychology Laboratory with the examiner as a social occasion.

1) Is There Cerebral Impairment?

Level of Performance: No Halstead Impairment Index was calculated due to his inability to complete either the TPT or the Category Test, which are indications of his impairment. His *T* score on Part B of the Trail Making Test was 24, which is impaired. This method of inference clearly indicates impairment. **(4-1)**

Pattern of Performance: The only available data relevant to Pattern of Performance are the VIQ (80) and PIQ (85). While the difference between them is not significant, the *T* scores of 15 and 27 do show a significant difference, supporting the presence of impairment. This is an indication of the importance of considering a patient's age and education.

Right/Left Differences: The limited sensory and motor testing data do not show any right/left differences, and therefore, this method of inference does not support the presence of impairment.

Pathognomonic Signs: No pathognomonic signs were seen in the limited sensory testing data available, but the Aphasia Screening Test revealed errors of dysnomia and spelling dyspraxia, which are clearly pathognomonic for a person with this patient's educational background. This is strong support for impairment. **(4-56)**

Overall, three of the four methods of inference support the presence of impairment, leaving no doubt about the answer to this question.

2) What is the Severity of Cerebral Dysfunction?

Level of Performance: This patient's inability to comprehend the instructions for several tests and his very poor performance on others indicates severe impairment. His Full Scale IQ of only 81 is probably at least 30 points below his premorbid level, also indicating severe impairment.

Pattern of Performance: The *T* scores of 15 and 27 for VIQ and PIQ suggest at least a moderately severe level of impairment.

Right/Left Differences: This method of inference does not contribute to answering this question in this case.

Pathognomonic Signs: The type of errors seen on the Aphasia Screening Test indicate a severe level of impairment for this patient.

3) Is the Lesion Progressive or Static?

Level of Performance: The low IQ and the severe difficulties on the Seashore Rhythm and Speech Sounds Perception tests suggest the possibility of a progressive lesion. As usual, the history is essential in regard to this question, and it indicates a progressive condition. **(6-7, 6-11)**

Pattern of Performance: This method of inference does not contribute to the answer of this question.

Right/Left Differences: This method of inference does not contribute to the answer of this question.

Pathognomonic Signs: The facts that this man has an awareness of his dysphasic problems, is disturbed by them, and has apparently not begun to compensate for them in any way all suggest that this may be a progressive condition.

Overall, one can say that the test data are consistent with a progressive condition, but they certainly do not provide a definite answer to this question. As usual, the history is much more helpful, and it makes it clear that this man's condition has been deteriorating over a period of several years.

4) Is the Lesion Diffuse or Lateralized?

Level of Performance: As usual, this method of inference does not contribute to the answer of this question.

Pattern of Performance: The 12-point difference in T scores for VIQ (15) and PIQ (27) is suggestive of more left-hemisphere impairment. **(4-10)**

Right/Left Differences: This method of inference contributes little to the answer of this question in this case since there is such limited sensory and motor data available.

Pathognomonic Signs: The aphasia signs indicate that there is significant left-hemisphere impairment. **(4-56)**

Overall, although the left hemisphere is clearly impaired, the general impairment of all cognitive functions and the lack of data from certain tests makes it difficult to say that there is a clearly lateralized lesion. Diffuse impairment seems more likely.

5) Is the Impairment in the Anterior or Posterior Part of the Cerebral Hemisphere?

Level of Performance: As usual, this method of inference does not contribute to the answer of this question.

Pattern of Performance: As usual, this method of inference does not contribute to the answer of this question.

Right/Left Differences: As usual, this method of inference does not contribute to the answer of this question.

Pathognomonic Signs: This patient had both receptive and expressive difficulties, and this does not contribute to the answer of this question.

Overall, there is nothing to indicate that there is any lesion of a focal nature.

6) What is the Most Likely Neuropathological Process?

There appears to be a severe, diffuse condition that has been progressing for several years at a relatively steady rate. Considering this man's age, a degenerative disease such as Alzheimer's disease appears to be the most likely neuropathological condition. A CT Scan of the brain revealed atrophy, which was considered to be consistent with Alzheimer's Disease.

7) What are the Implications for Everyday Functioning and Treatment?

Unfortunately, there is no definitive treatment for this disease, and this man will need nursing-home care at some point. At the present time, he is able to feed himself and dress himself appropriately, although he is not able to live independently. The major question is how much support his family is able to provide for him. Counseling was offered to his wife to assist her in deciding when she would need to find an appropriate nursing home for him, and she was referred to a support group for caregivers of Alzheimer's disease patients.

Case 2

This is a 29-year-old, white, right-handed male carpenter with 10 years of education. On two additional tests, his performances were as follows: On the Benton Judgment of Line Orientation Test (JOLO) his score of 26 was in the average range; on the Russell Revision of the Wechsler Memory Scale (RRWMS) his scores for both immediate and delayed verbal memory were severely impaired, while his scores for visual memory were only mildly impaired.

1) Is There Cerebral Impairment?

Level of Performance: His Halstead Impairment Index yields a *T* score of only 2, which is severely impaired. His *T* score of 43 for the Category Test is just slightly below average, while his *T* score of 46 on the TPT Location component is in the average range. His *T* score of 22 on Part B of the Trail Making Test is moderately-to-severely impaired. With two of the four most sensitive indicators being severely impaired, this method of inference suggests impairment.

Pattern of Performance: The VIQ *T* score of 26 is just one standard deviation lower than the PIQ *T* score of 36. As noted earlier, his verbal memory is significantly more impaired than his visual memory. This method of inference, then, also suggests impairment.

Right/Left Differences: His strength of grip with his dominant hand is weaker than his nondominant hand, and the possible lateralizing significance of this is indicated by the L next to the *T* score on the first page of the Norms printout. The relationships for Tapping and TPT are normal. Note that although the *T* scores for Sensory Perceptual errors on the right and left are 44 and 68, this is based on a total of only three errors and must be viewed with caution. Similarly, although the Tactile Form Recognition Time has an L next to it, this represents a difference of only 2 seconds between the total times for the two hands. Overall, this method of inference provides only modest support for impairment.

Pathognomonic Signs: A right homonymous hemianopsia was noted on the examination of visual fields. On the Aphasia Screening Test, there were numerous errors of both receptive and expressive types. In addition, severe word-finding problems were noted on all verbal tests, during interviews, and in everyday conversation. These multiple pathognomonic signs leave no doubt about the presence of impairment.

2) What is the Severity of Cerebral Dysfunction?

Level of Performance: The level of performance ranges from average, or normal, on some tests to quite severely impaired on others such as the Trail Making Test.

HRB NORMS PROGRAM
Raw Score Transformations

Name: Case2   Sex: M
Age: 29   Years of Educ: 10
Date: 02/26/93   File Name: CASE2
Handedness: Right

Measure	Abbreviation	Raw Scores	Scaled Scores	T Scores
HALSTEAD REITAN				
BATTERY SCORES				
Halstead Impairment Index	HII	1.0	1	3#
Average Impairment Rating	AIR			
Category Test	CAT ERROR	55	8	43
Trail Making Test-A (secs)	TRAIL A	100	1	12#
Trail Making Test-B (secs)	TRAIL B	275	3	22#
Tact Perf Test-Time (min/blk)	TPT TIME	.586	8	40
Tact Perf Test-Memory (correct)	TPT MEM	5	6	33#
Tact Perf Test-Location (correct)	TPT LOC	4	10	46
Seashore Rhythm (correct)	SSHOR RHYM	20	5	33#
Speech Perception (errors)	SPCH PERC			
Aphasia Screening (errors)	APHAS SCRN	24	2	21#
Spatial Relations (rating)	SPAT REL	3	9	47
Sensory-Perceptual Total (errors)	SP TOTAL	3	10	54
LATERALIZED SENSORIMOTOR/				
PSYCHOMOTOR INDICES				
Finger Tapping-Dom (taps)	TAP DH	53.2	11	49
Finger Tapping-Non-dom (taps)	TAP NDH	48.8	11	52
Hand Dynamometer-Dom (kgs)	GRIP DH	47.7	11	48L
Hand Dynamometer-Non-dom (kgs)	GRIP NDH	49.3	12	49
Grooved Pegboard-Dom (secs)	PEG DH	83	6	31#
Grooved Pegboard-Non-dom (secs)	PEG NDH	91	6	30#
Tact Perf Test-Dom (min/blk)	TPT DH	.67	8	40
Tact Perf Test-Non-dom (min/blk)	TPT NDH	.57	8	44
Tact Perf Test-Both Hands (min/blk)	TPT BOTH	.52	7	37#
Sensory-Perceptual-Right (errors)	SP R	0	16	68
Sensory-Perceptual-Left (errors)	SP L	3	7	44
Tactile Form Recog-Right (secs)	TFR R	14	9	46
Tactile Form Recog-Left (secs)	TFR L	16	7	40L

\# = Impaired
L = Right-left difference, with possible lateralizing significance

Figure 4. Case 2.

```
                          HRB NORMS PROGRAM
                       Raw Score Transformations

                               Page 2

Name:        Case2                              Sex:       M
Age:         29                       Years of Educ:       10
Date:        02/26/93                     File Name:       CASE2
Handedness: Right
```

| | | Raw | Scaled | T |
Measure	Abbreviation	Scores	Scores	Scores
WAIS-R SCORES				
Verbal IQ (VIQ)	VIQ	66	3	26#
Performance IQ (PIQ)	PIQ	72	5	36#
Full Scale IQ (FSIQ)	FSIQ	67	4	31#
Information	INFO	2	2	24#
Digit Span	DIGIT SPAN	1	2	21#
Vocabulary	VOCAB	5	5	38#
Arithmetic	ARITH	6	6	39#
Comprehension	COMP	6	6	42
Similarities	SIMIL	3	3	31#
Picture Completion	PICT COMP	8	8	46
Picture Arrangement	PICT ARR	6	6	38#
Block Design	BLOCK DESGN	6	6	37#
Object Assembly	OBJ ASSMB	3	3	27#
Digit Symbol	DIGIT SYMB	4	4	33#

= Impaired

Figure 4. Case 2 (continued).

Name: Case2   Sex: M
Age: 29   Years of Educ: 10
Date: 02/26/93   File Name: CASE2
Handedness: Right

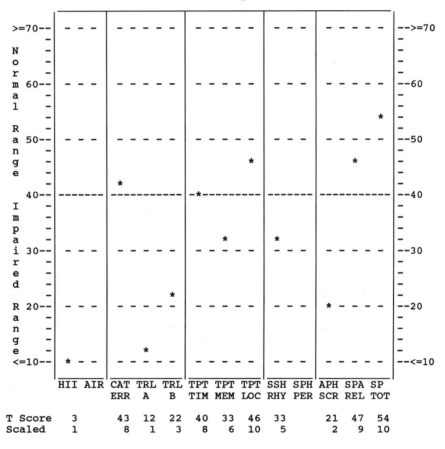

Figure 4. Case 2 (continued).

Page 4

```
Name:        Case2                              Sex:     M
Age:         29                        Yrs of Educ:      10
Date:        02/26/93                    File Name:      CASE2
Handedness:  Right
```

Lateralized Sensorimotor/Psychomotor T Score Profile

```
>=70--  - - -   - - -   - - -   - - - - -   - - -   - - -   -->=70
     -                                         *
N    -
o    -
r    -
m  60--  - - -   - - -   - - -   - - - - -   - - -   - - -   --60
a    -
l    -
     -
R    -           *
a  50--  - - -   - - -   - - -   - - - - -   - - -   - - -   --50
n    -  *        *   *
g    -                                                 *
e    -                           *             *
     -
    40--  -------  -------  -------  -*---------  -------  ------*-  --40
I    -
m    -                                   *
p    -
a    -
i  30--  - - -   - - -   * - *   - - - - -   - - -   - - -   --30
r    -
e    -
d    -
     -
R  20--  - - -   - - -   - - -   - - - - -   - - -   - - -   --20
a    -
n    -
g    -
e    -
<=10--  - - -   - - -   - - -   - - - - -   - - -   - - -   --<=10
```

	TAP DH	TAP NDH	GRP DH	GRP NDH	PEG DH	PEG NDH	TPT DH	TPT NDH	TPT BTH	SP R	SP L	TFR R	TFR L
T Score	49	52	48	49	31	30	40	44	37	68	44	46	40
Scaled	11	11	11	12	6	6	8	8	7	16	7	9	7

Figure 4. Case 2 (continued).

Name: Case2   Sex: M
Age: 29   Yrs of Educ: 10
Date: 02/26/93   File Name: CASE2
Handedness: Right

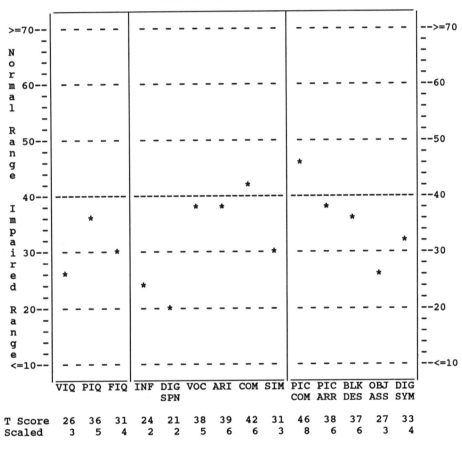

WAIS-R T Score Profile

	VIQ	PIQ	FIQ	INF	DIG SPN	VOC	ARI	COM	SIM	PIC COM	PIC ARR	BLK DES	OBJ ASS	DIG SYM
T Score	26	36	31	24	21	38	39	42	31	46	38	37	27	33
Scaled	3	5	4	2	2	5	6	6	3	8	6	6	3	4

Figure 4. Case 2 (continued).

SENSORY—PERCEPTUAL EXAMINATION   **Case 2**

Indicate Instance in which stimulus is not perceived or is incorrectly perceived.

	Error Totals

Tactile: *Had to practice saying "face"*
"cheek" was in hand - didn't know what cheek was

Right Hand/Left Hand — RH ☐☐☐   LH ☐☐☐   Both: RH ☐☐☐   LH ☐☐☐   RH _0_ LH _0_

Right Hand/Left Face — RH ☐☐☐   LF ☐☐☐   Both: RH ☐☐☐   LF ☐☐☐   RH _0_ LF _0_

Left Hand/Right Face — LH ☐☐☐   RF ☐☐☐   Both: LH ☐☐☐   RF ☐☐☐   RF _0_ LH _0_

Auditory: *S said of*   *@ first*

Right Ear/Left Ear — RE ☐☐☐   LE ☐☐☐   Both: RE ☐☐☐   LE ☒☒☒   RE _0_ LE _3_

Visual:

Above eye level
Eye level   { RV ☒☒☒☒ LV ☐☐☐☐   Both: RV ☒☒☒☒ LV ☐☐☐☐   RV _24_ LV _0_
Below eye level

Finger Agnosia:

Right: 1 ☐☐☐   2 ☐☐☐   3 ☐☐☐   4 ☐☐☐   5 ☐☐☐   R _0/_
Left: 1 ☐☐☐   2 ☐☐☐   3 ☐☐☐   4 ☐☐☐   5 ☐☐☐   L _0/_

Finger-tip Number Writing Perception: *Counts up (& answer) silently - just lip movement.*

Right: | 4 | 6 | 3 | 5 | | 3 | 5 | 4 | 6 | | 6 | 5 | 4 | 3 | | 5 | 4 | 6 | 3 | | 6 | 3 | 5 | 4 | R _0/_
Left: L _0/_

Astereognosis:

Right: | P | N | D | / | P | Left: | D | N | P | Both: Right: | N | P | D | / P | R _2_
                                                   Left: | 10 | L _1_

Tactile Form Recognition:

Errors: RH | ○ | □ | △ | ✛ | LH | △ | ✛ | ○ | □ | RH | ✛ | ○ | □ | △ | LH | □ | △ | ✛ | ○ | R _0_
Response Time: | 2 | 2 | 2 | 3 | | 2 | 2 | 2 | 2 | | 2 | 1 | 1 | 1 | | 4 | 1 | 1 | 2 | L _0_
             9   8   *oh, you're seeing* 5   8
                                          how fast Total Time: R _14_   L _16_

Visual Fields: Left   Right

Figure 4. Case 2 (continued).

APHASIA SCREENING TEST   Case 2

Form for Adults and Older Children

Name: _____ Age: **29** Date: **6/9/83** Examiner: _____

1. Copy SQUARE	17. Repeat TRIANGLE
2. Name SQUARE *IT'S A - IT'S A - A - I DON'T KNOW. WHAT DOES IT START STATE? THAT'S A - A PICTURE- A - A STRAIGHT RIGHT - A - I DON'T KNOW HOW TO SAY IT. OH. THAT'S A THING THAT GOES AROUND IN A SQUARE. I DON'T KNOW HOW THAT CAME OUT! (laughs)*	18. Repeat MASSACHUSETTS *MESHATUSHLESS*
3. Spell SQUARE *SQUARE - IT STARTS WITH A CIRCLE - O - AND THEN I DON'T KNOW*	19. Repeat METHODIST EPISCOPAL *MAKATIS ETUSITAL*
4. Copy CROSS	20. Write SQUARE *(Printed, then attempted to write - scribbled over it)*
5. Name CROSS *IT'S - WRITE - CIRCLE. NO. NO CIRCLE. IT'S A - WRITING A - NOT A CIRCLE. BUT A - I DON'T KNOW. A - IT MEANS ABOUT - IT'S A GOOD ONE - FOR GOD. (Looks at cross he wears around his neck) I DON'T KNOW.*	21. Read SEVEN
6. Spell CROSS *OH, YEAH! CROSS - CROSS - THAT'S A C - A. NO. I DON'T KNOW.*	22. Repeat SEVEN
7. Copy TRIANGLE	23. Repeat/Explain HE SHOUTED THE WARNING. *A WO-MAN? (R) HE SHOUSSES A WO-MAN. (Q) MEANS YOU'RE - SOMEBODY YELLED TO LET YOU KNOW SOMEBODY'S LEAVING OR SOMETHING'S HAPPENING.*
8. Name TRIANGLE *THAT'S A RAN'FENCEE. NO. KEEFAH - NO. I DON'T KNOW. - IT'S A - STARTS WITH A CIRCLE. PROBABLY NOT - NO. THAT STARTS WITH A RODNEY - LET ME THINK (pause) (Q) 3 SIDES.*	24. Write HE SHOUTED THE WARNING. *(Printed 'A') NO, I'LL JUST LEAVE THAT - THAT'S 'A.'*
9. Spell TRIANGLE *(E: It's a tri-) TRIUNKLE. (E) (E began saying tri-) S: "TRIUNCLE" (spell triangle) I DON'T KNOW*	25. Compute 85 − 27 = *112*
10. Name BABY *A BABY. SOME WORDS COME OUT OK.*	26. Compute 17 X 3 = *SAY AGAIN (R) WHAT IS IT ALTOGETHER? (uses fingers) 36 (4 x 3?) SAY IT SLOWER. (R) 16.*
11. Write CLOCK *(Wrote TI). NO. THAT'S NOT RIGHT.*	27. Name KEY *IT'S A THING THAT CAN BE LOCKED. (points toward the door) SOMEBODY COULD LET ME OUT.*
12. Name FORK *WOOF - I MEAN WITH - WIFF. IT AIN'T COMING OUT RIGHT. WOOF. WIFF. (E: TRY SAYING. "I EAT WITH A___.") I EAT WITH A WIFF. I'M HUNGRY: LET ME HAVE YOUR WOOF...*	28. Demonstrate use of KEY *OK.*
13. Read 7 SIX 2 *THAT IS - SHOULD I SAY IT? SIXTH - SIX - SEVENTH - IS THAT ALL? OH. THERE'S MORE. I DIDN'T LOOK (R homomynous hemianopsia) 7 6 2.*	29. Draw KEY *(Put in shading & detail without being prompted) I SHOULD'VE MADE IT ABOUT HALF THE SIZE (pointing) (E: In here?) YEAH. IT SHOULDN'T HAVE BEEN SO WIDE.*
14. Read M G W *THAT'S A CAR. ISN'T IT? WAUF 'INSIN. I CAN'T SAY THAT. H. F. IS THAT F - F? OH. I DON'T KNOW.*	30. Read PLACE LEFT HAND TO RIGHT EAR. *WHAT DOES IT SAY? IT SAYS YOUR LEFT NOSE. NOT YOUR NOSE BUT YOUR EAR - OR SOMETHING LIKE THAT. THAT'S ALL I KNOW OR CAN FIGURE.*
15. Reading I *DARK - OLD - DOG - I MEAN. BLACK DOG - BLOCK DOG - BLACK DOG. (E: There's a line above that one.) I DON'T KNOW WHAT IT SAYS. OH. "THE END."*	31. Place LEFT HAND TO RIGHT EAR *(E read instruction) (RH to R ear and LH to nose. Pt. was able to perform correctly when E gave instructions one step at a time)*
16. Reading II *FRIENDS - CAN'T - WHEN IT'S COLD AND - I DON'T KNOW WHAT THAT'S SAYING. FRIENDS. IS THAT RIGHT? NO. (smiles)*	32. Place LEFT HAND TO LEFT ELBOW *(RH to L ear)*

Figure 4. Case 2 (continued).

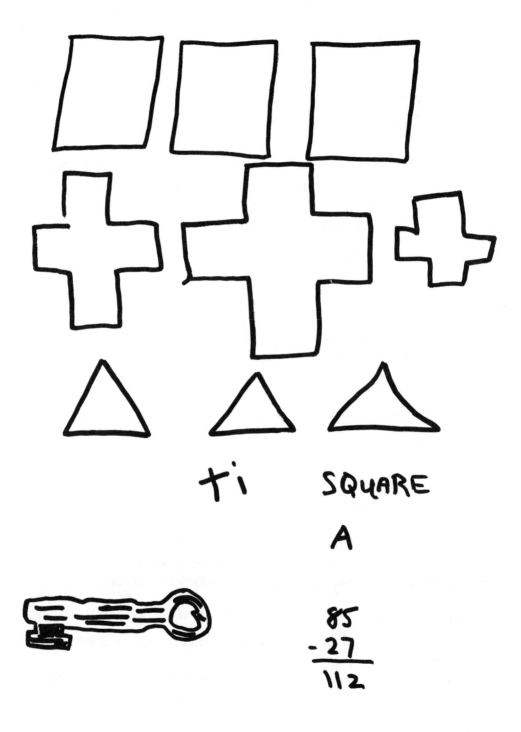

Figure 4. Case 2 (continued).

Pattern of Performance: This method of inference does not contribute to answering this question in this case.

Right/Left Differences: This method of inference does not contribute to answering this question in this case.

Pathognomonic Signs: The errors seen on the Aphasia Screening Test and the right homonymous hemianopsia indicate a severe level of impairment in some areas, but the adequate functioning in other areas makes it clear that the severity of impairment is quite variable in different locations of the brain. **(4-56, 4-69)**

3) Is the Lesion Progressive or Static?

Level of Performance: The significant impairment seen on Seashore Rhythm and Digit Span reflect possible attention deficits, which could be associated with a progressive lesion, but the relatively good performance on several other tests makes that rather unlikely. **(6-11)**

Pattern of Performance: This method of inference does not contribute to the answer of this question.

Right/Left Differences: This method of inference does not contribute to the answer of this question.

Pathognomonic Signs: This method of inference does not contribute to the answer of this question in this case.

Overall, there is little in the test data that helps answer this question. A history, or repeat testing would be required to answer this question.

4) Is the Lesion Diffuse or Lateralized?

Level of Performance: As usual, this method of inference does not contribute to the answer of this question.

Pattern of Performance: The 10-point difference in T scores for VIQ (26) and PIQ (36) is consistent with more left-hemisphere impairment, as is the significantly greater impairment of verbal memory compared to visual memory. **(4-10)**

Right/Left Differences: The weaker strength of grip with the dominant hand suggests more impairment of the left hemisphere. **(5-11)**

Pathognomonic Signs: Both the right homonymous hemianopsia and the aphasia signs indicate that there is significant left-hemisphere impairment. **(4-56)**

Overall, it is clear that there is a lesion lateralized to the left hemisphere.

5) Is the Impairment in the Anterior or Posterior Part of the Cerebral Hemisphere?

Level of Performance: As usual, this method of inference does not contribute to the answer of this question.

Pattern of Performance: There is not a significant difference between performance on the TPT and Finger Tapping. The severe verbal memory deficits suggest temporal lobe impairment.

Right/Left Differences: As usual, this method of inference does not contribute to the answer of this question.

Pathognomonic Signs: Both receptive and expressive aphasic errors were present, indicating both posterior (temporal lobe) and anterior impairment. The right homonymous hemianopsia indicates that there is a lesion posterior to the optic chiasm. **(4-58, 4-59, 4-69)**

Overall, it appears that there is damage to the frontal, temporal, and parietal lobes in the left hemisphere.

6) What is the Most Likely Neuropathological Process?

There is damage to the frontal, temporal, and parietal lobes of the left hemisphere with the right hemisphere being generally spared. Although closed head injuries are the most common cause of brain injuries for male adults in this age range, the damage is much more highly lateralized than is usually the case with a closed head injury. Both the relative sparing of the right hemisphere and the patient's age make either a tumor or a CVA unlikely. A penetrating head injury could account for this picture.

This man suffered an accidental gunshot wound with the point of entry in the left frontal region and the exit in the left occipital region.

7) What are the Implications for Everyday Functioning and Treatment?

This man's aphasic problems caused him a great deal of difficulty in most types of interactions with other people. Treatment by a speech/language therapist helped him somewhat, but his residual deficits caused him a great deal of embarrassment; he was afraid people would think he was stupid when he had difficulty communicating. He was provided with a laminated card explaining that his communication problems were caused by a head injury, and he felt somewhat better having it. His right homonymous hemianopsia resulted in numerous minor injuries from bumping into things on his right side. Training in scanning to the right helped somewhat, but he had difficulty remembering to look to the right in new situations. He was not able to return to his former job as a carpenter, and he was placed in a sheltered workshop.

Case 3

This is a 57-year-old, white, right-handed male with a college education. He frequently got lost in familiar surroundings. He had previously enjoyed reading, both in connection with his work and for recreation. At the time of this evaluation, however, he complained that he could not read anymore and was frustrated and depressed by this. After spending a long time trying to read quite simple material, he had no comprehension of what he had read. The onset of these symptoms had been acute.

Additional tests administered were the Russell Revision of the Wechsler Memory Scale (RRWMS) and the Benton Judgment of Line Orientation Test (JOLO).

1) Is there Cerebral Impairment?

Level of Performance: His Halstead Impairment Index yields a *T* score of only 9, which is severely impaired. His *T* scores of 34 for the Category Test, 34 on the TPT

HRB NORMS PROGRAM
Raw Score Transformations

Name:	Case3		Sex:	M
Age:	57		Years of Educ:	16
Date:	02/26/93		File Name:	CASE3
Handedness:	Right			

Measure	Abbreviation	Raw Scores	Scaled Scores	T Scores
HALSTEAD REITAN BATTERY SCORES				
Halstead Impairment Index	HII	1.0	1	9#
Average Impairment Rating	AIR			
Category Test	CAT ERROR	98	4	34#
Trail Making Test-A (secs)	TRAIL A	68	4	29#
Trail Making Test-B (secs)	TRAIL B	160	5	32#
Tact Perf Test-Time (min/blk)	TPT TIME	.97	5	35#
Tact Perf Test-Memory (correct)	TPT MEM	5	6	35#
Tact Perf Test-Location (correct)	TPT LOC	0	5	34#
Seashore Rhythm (correct)	SSHOR RHYM	19	5	35#
Speech Perception (errors)	SPCH PERC	13	5	31#
Aphasia Screening (errors)	APHAS SCRN	5	8	42
Spatial Relations (rating)	SPAT REL	7	1	0#
Sensory-Perceptual Total (errors)	SP TOTAL	27	3	34#
LATERALIZED SENSORIMOTOR/ PSYCHOMOTOR INDICES				
Finger Tapping-Dom (taps)	TAP DH	44	8	40
Finger Tapping-Non-dom (taps)	TAP NDH	33.8	5	28#L
Hand Dynamometer-Dom (kgs)	GRIP DH	39.7	9	39#
Hand Dynamometer-Non-dom (kgs)	GRIP NDH	33	9	40L
Grooved Pegboard-Dom (secs)	PEG DH	88	6	39#
Grooved Pegboard-Non-dom (secs)	PEG NDH	163	3	29#L
Tact Perf Test-Dom (min/blk)	TPT DH	.75	8	48
Tact Perf Test-Non-dom (min/blk)	TPT NDH	2	4	31#L
Tact Perf Test-Both Hands (min/blk)	TPT BOTH	.67	6	38#
Sensory-Perceptual-Right (errors)	SP R	10	5	37#
Sensory-Perceptual-Left (errors)	SP L	16	3	26#
Tactile Form Recog-Right (secs)	TFR R	11	10	46
Tactile Form Recog-Left (secs)	TFR L	18	6	32#L

\# = Impaired
L = Right-left difference, with possible lateralizing significance

Figure 5. Case 3.

HRB NORMS PROGRAM
Raw Score Transformations

Page 2

Name:	Case3		Sex:	M
Age:	57		Years of Educ:	16
Date:	02/26/93		File Name:	CASE3
Handedness:	Right			

Measure	Abbreviation	Raw Scores	Scaled Scores	T Scores
WAIS-R SCORES				
Verbal IQ (VIQ)	VIQ	112	12	41
Performance IQ (PIQ)	PIQ	77	6	24#
Full Scale IQ (FSIQ)	FSIQ	95	9	29#
Information	INFO	13	13	49
Digit Span	DIGIT SPAN	9	10	42
Vocabulary	VOCAB	13	13	50
Arithmetic	ARITH	7	7	27#
Comprehension	COMP	12	12	47
Similarities	SIMIL	13	13	55
Picture Completion	PICT COMP	5	5	30#
Picture Arrangement	PICT ARR	4	4	28#
Block Design	BLOCK DESGN	4	4	28#
Object Assembly	OBJ ASSMB	4	4	29#
Digit Symbol	DIGIT SYMB	4	4	34#

= Impaired

Figure 5. Case 3 (continued).

Name: Case3   Sex: M
Age: 57   Years of Educ: 16
Date: 02/26/93   File Name: CASE3
Handedness: Right

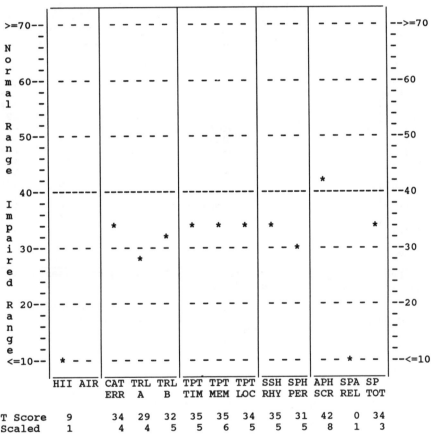

Halstead-Reitan Battery T Score Profile

	HII	AIR	CAT ERR	TRL A	TRL B	TPT TIM	TPT MEM	TPT LOC	SSH RHY	SPH PER	APH SCR	SPA REL	SP TOT
T Score	9		34	29	32	35	35	34	35	31	42	0	34
Scaled	1		4	4	5	5	6	5	5	5	8	1	3

Figure 5. Case 3 (continued).

Page 4

Name: Case3   Sex: M
Age: 57   Yrs of Educ: 16
Date: 02/26/93   File Name: CASE3
Handedness: Right

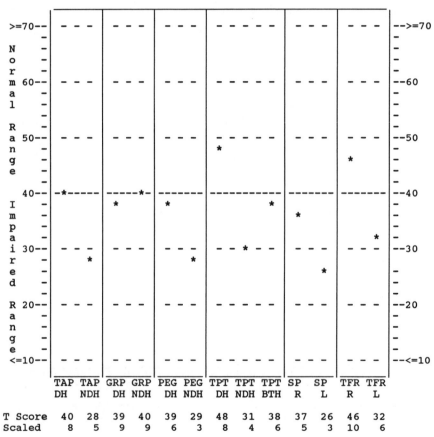

Figure 5. Case 3 (continued).

Page 5

Name: Case3   Sex: M
Age: 57   Yrs of Educ: 16
Date: 02/26/93   File Name: CASE3
Handedness: Right

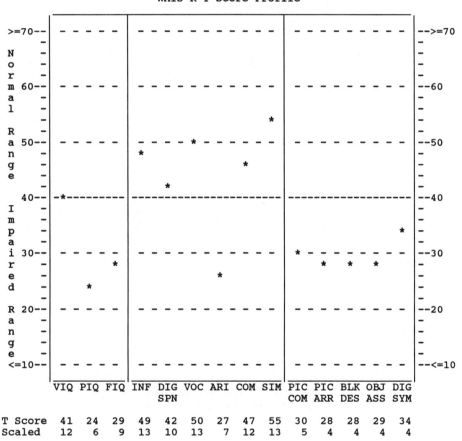

WAIS-R T Score Profile

	VIQ	PIQ	FIQ	INF	DIG SPN	VOC	ARI	COM	SIM	PIC COM	PIC ARR	BLK DES	OBJ ASS	DIG SYM
T Score	41	24	29	49	42	50	27	47	55	30	28	28	29	34
Scaled	12	6	9	13	10	13	7	12	13	5	4	4	4	4

Figure 5. Case 3 (continued).

SENSORY—PERCEPTUAL EXAMINATION   Case 3

Indicate Instance in which stimulus is not perceived or is incorrectly perceived.

Error Totals

Tactile:

Right Hand/Left Hand — RH [| | |]   LH [| | |]   Both: RH [| | |]   LH [X|X|X|X]   RH _0_   LH _4_

Right Hand/Left Face — RH [| | |]   LF [| | |]   Both: RH [| | |]   LF [X|X| |X]   RH _0_   LF ____

Left Hand/Right Face — LH [| | |]   RF [| | |]   Both: LH [X|X|X|X]   RF [| | |]   RF _0_   LH _4_

Auditory:

Right Ear/Left Ear — RE [| | |]   LE [| | |]   Both: RE [X|X| |X]   LE [| | |]   RE ____   LE ____

Visual: *L Hom Hemianopsia*

Above eye level   {   RV [ ]   LV [X|X|X|X]   Both: RV [|X|X|]   LV [ ]   RV _0_   LV _22_
Eye level
Below eye level

Finger Agnosia:

Right: 1 [ ]   2 [ ]   3 [ ]   4 [5]   5 [ ]   R _1 /_
Left: 1 [ ]   2 [1]   3 [ ]   4 [ ]   5 [ ]   L _1 /_

Finger-tip Number Writing Perception:

Right: [4 6 3 5 / 6 5]   [3 5 4 6 / 3]   [6 5 4 3 / 3 5]   [5 4 6 3 / 3]   [6 3 5 4 / 6]   R _6 /_
Left: [/ ok]   [/ 3]   [/]   [/ 2]   [/ 3]   L _4 /_

Astereognosis:

Right: [P | N | D]   *Button? (E)*   Left: [D | N | P / N | P] *Looked...*   Both: Right: [N | P | D]   R _0_
           Left: L _3_

Tactile Form Recognition:

Errors: RH [○ □ △ ✚]   LH [△ ✚ ○ □ / □]   RH [✚ ○ □ △]   LH [□ △ ✚ ○]   R _0_
Response Time: [2 | 1 | 1 | 2]   [4 | 3 | 3 | 1]   [1 | 2 | 1 | 1]   [3 | 2 | 1 | 1]   L _1_

Total Time: R _11_   L _18_

Visual Fields: Left   Right

Figure 5. Case 3 (continued).

APHASIA SCREENING TEST   **Case 3**

Form for Adults and Older Children

Name: _____ Age: __57__ Date: __11/13/87__ Examiner: _____

1. Copy SQUARE	17. Repeat TRIANGLE
2. Name SQUARE	18. Repeat MASSACHUSETTS
3. Spell SQUARE	19. Repeat METHODIST EPISCOPAL
4. Copy CROSS	20. Write SQUARE
5. Name CROSS	21. Read SEVEN
6. Spell CROSS	22. Repeat SEVEN
7. Copy TRIANGLE	23. Repeat/Explain HE SHOUTED THE WARNING. *SOMETHING WAS GONNA HAPPEN - LIKE A TREE WAS GONNA FALL - THIS PERSON WAS NOTIFYING OTHERS AROUND HIM THAT SOMETHING WAS GONNA HAPPEN*
8. Name TRIANGLE	24. Write HE SHOUTED THE WARNING. *(See)*
9. Spell TRIANGLE	25. Compute 85 − 27 =
10. Name BABY	26. Compute 17 X 3 =
11. Write CLOCK	27. Name KEY
12. Name FORK	28. Demonstrate use of KEY
13. Read 7 SIX 2 *SIX SIX 2* *(E - Look at the whole card) OK - SEVEN SIX TWO. IT'S THAT LEFT HAND DEAL AGAIN*	29. Draw KEY *(E prompted for untimed detail)*
14. Read M G W	30. Read PLACE LEFT HAND TO RIGHT EAR.
15. Reading I	31. Place LEFT HAND TO RIGHT EAR ↓ *ON*
16. Reading II *A FAMOUS DOG - A FAMOUS WINNER OF . . . " THAT LEFT HAND DEAL KEEPS CROPPING UP."*	32. Place LEFT HAND TO LEFT ELBOW *(pause) I CAN'T DO THAT*

Figure 5. Case 3 (continued).

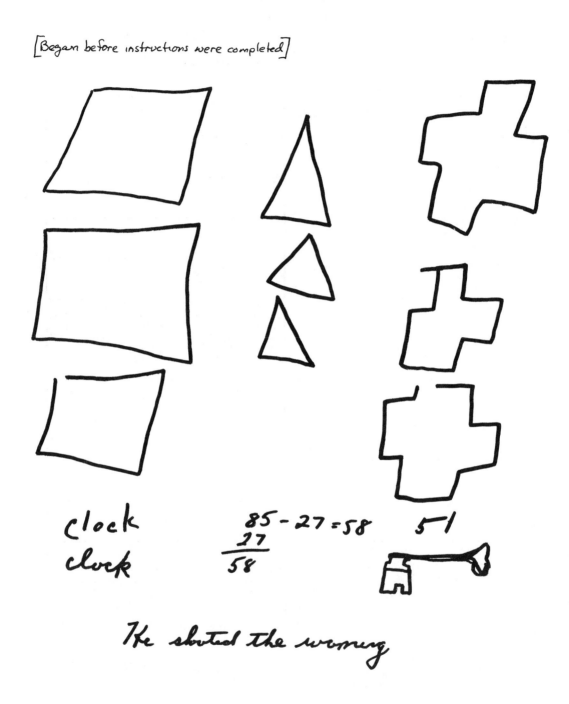

Figure 5. Case 3 (continued).

Location component, and 32 on Part B of the Trail Making Test are all significantly impaired. Thus, this method of inference strongly supports cerebral impairment. **(4-1)**

Pattern of Performance: The VIQ *T* score of 112 is in the average range for his age and education, but his PIQ is significantly impaired. Similarly, his verbal memory on the RRWMS is normal, while his spatial memory is severely impaired. Also note that his *T* score of 42 on Aphasia Screening is in the normal range, but his *T* score of 0 on Spatial Relations is very severely impaired. This method of inference also strongly supports cerebral impairment. **(4-10, 5-19)**

Right/Left Differences: His strength of grip shows the normal relationship between the two hands, but on Finger Tapping, the Grooved Pegboard, and TPT the left hand is significantly impaired in comparison to the right hand. In addition, he made significantly more sensory perceptual errors on the left side of the body than on the right side, and his time on TFR was significantly slower with the left hand than with the right hand. These differences strongly support the presence of impairment. **(5-11)**

Pathognomonic Signs: A left homonymous hemianopsia was noted on the examination of visual fields. In addition, he had 11 tactile suppressions and three auditory suppressions on the left side. These multiple pathognomonic signs leave no doubt about the presence of impairment.

Overall, the presence of impairment is very clear, with support from all four methods of inference.

2) What is the Severity of Cerebral Dysfunction?

Level of Performance: The level of performance is quite severely impaired, with only verbal skills such as those seen on VIQ and the Aphasia Screening Test remaining adequate.

Pattern of Performance: This method of inference does not usually contribute much to answering this question, but in this case the differences between VIQ and PIQ and verbal and visual memory are so great that it seems clear that the impairment is severe.

Right/Left Differences: This method of inference does not contribute much to answering this question in this case.

Pathognomonic Signs: The left homonymous hemianopsia indicates a severe level of impairment. The adverse effect it has on this man's reading ability makes it clear that his everyday functioning is severely impaired. **(4-73)**

3) Is the Lesion Progressive or Static?

Level of Performance: The significant impairment seen on the Seashore Rhythm and Speech Sounds Perception tests reflects possible attention deficits which could be associated with a progressive lesion. **(6-11)**

Pattern of Performance: This method of inference does not usually contribute much to the answer of this question, but the very significant difference between VIQ and PIQ would be consistent with a progressive, or fairly acute lesion. **(6-8)**

Right/Left Differences: This method of inference does not contribute to the answer of this question.

Pathognomonic Signs: This method of inference does not contribute to the answer of this question in this case.

Overall, there is a possibility of a progressive or acute lesion, although this would not be certain without the information about the acute onset of his symptoms.

4) Is the Lesion Diffuse or Lateralized?

Level of Performance: As usual, this method of inference dose not contribute to the answer of this question.

Pattern of Performance: The differences between VIQ and PIQ and verbal and visual memory are consistent with more impairment of the right hemisphere. **(5-8, 5-19)**

Right/Left Differences: The impairment of the left side of the body on motor and sensory perceptual testing noted above makes impairment of the right hemisphere clear.

Pathognomonic Signs: Both the left homonymous hemianopsia and the tactile and auditory suppressions on the left side of the body indicate that there is significant right-hemisphere impairment.

Overall, it is clear that there is a lesion lateralized to the right hemisphere.

5) Is the Impairment in the Anterior or Posterior Part of the Cerebral Hemisphere?

Level of Performance: As usual, this method of inference does not contribute to the answer of this question.

Pattern of Performance: There are generally no significant differences between performance on motor and sensory tests; performance on both is impaired, with the exception of strength of grip. The sparing of strength of grip suggests that the posterior impairment may be greater. This is supported by the very severely impaired performance on the JOLO, which is particularly sensitive to posterior right-hemisphere lesions. **(5-32, 5-54)**

Right/Left Differences: As usual, this method of inference does not contribute to the answer of this question.

Pathognomonic Signs: The right homonymous hemianopsia indicates that there is a lesion posterior to the optic chiasm (see Appendix C).

Overall, it is clear that the posterior portion of the right hemisphere is most severely impaired, with impairment of the anterior portion of the right hemisphere and the left hemisphere being much less impaired.

6) What is the Most Likely Neuropathological Process?

This is a 57-year-old man with a fairly focal lesion of the posterior part of the right hemisphere with acute onset of symptoms and some additional impairment in the more anterior part of the right hemisphere. Impairment of the left hemisphere cannot be completely ruled out, although it is much less severe. The preservation of certain functions such as VIQ and verbal memory, along with the acute onset make a neoplasm unlikely. The remaining possibility is a CVA, which is what he had suffered.

7) What are the Implications for Everyday Functioning and Treatment?

The fact that this man got lost in familiar surroundings created significant limitations on his ability to function independently. His inability to read with comprehension prevented him from doing any type of work that he might have previously been able to do and generally caused him a great deal of distress. This is the patient whose rehabilitation program is described in Case 2 in chapter 11.

Case 4

This is a 28-year-old, white, right-handed male with 8 years of education who is a semiskilled construction worker. He has a history of sudden explosive outbursts in which he has injured others and damaged property, including driving his car through the front of a building on one occasion. Following that incident, laboratory tests failed to show the presence of alcohol or other drugs in his blood, and he denied significant alcohol or drug abuse at any time, although this could not be verified by independent sources. Following his most serious episodes, he stated that he was puzzled by his behavior and was remorseful about it.

Additional tests administered were the Russell Revision of the Wechsler Memory Scale (RRWMS), on which both verbal and visual memory were above average, and the Benton Judgment of Line Orientation Test (JOLO), on which his performance was in the average range.

1) Is There Cerebral Impairment?

Level of Performance: The Halstead Impairment Index, the Category Test, the TPT Location component, and Part B of the Trail Making Test are all in the average range. Thus, this method of inference does not support the presence of cerebral impairment.

Pattern of Performance: The VIQ/PIQ and verbal/visual memory relationships are both normal. The relationship between the Aphasia *T* score of 58 and the Spatial Relations *T* score of 13 is suggestive of impairment. This method of inference lends only weak support for the presence of cerebral impairment.

Right/Left Differences: The expected right/left relationship is seen on all of the motor tests. The Sensory Perceptual Right *T* score is 36, while the corresponding *T* score on the Left is 59. It is important to note that this is a result, primarily, of eight errors on Finger Tip Number Writing Perception on the right hand and only one error on the left hand. Again, this lends fairly weak support for the presence of cerebral impairment.

Pathognomonic Signs: There were no pathognomonic signs.

Overall, there is rather weak support for the presence of impairment.

2) What is the Severity of Cerebral Dysfunction?

Level of Performance: The level of performance is generally quite adequate, which suggests that if there is any impairment, it is mild.

Pattern of Performance: This method of inference does not contribute much to answering this question.

HRB NORMS PROGRAM
Raw Score Transformations

Name: Case4   Sex: M
Age: 28   Years of Educ: 8
Date: 02/26/93   File Name: CASE4
Handedness: Right

Measure	Abbreviation	Raw Scores	Scaled Scores	T Scores
HALSTEAD REITAN BATTERY SCORES				
Halstead Impairment Index	HII	0	13	66
Average Impairment Rating	AIR			
Category Test	CAT ERROR	33	10	54
Trail Making Test-A (secs)	TRAIL A	22	11	55
Trail Making Test-B (secs)	TRAIL B	56	11	58
Tact Perf Test-Time (min/blk)	TPT TIME	.21	16	73
Tact Perf Test-Memory (correct)	TPT MEM	9	14	63
Tact Perf Test-Location (correct)	TPT LOC	7	14	62
Seashore Rhythm (correct)	SSHOR RHYM	28	12	56
Speech Perception (errors)	SPCH PERC	6	9	49
Aphasia Screening (errors)	APHAS SCRN	2	10	58
Spatial Relations (rating)	SPAT REL	6	3	13#
Sensory-Perceptual Total (errors)	SP TOTAL	10	6	42
LATERALIZED SENSORIMOTOR/ PSYCHOMOTOR INDICES				
Finger Tapping-Dom (taps)	TAP DH	51.4	10	46
Finger Tapping-Non-dom (taps)	TAP NDH	45.8	10	49
Hand Dynamometer-Dom (kgs)	GRIP DH	58.3	13	59
Hand Dynamometer-Non-dom (kgs)	GRIP NDH	54.0	13	55
Grooved Pegboard-Dom (secs)	PEG DH	60	11	55
Grooved Pegboard-Non-dom (secs)	PEG NDH	61	12	55
Tact Perf Test-Dom (min/blk)	TPT DH	.34	13	59
Tact Perf Test-Non-dom (min/blk)	TPT NDH	.20	15	73
Tact Perf Test-Both Hands (min/blk)	TPT BOTH	.10	15	72
Sensory-Perceptual-Right (errors)	SP R	9	5	36#L
Sensory-Perceptual-Left (errors)	SP L	1	10	59
Tactile Form Recog-Right (secs)	TFR R			
Tactile Form Recog-Left (secs)	TFR L			

# = Impaired
L = Right-left difference, with possible lateralizing significance

Figure 6. Case 4.

HRB NORMS PROGRAM
Raw Score Transformations

Page 2

Name:	Case4	Sex:	M
Age:	28	Years of Educ:	8
Date:	02/26/93	File Name:	CASE4
Handedness:	Right		

Measure	Abbreviation	Raw Scores	Scaled Scores	T Scores
WAIS-R SCORES				
Verbal IQ (VIQ)	VIQ	103	11	68
Performance IQ (PIQ)	PIQ	93	9	55
Full Scale IQ (FSIQ)	FSIQ	98	10	62
Information	INFO	8	8	55
Digit Span	DIGIT SPAN	9	10	56
Vocabulary	VOCAB	10	10	65
Arithmetic	ARITH	11	11	64
Comprehension	COMP	14	14	78
Similarities	SIMIL	14	14	77
Picture Completion	PICT COMP	10	10	57
Picture Arrangement	PICT ARR	15	15	75
Block Design	BLOCK DESGN	7	7	45
Object Assembly	OBJ ASSMB	7	7	45
Digit Symbol	DIGIT SYMB	6	6	45

= Impaired

Figure 6. Case 4 (continued).

```
Name:        Case4                          Sex:         M
Age:         28                     Years of Educ:       8
Date:        02/26/93                   File Name:       CASE4
Handedness:  Right
```

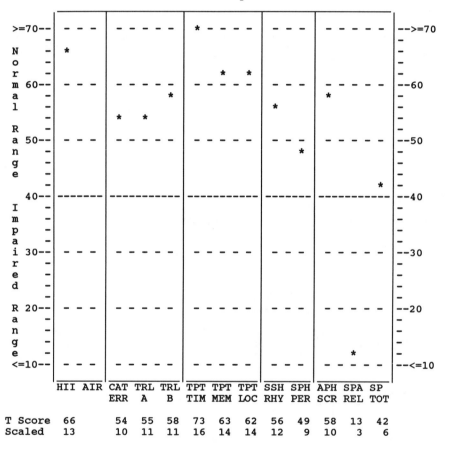

Figure 6. Case 4 (continued).

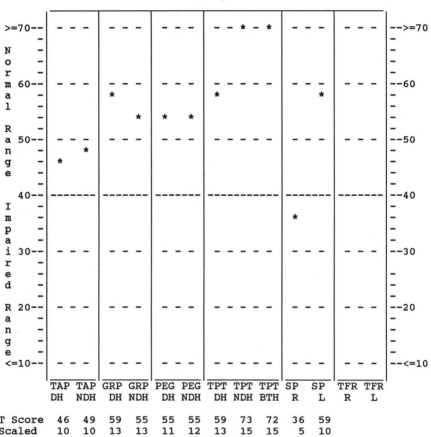

Figure 6. Case 4 (continued).

Page 5

Name: Case4   Sex: M
Age: 28   Yrs of Educ: 8
Date: 02/26/93   File Name: CASE4
Handedness: Right

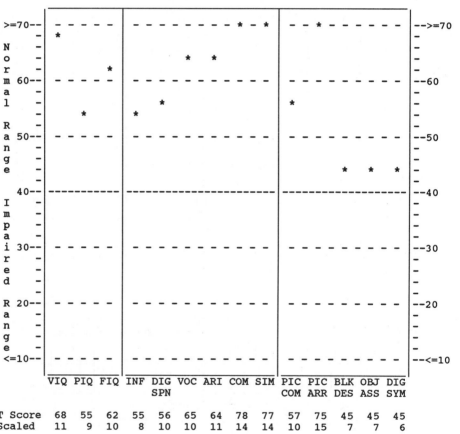

WAIS-R T Score Profile

	VIQ	PIQ	FIQ	INF	DIG SPN	VOC	ARI	COM	SIM	PIC COM	PIC ARR	BLK DES	OBJ ASS	DIG SYM
T Score	68	55	62	55	56	65	64	78	77	57	75	45	45	45
Scaled	11	9	10	8	10	10	11	14	14	10	15	7	7	6

Figure 6. Case 4 (continued).

SENSORY—PERCEPTUAL EXAMINATION   Case 4

Indicate Instance in which stimulus is not perceived or is incorrectly perceived.

Error Totals

Tactile:

Right Hand/Left Hand — RH ▢▢▢   LH ▢▢▢   Both: RH ▢▢▢   LH ▢▢▢   RH _0_ LH _0_

Right Hand/Left Face — RH ▢▢▢   LF ▢▢▢   Both: RH ▢▢▢   LF ▢▢▢   RH _0_ LF _0_

Left Hand/Right Face — LH ▢▢▢   RF ▢▢▢   Both: LH ▢▢▢   RF ▢▢▢   RF _0_ LH _0_

Auditory:

Right Ear/Left Ear — RE ▢▢▢   LE ▢▢▢   Both: RE ▢▢▢   LE ▢▢▢   RE _0_ LE _0_

Visual:

Above eye level
Eye level   { RV   LV   Both: RV   LV   RV _0_ LV _0_
Below eye level

Finger Agnosia:

Right: 1 ▢▢▢   2 ▢▢▢   3 ▢▢▢   4 [3]▢▢   5 ▢▢▢   R _1/_
Left: 1 ▢▢▢   2 ▢▢▢   3 ▢▢▢   4 ▢▢▢   5 ▢▢▢   L _0/_

Finger tips heavily calloused from his work.
Finger-tip Number Writing Perception: *Hasn't worked in a month –*

Right: |4|6|3|5| |3|5|4|6| |6|5|4|3| |5|4|6|3| |6|3|5|4| R _8/_
         |5|4| |5|4| |4| |4| |5|3|
Left: |6| L _1/_

I can feel pressure but not feel shape - Thinks both hands should be calloused–
Astereognosis: *Never wears gloves. His numbness in R hand, but doesn't think its affecting palm.*

                                                           |N|P|D|
Right: |P|N|D| Left: |D|N|P| Both: Right: |Q| R _2_
       |D| |P| Left: L _1_

Commented that it felt like one side of penny was
Tactile Form Recognition: *up and one down-odd if callousing is?*

Errors: RH |○|□|△|✚| LH |△|✚|○|□| RH |✚|○|□|△| LH |□|△|✚|○| R _0_
Response Time: |1|1|1|1| |2|1|1|2| |1|2|2|1| |2|2|2|2| L _0_

Total Time: R _10_   L _14_

Visual Fields: Left   Right

Figure 6. Case 4 (continued).

APHASIA SCREENING TEST   Case 4

Form for Adults and Older Children

Name: _____ Age: __28__ Date: __9/9/83__ Examiner: _____

1. Copy SQUARE	17. Repeat TRIANGLE
2. Name SQUARE	18. Repeat MASSACHUSETTS
3. Spell SQUARE	19. Repeat METHODIST EPISCOPAL
4. Copy CROSS	20. Write SQUARE
5. Name CROSS	21. Read SEVEN
6. Spell CROSS	22. Repeat SEVEN
7. Copy TRIANGLE	23. Repeat/Explain HE SHOUTED THE WARNING. *GET BACK!.*
8. Name TRIANGLE	24. Write HE SHOUTED THE WARNING. *(Wrote "He h" & then changed h to S & completed)*
9. Spell TRIANGLE *OK. T - R - I --ANG - ANGLE*	25. Compute 85 – 27 = *DO YOU WANT AN ANSWER? (Before E finished instruction)*
10. Name BABY *(Tilts head) "IT'S A BABY"*	26. Compute 17 X 3 =
11. Write CLOCK *(printed 1st)*	27. Name KEY *IT'S A SKELETON KEY.*
12. Name FORK *(Joked) "IT'S A FLYING SAUCER" (laughs) OK.*	28. Demonstrate use of KEY *P & T*
13. Read 7 SIX 2	29. Draw KEY *THAT AIN'T GONNA WORK. (Started over)*
14. Read M G W	30. Read PLACE LEFT HAND TO RIGHT EAR. *"over"*
15. Reading I	31. Place LEFT HAND TO RIGHT EAR
16. Reading II	32. Place LEFT HAND TO LEFT ELBOW *LH to RE*

Figure 6. Case 4 (continued).

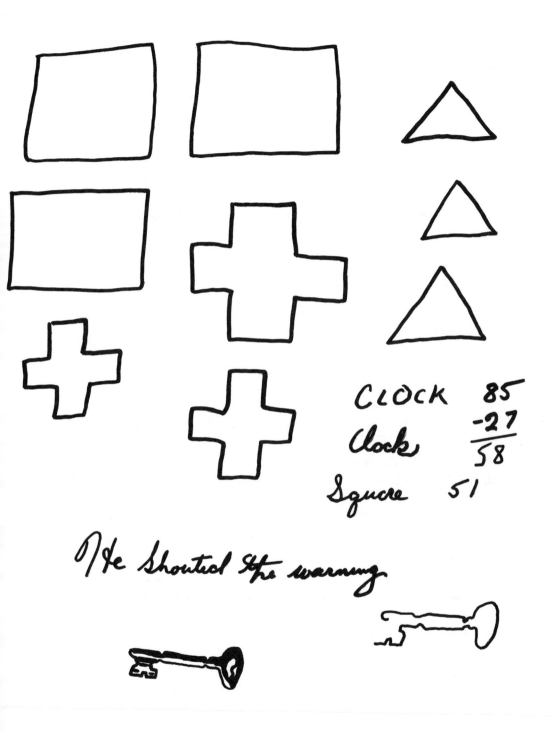

Figure 6. Case 4 (continued).

Right/Left Differences: This method of inference does not contribute much to answering this question in this case.

Pathognomonic Signs: There were no pathognomonic signs.

Overall, the evidence suggests that if there is any impairment, it is mild.

3) Is the Lesion Progressive or Static?

Level of Performance: There is nothing about the level of performance that helps answer this question.

Pattern of Performance: This method of inference does not usually contribute much to the answer of this question.

Right/Left Differences: This method of inference does not contribute much to the answer of this question.

Pathognomonic Signs: This method of inference does not contribute to the answer of this question in this case.

Overall, it is not possible to say much about this question in this case.

4) Is the Lesion Diffuse or Lateralized?

Level of Performance: As usual, this method of inference dose not contribute to the answer of this question.

Pattern of Performance: The relationship between the Aphasia Screening *T* score of 58 and the Spatial Relations *T* score of 13 is suggestive of more impairment of the right hemisphere.

Right/Left Differences: The finding of eight errors on Finger Tip Number Writing Perception on the right hand with only one error on the left hand is suggestive of more impairment of the right hemisphere.

Pathognomonic Signs: There were no pathognomonic signs.

Overall, it is clear that if there is a lesion, it is lateralized to the right hemisphere.

5) Is the Impairment in the Anterior or Posterior Part of the Cerebral Hemisphere?

Level of Performance: As usual, this method of inference dose not contribute to the answer of this question.

Pattern of Performance: The errors on Finger Tip Number Writing, in the absence of any motor problems, suggest that if there is a lesion, it is in the sensory strip region of the parietal lobe. **(4-75)**

Right/Left Differences: As usual, this method of inference does not contribute to the answer of this question.

Pathognomonic Signs: There were no pathognomonic signs.

Overall, it is clear that if there is a lesion, it is in the in the sensory strip region of the parietal lobe. **(However, also see 5-46)**

6) What is the Most Likely Neuropathological Process?

If there is a lesion, it is a focal one in the sensory strip region of the parietal lobe. The absence of any suppressions or visual field defects suggests that it does not involve any actual destruction of tissue. Seizure disorders sometimes result from such lesions, and in this case a partial complex seizure disorder could account for the explosive outbursts described in the history.

Because the evidence for cerebral impairment was weak in this case and depended heavily on the results of the Sensory Perceptual Examination, that examination was repeated. The results were the same as on the initial examination: There were eight errors on Finger Tip Number Writing Perception on the right hand and only one error on the left hand. This replication supported the hypothesis of a seizure disorder.

7) What are the Implications for Everyday Functioning and Treatment?

An EEG with nasopharingial leads was performed, and even though the results were equivocal, the patient was started on Tegretol, an anticonvulsant medication. Follow-up after 11 months revealed that he had not had any more explosive outbursts.

Case 5

This is a 20-year-old, white, right-handed male with 11 years of education and a GED who was a cosmetology student. Additional tests administered were the Russell Revision of the Wechsler Memory Scale (RRWMS), on which both verbal and visual memory very severely impaired, and the Benton Judgment of Line Orientation Test (JOLO), on which his performance was in the average range.

1) Is There Cerebral Impairment?

Level of Performance: The Halstead Impairment Index, the Category Test, and Part B of the Trail Making Test are all in the average range. His T score of 30 on the TPT Location was in the impaired range. This method of inference lends slight support for the presence of cerebral impairment.

Pattern of Performance: The VIQ/PIQ and verbal/visual memory relationships are both normal. The relationship between the Aphasia Screening T score of 55 and the Spatial Relations T score of 58 is also normal. This method of inference lends no support for the presence of cerebral impairment.

Right/Left Differences: The expected right/left relationship is seen on all of the motor tests. The Sensory Perceptual Right T score is 51, while the corresponding T score on the Left is 28. This is a result, primarily, of two errors on Finger Tip Number Writing Perception on the right hand and five errors on the left hand. This lends only weak support for the presence of cerebral impairment.

Pathognomonic Signs: There were no pathognomonic signs.

Overall, there is only weak support for the presence of impairment.

2) What is the Severity of Cerebral Dysfunction?

Level of Performance: The level of performance is generally quite adequate, which suggests that if there is any impairment, it is mild, except in the area of memory where the impairment is severe.

HRB NORMS PROGRAM
Raw Score Transformations

Name:	Case5		Sex:	M
Age:	20	Years of Educ:		11
Date:	02/26/93	File Name:		CASE5
Handedness: Right				

Measure	Abbreviation	Raw Scores	Scaled Scores	T Scores
HALSTEAD REITAN BATTERY SCORES				
Halstead Impairment Index	HII	0.3	10	47
Average Impairment Rating	AIR			
Category Test	CAT ERROR	26	11	55
Trail Making Test-A (secs)	TRAIL A	28	9	44
Trail Making Test-B (secs)	TRAIL B	48	12	59
Tact Perf Test-Time (min/blk)	TPT TIME	.686	7	36#
Tact Perf Test-Memory (correct)	TPT MEM	8	11	50
Tact Perf Test-Location (correct)	TPT LOC	1	6	30#
Seashore Rhythm (correct)	SSHOR RHYM	29	14	60
Speech Perception (errors)	SPCH PERC	3	12	56
Aphasia Screening (errors)	APHAS SCRN	3	10	55
Spatial Relations (rating)	SPAT REL	2	11	58
Sensory-Perceptual Total (errors)	SP TOTAL	9	7	44
LATERALIZED SENSORIMOTOR/ PSYCHOMOTOR INDICES				
Finger Tapping-Dom (taps)	TAP DH	51.8	10	45
Finger Tapping-Non-dom (taps)	TAP NDH	43.8	9	44
Hand Dynamometer-Dom (kgs)	GRIP DH	49.7	11	48
Hand Dynamometer-Non-dom (kgs)	GRIP NDH	47	12	49
Grooved Pegboard-Dom (secs)	PEG DH	68	9	44
Grooved Pegboard-Non-dom (secs)	PEG NDH	72	9	42
Tact Perf Test-Dom (min/blk)	TPT DH	.77	8	40
Tact Perf Test-Non-dom (min/blk)	TPT NDH	.62	8	44
Tact Perf Test-Both Hands (min/blk)	TPT BOTH	.67	6	32#
Sensory-Perceptual-Right (errors)	SP R	2	10	51
Sensory-Perceptual-Left (errors)	SP L	7	4	28#L
Tactile Form Recog-Right (secs)	TFR R	9	12	56
Tactile Form Recog-Left (secs)	TFR L	8	12	56

\# = Impaired
L = Right-left difference, with possible lateralizing significance

Figure 7. Case 5.

```
                        HRB NORMS PROGRAM
                     Raw Score Transformations

                            Page 2

Name:       Case5                          Sex:      M
Age:        20                   Years of Educ:      11
Date:       02/26/93                  File Name:      CASE5
Handedness: Right
```

Measure	Abbreviation	Raw Scores	Scaled Scores	T Scores
WAIS-R SCORES				
Verbal IQ (VIQ)	VIQ	99	10	57
Performance IQ (PIQ)	PIQ	98	10	55
Full Scale IQ (FSIQ)	FSIQ	99	10	56
Information	INFO	8	8	49
Digit Span	DIGIT SPAN	16	18	83
Vocabulary	VOCAB	6	6	43
Arithmetic	ARITH	11	11	59
Comprehension	COMP	9	9	54
Similarities	SIMIL	9	9	53
Picture Completion	PICT COMP	11	11	57
Picture Arrangement	PICT ARR	12	12	61
Block Design	BLOCK DESGN	11	11	57
Object Assembly	OBJ ASSMB	10	10	54
Digit Symbol	DIGIT SYMB	07	7	45

\# = Impaired

Figure 7. Case 5 (continued).

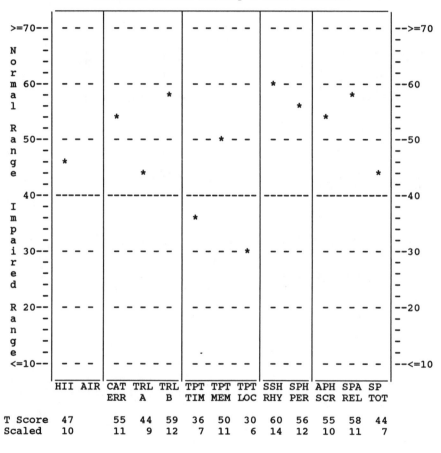

Figure 7. Case 5 (continued).

Page 4

Name: Case5   Sex: M
Age: 20   Yrs of Educ: 11
Date: 02/26/93   File Name: CASE5
Handedness: Right

Lateralized Sensorimotor/Psychomotor T Score Profile

	TAP DH	TAP NDH	GRP DH	GRP NDH	PEG DH	PEG NDH	TPT DH	TPT NDH	TPT BTH	SP R	SP L	TFR R	TFR L
T Score	45	44	48	49	44	42	40	44	32	51	28	56	56
Scaled	10	9	11	12	9	9	8	8	6	10	4	12	12

Figure 7. Case 5 (continued).

Page 5

Name: Case5   Sex: M
Age: 20   Yrs of Educ: 11
Date: 02/26/93   File Name: CASE5
Handedness: Right

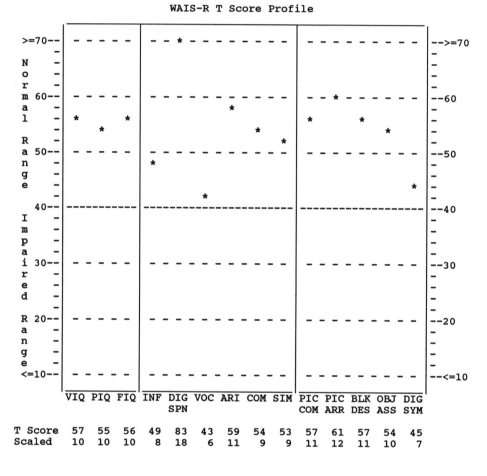

Figure 7. Case 5 (continued).

SENSORY—PERCEPTUAL EXAMINATION Case 5

Indicate Instance in which stimulus is not perceived or is incorrectly perceived.

Figure 7. Case 5 (continued).

APHASIA SCREENING TEST   Case 5

Form for Adults and Older Children

Name: _____ Age: __*20*__ Date: __*9/25/86*__ Examiner: _____

1. Copy SQUARE	17. Repeat TRIANGLE
2. Name SQUARE	18. Repeat MASSACHUSETTS
3. Spell SQUARE	19. Repeat METHODIST EPISCOPAL
4. Copy CROSS	20. Write SQUARE *SQUARE. IN CURSIVE?*
5. Name CROSS	21. Read SEVEN
6. Spell CROSS	22. Repeat SEVEN
7. Copy TRIANGLE	23. Repeat/Explain HE SHOUTED THE WARNING. *HE WAS CALLING FOR A SIGNAL (Q) INCIDENT -* *TRAGIC ACCIDENT*
8. Name TRIANGLE	24. Write HE SHOUTED THE WARNING.
9. Spell TRIANGLE	25. Compute 85 – 27 =
10. Name BABY	26. Compute 17 X 3 =
11. Write CLOCK *WRITE IT? LIKE WRITE IT DOWN? (printed 1st)*	27. Name KEY
12. Name FORK	28. Demonstrate use of KEY
13. Read 7 SIX 2	29. Draw KEY
14. Read M G W	30. Read PLACE LEFT HAND TO RIGHT EAR.
15. Reading I	31. Place LEFT HAND TO RIGHT EAR
16. Reading II	32. Place LEFT HAND TO LEFT ELBOW *WHAT'S THAT! (laughs)*

Figure 7. Case 5 (continued).

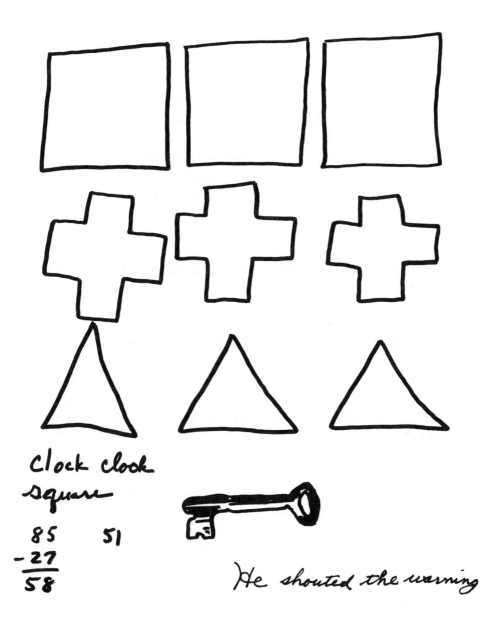

Figure 7. Case 5 (continued).

Pattern of Performance: This method of inference does not contribute much to answering this question.

Right/Left Differences: This method of inference does not contribute much to answering this question in this case.

Pathognomonic Signs: There were no pathognomonic signs.

Overall, the evidence suggests that if there is any impairment, it is mild, except in the area of memory where the impairment is severe.

3) Is the Lesion Progressive or Static?

Level of Performance: Scores on the Seashore Rhythm and Speech Sounds Perception tests are quite good, and the IQ is apparently unimpaired; therefore, it seems unlikely that there is any progressive lesion. **(6-11)**

Pattern of Performance: This method of inference does not usually contribute much to the answer of this question.

Right/Left Differences: This method of inference does not contribute much to the answer of this question.

Pathognomonic Signs: This method of inference does not contribute to the answer of this question in this case.

Overall, there is nothing to suggest that there is any progressive lesion, but this cannot be ruled out without an adequate history or repeat testing.

4) Is the Lesion Diffuse or Lateralized?

Level of Performance: As usual, this method of inference does not contribute to the answer of this question.

Pattern of Performance: The relationships between the VIQ and PIQ, verbal and visual memory, and Aphasia and Spatial Relations are all normal. This does not suggest any lateralization. The severe impairment of both verbal and visual memory suggests bilateral impairment.

Right/Left Differences: The finding of two errors on Finger Tip Number Writing Perception on the right hand with five errors on the left hand provides the only suggestion of more impairment of the right hemisphere, and this is quite weak in the face of the normal right/left relationship on all motor tests.

Pathognomonic Signs: There were no pathognomonic signs.

Overall, it is clear that the impairment is bilateral, with only a weak indication of slightly more impairment of the right hemisphere.

5) Is the Impairment in the Anterior or Posterior Part of the Cerebral Hemisphere?

Level of Performance: As usual, this method of inference does not contribute to the answer of this question.

Pattern of Performance: The errors on Finger Tip Number Writing, in the absence of any motor problems, suggests that there may be slightly more posterior impairment, but the evidence is weak. Note also that the Picture Arrangement, Block Design, and JOLO scores are quite adequate. The severe deficits in both verbal and visual memory suggest impairment of the medial portion of both temporal lobes.

Right/Left Differences: As usual, this method of inference does not contribute to the answer of this question.

Pathognomonic Signs: There were no pathognomonic signs.

Overall, there is very little evidence to suggest a focal lesion other than the temporal lobe impairment reflected by the severe memory deficits.

6) What is the Most Likely Neuropathological Process?

This is a picture of bilateral temporal lobe impairment with little evidence of any other damage. Overall impairment is very mild except for memory impairment, which is severe. Any type of lateralized lesion is ruled out. A closed head injury would have caused more generalized impairment, affecting motor skills, for example. The striking memory deficits point toward the possibility of anoxia as the pathological process.

Three months prior to this evaluation, he had been found unconscious in his apartment as a result of a defective furnace. He was reportedly comatose for about 1 week, although Glasgow Coma Scale scores were not available, and he was hospitalized for 1 month.

7) What are the Implications for Everyday Functioning and Treatment?

At the time of this evaluation, his memory problems obviously precluded his successful return to school. Since it had been such a short time since his injury, more comprehensive testing of memory was recommended in another 3-6 months. At that time, training in the use of compensatory mnemonic techniques could be considered. As indicated in chapter 11, "memory training" is not likely to be helpful.

Case 6

This is a 46-year-old, white, left-handed woman with a 2-year college degree in accounting who had reportedly worked very successfully as an accountant for 20 years. She was referred for neuropsychological evaluation by a psychiatrist who was treating her for a schizophrenic disorder because he was concerned about her apparent memory problems. Her psychiatric symptoms consisted mainly of delusions that she was being persecuted by the Internal Revenue Service because she had discovered that the income tax laws were unconstitutional. No further details of her psychiatric history were available at the time of referral.

Additional tests administered were: The Wechsler Memory Scale-Revised (WMS-R) on which her scores were: Verbal Memory Index, 106; Visual Memory Index, 80; General Memory Index, 94; Attention/Concentration Index, 81; and Delayed Recall Index, 67.

The Rey Auditory Verbal Learning Test (RAVLT) (Lezak, 1983) on which she learned 2 words on trial 1; 5 words on trial 2; 4 words on trial 3; 7 words on trial 4; 9 words on trial 5; 3 words from List B; 5 words from the original list on trial 6; and recognized 12 words on the recognition trial, but at the expense of including 9 incorrect words. This is at least a moderately severely impaired performance.

The Benton Judgment of Line Orientation Test (JOLO) (Benton, et al., 1978), on which her performance was in the average range.

```
                        HRB NORMS PROGRAM
                      Raw Score Transformations


     Name:      Case6                         Sex:    F
     Age:       46                   Years of Educ:   14
     Date:      02/26/93                 File Name:    CASE6
     Handedness: Left
```

Measure	Abbreviation	Raw Scores	Scaled Scores	T Scores
HALSTEAD REITAN				
BATTERY SCORES				
Halstead Impairment Index	HII	0.9	4	23#
Average Impairment Rating	AIR			
Category Test	CAT ERROR	77	6	34#
Trail Making Test-A (secs)	TRAIL A	58	5	30#
Trail Making Test-B (secs)	TRAIL B	215	4	24#
Tact Perf Test-Time (min/blk)	TPT TIME	1.61	4	27#
Tact Perf Test-Memory (correct)	TPT MEM	0	1	14#
Tact Perf Test-Location (correct)	TPT LOC	0	5	30#
Seashore Rhythm (correct)	SSHOR RHYM	26	10	48
Speech Perception (errors)	SPCH PERC	10	6	34#
Aphasia Screening (errors)	APHAS SCRN	3	10	49
Spatial Relations (rating)	SPAT REL	2	11	56
Sensory-Perceptual Total (errors)	SP TOTAL	3	10	45
LATERALIZED SENSORIMOTOR/				
PSYCHOMOTOR INDICES				
Finger Tapping-Dom (taps)	TAP DH	34	5	37#
Finger Tapping-Non-dom (taps)	TAP NDH	27	3	30#L
Hand Dynamometer-Dom (kgs)	GRIP DH	31	8	54
Hand Dynamometer-Non-dom (kgs)	GRIP NDH	23.7	7	49L
Grooved Pegboard-Dom (secs)	PEG DH	123	3	14#L
Grooved Pegboard-Non-dom (secs)	PEG NDH	101	5	28#
Tact Perf Test-Dom (min/blk)	TPT DH	2.5	3	25#
Tact Perf Test-Non-dom (min/blk)	TPT NDH	2.5	4	26#
Tact Perf Test-Both Hands (min/blk)	TPT BOTH	.89	5	31#
Sensory-Perceptual-Right (errors)	SP R	2	10	45
Sensory-Perceptual-Left (errors)	SP L	1	10	53
Tactile Form Recog-Right (secs)	TFR R	15.5	8	46L
Tactile Form Recog-Left (secs)	TFR L	10.5	10	52

```
# = Impaired
L = Right-left difference, with possible lateralizing significance
```

Figure 8. Case 6.

HRB NORMS PROGRAM
Raw Score Transformations

Page 2

Name:	Case6		Sex:	F
Age:	46		Years of Educ:	14
Date:	02/26/93		File Name:	CASE6
Handedness:	Left			

Measure	Abbreviation	Raw Scores	Scaled Scores	T Scores
ADDITIONAL TEST SCORES				
Thurstone Word Fluency (correct)	WORD FLUEN	28	6	33#
Boston Naming (correct)	BSTN NAME			
BDAE Complex Material (correct)	BDAE COMP			
WCST Perseverative Responses	WCST PSVR	18	9	46
Seashore Tonal Memory (correct)	SSHOR TONAL			
Digit Vigilance Time (sec)	DIGIT TIME			
Digit Vigilance Errors	DIGIT ERROR			
Story Learning (points/trials)	STORY LEARN			
Story Memory (% loss)	STORY LOSS			
Figure Learning (points/trial)	FIGUR LEARN			
Figure Memory (% loss)	FIGUR LOSS			
PIAT Reading Recog (percentile)	PIAT RECOG			
PIAT Reading Comp (percentile)	PIAT COMP			
PIAT Spelling (percentile)	PIAT SPELL			
WAIS-R SCORES				
Verbal IQ (VIQ)	VIQ	89	8	33#
Performance IQ (PIQ)	PIQ	85	7	33#
Full Scale IQ (FSIQ)	FSIQ	86	7	30#
Information	INFO	10	10	46
Digit Span	DIGIT SPAN	8	10	43
Vocabulary	VOCAB	9	9	40
Arithmetic	ARITH	9	9	44
Comprehension	COMP	5	5	26#
Similarities	SIMIL	5	5	29#
Picture Completion	PICT COMP	5	5	33#
Picture Arrangement	PICT ARR	7	7	42
Block Design	BLOCK DESGN	5	5	32#
Object Assembly	OBJ ASSMB	8	8	45
Digit Symbol	DIGIT SYMB	6	6	35#

= Impaired

Figure 8. Case 6 (continued).

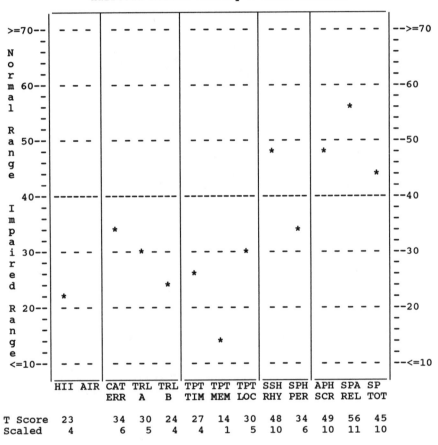

Figure 8. Case 6 (continued).

Page 4

Name: Case6   Sex: F
Age: 46   Yrs of Educ: 14
Date: 02/26/93   File Name: CASE6
Handedness: Left

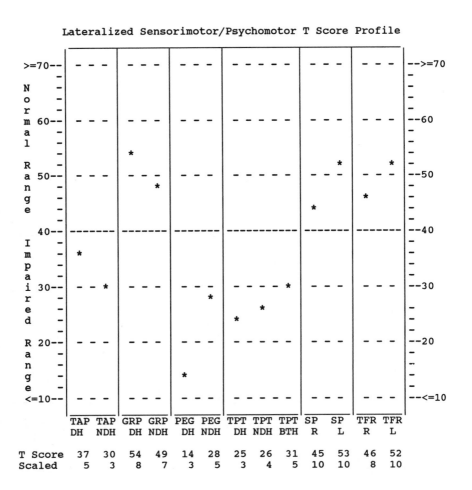

Lateralized Sensorimotor/Psychomotor T Score Profile

	TAP DH	TAP NDH	GRP DH	GRP NDH	PEG DH	PEG NDH	TPT DH	TPT NDH	TPT BTH	SP R	SP L	TFR R	TFR L
T Score	37	30	54	49	14	28	25	26	31	45	53	46	52
Scaled	5	3	8	7	3	5	3	4	5	10	10	8	10

Figure 8. Case 6 (continued).

Name: Case6   Sex: F
Age: 46   Yrs of Educ: 14
Date: 02/26/93   File Name: CASE6
Handedness: Left

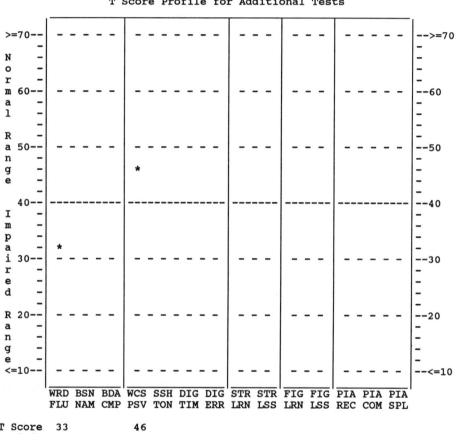

T Score Profile for Additional Tests

Figure 8. Case 6 (continued).

Page 6

Name: Case6   Sex: F
Age: 46   Yrs of Educ: 14
Date: 02/26/93   File Name: CASE6
Handedness: Left

WAIS-R T Score Profile

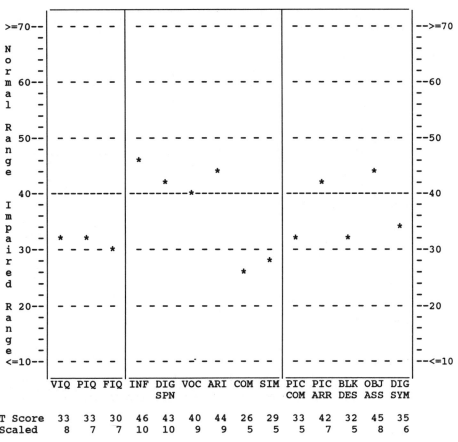

	VIQ	PIQ	FIQ	INF	DIG SPN	VOC	ARI	COM	SIM	PIC COM	PIC ARR	BLK DES	OBJ ASS	DIG SYM
T Score	33	33	30	46	43	40	44	26	29	33	42	32	45	35
Scaled	8	7	7	10	10	9	9	5	5	5	7	5	8	6

Figure 8. Case 6 (continued).

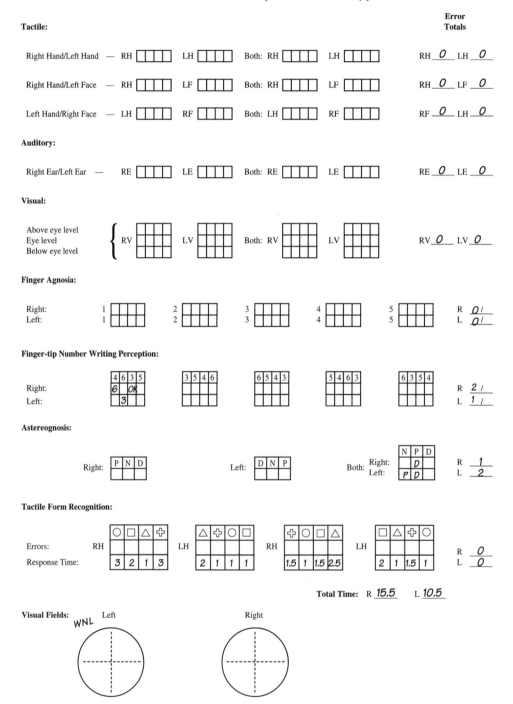

Figure 8. Case 6 (continued).

APHASIA SCREENING TEST Case 6

Form for Adults and Older Children

Name: _____ Age: _46_ Date: _10/9/92_ Examiner: _____

1. Copy SQUARE	17. Repeat TRIANGLE
2. Name SQUARE *RECTANGLE (Q) SQUARE*	18. Repeat MASSACHUSETTS *" TUSHETS*
3. Spell SQUARE	19. Repeat METHODIST EPISCOPAL
4. Copy CROSS	20. Write SQUARE *Says "SQUARE," Then writes*
5. Name CROSS	21. Read SEVEN
6. Spell CROSS	22. Repeat SEVEN
7. Copy TRIANGLE	23. Repeat/Explain HE SHOUTED THE WARNING. *MEANS HE SHOUTED THE WARNING - COULD'VE BEEN SOME DANGER THERE -*
8. Name TRIANGLE	24. Write HE SHOUTED THE WARNING.
9. Spell TRIANGLE *TRI - ANG - LE*	25. Compute 85 − 27 =
10. Name BABY	26. Compute 17 X 3 = *IS 51 (Very quick response)*
11. Write CLOCK *WRITE IT? CLOCK?*	27. Name KEY
12. Name FORK	28. Demonstrate use of KEY *IN THE DOOR (show me) TURN ONLY*
13. Read 7 SIX 2	29. Draw KEY
14. Read M G W	30. Read PLACE LEFT HAND TO RIGHT EAR. *PLACE LH AT THE BACK OF R EAR.*
15. Reading I	31. Place LEFT HAND TO RIGHT EAR *LH to R ear lobe, then L hand to L ear lobe -*
16. Reading II	32. Place LEFT HAND TO LEFT ELBOW *LH ON L ELBOW! (laughs)*

Figure 8. Case 6 (continued).

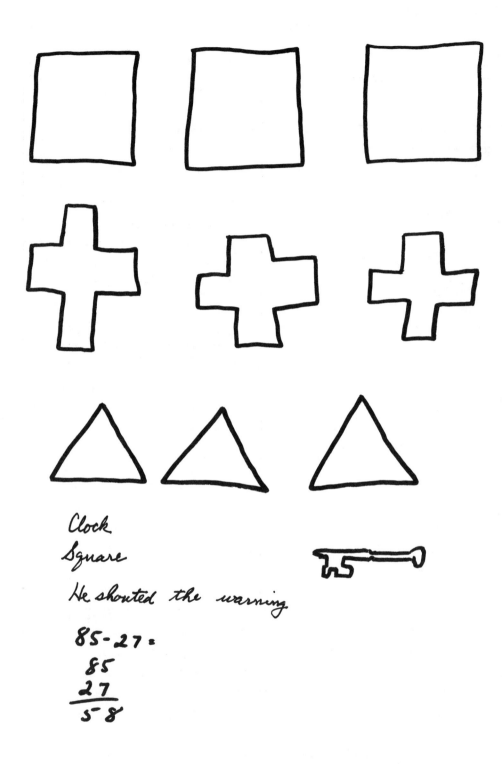

Figure 8. Case 6 (continued).

1) Is There Cerebral Impairment?

Level of Performance: The Halstead Impairment Index, the Category Test, the TPT Location score, and Part B of the Trail Making Test are all in the impaired range. This method of inference clearly lends support for the presence of cerebral impairment. **(4-1)**

Pattern of Performance: The VIQ/PIQ and the Aphasia/Spatial Relations relationships are normal, but her Visual Memory Index is significantly more impaired than her Verbal Memory Index on the WMS-R. This method of inference lends only rather weak support for the presence of cerebral impairment. **(5-25)**

Right/Left Differences: The relationships between the two hands on Finger Tapping, the Grooved Peg Board, and sensory perceptual errors all have possible lateralizing significance as indicated by the Ls next to them on the HRB Norms Transformation. This lends support for the presence of cerebral impairment. **(5-11)**

Pathognomonic Signs: There were no pathognomonic signs.

Overall, there is fairly strong support for the presence of impairment, although the fact that this woman reportedly has a schizophrenic disorder complicates the picture. A more detailed psychiatric history would be helpful.

2) What is the Severity of Cerebral Dysfunction?

Level of Performance: The level of performance is at least moderately severely impaired. Note, for example, that her *T* scores for most of the test of the HRB are below 40. In addition, her FSIQ of 85 is lower than would be expected in view of her reported work history.

Pattern of Performance: This method of inference does not contribute much to answering this question.

Right/Left Differences: This method of inference does not contribute much to answering this question in this case.

Pathognomonic Signs: There were no pathognomonic signs.

Overall, the evidence suggests that if there is any impairment, it is at least moderately severe. However, the lack of certainty about her history creates a problem in interpreting the data.

3) Is the Lesion Progressive or Static?

Level of Performance: Her adequate performance on the Seashore Rhythm Test argues against a rapidly progressive lesion. **(6-11)**

Pattern of Performance: This method of inference does not usually contribute much to the answer of this question.

Right/Left Differences: This method of inference does not contribute much to the answer of this question.

Pathognomonic Signs: This method of inference does not contribute to the answer of this question in this case.

Overall, there is nothing to suggest that there is any progressive lesion.

4) Is the Lesion Diffuse or Lateralized?

Level of Performance: As usual, this method of inference does not contribute to the answer of this question.

Pattern of Performance: The relationships between the VIQ and PIQ and Aphasia and Spatial Relations are normal. The significant difference between Verbal and Visual Memory is suggestive of more impairment of the right hemisphere. **(5-25)**

Right/Left Differences: The right/left relationship on finger tapping suggests impairment of the left hemisphere; the relationship on the grooved peg board suggests impairment of the right hemisphere; and the TFR time relationship suggests left-hemisphere impairment. Overall, this looks like a pattern of spotty or bilateral impairment.

Pathognomonic Signs: There were no pathognomonic signs.

Overall, it appears that the impairment is spotty or bilateral.

5) Is the Impairment in the Anterior or Posterior Part of the Cerebral Hemisphere?

Level of Performance: As usual, this method of inference does not contribute to the answer of this question.

Pattern of Performance: The most significant data in regard to this question in this case is that from the Wisconsin Card Sorting Test. Although her *T* score is 46, it is essential to note that this score is based on perseverative responses; it does not take into account the fact that she never achieved a single category. When that is considered, it is clear that her performance is very severely impaired, and there is an indication of impairment of one or both frontal lobes. The significant impairment of visual memory with adequate verbal memory suggests impairment of the right temporal lobe. **(5-37, 5-19)**

Right/Left Differences: As usual, this method of inference does not contribute to the answer of this question.

Pathognomonic Signs: There were no pathognomonic signs.

Overall, there appears to be spotty or bilateral impairment with the frontal lobes and right temporal lobe showing significant problems.

6) What is the Most Likely Neuropathological Process?

The pattern of impairment seen rules out any process involving a single focal lesion. The reasonably adequate attention abilities make a destructive process like multiple metasteses unlikely. The lack of errors on the Sensory Perceptual Examination makes MS unlikely, and no other signs or symptoms consistent with that disease were noted on the physical examination by the referring physician. The type of spotty picture found in this case, particularly with significant frontal and temporal lobe impairment is frequently seen with closed head injuries.

This case was complicated by this woman's psychiatric disorder and the vague, incomplete history available at the time of the referral. It was eventually possible to locate two brothers of the patient who verified her education and work history. They also revealed that the patient's psychiatric problems had first become apparent about 4 years prior to this evaluation, after she had suffered a closed head injury in a motor vehicle accident. They reported that she had been in a coma for several days and had remained hospitalized for over a month.

7) What are the Implications for Everyday Functioning and Treatment?

As a result of the new information, the patient's psychiatrist changed her psychiatric diagnosis to Organic Delusional Disorder and decided to minimize the use of neuroleptic medications. Insight-oriented psychotherapy was not thought likely to be helpful because of her very limited concept formation abilities; a reality-oriented, problem-solving approach was instituted instead, with an operant-based behavioral treatment program considered if that was not helpful. It seemed most unlikely that she would be able to return to her former work as an accountant. In fact, it appeared that the problems she experienced when she tried to do so a few months after her injury had led to the development of her delusions. A vocational evaluation was deferred pending evaluation of her psychiatric treatment progress.

Case 7

This is a 35-year-old, white, right-handed male attorney with 20 years of education. He is a successful trial lawyer and a partner in a large law firm. Two months prior to this evaluation, he received a closed head injury in a motor vehicle accident in which he was the restrained driver of a Mercedes sedan. If he lost consciousness, it was for only a few minutes, since he had extracted himself from his car and appeared alert and fully oriented by the time the ambulance arrived. His memory for the details of the accident was somewhat vague. He was examined at a local hospital and released after 4 hours. The neurological examination was normal, and a CT scan of the head on the day of the accident was normal, as was another one 1 month later. An EEG 1 month after the accident was normal. He suffered muscle strains in the neck and back, which seemed to be responding well to physical therapy.

At the time of this evaluation, he complained of memory problems: occasional difficulty with spatial orientation when driving; difficulty reading complex material with comprehension; and difficulty concentrating on the details of the complex issues involved in his work, particularly if there were any distractions present. He had not appeared in court since the accident and was concerned that he would not be able to handle that aspect of his work as well as he had in the past because he didn't believe he could "think on my feet any more." There was a potential threat of a law suit over the accident, but his main concern was whether his memory problems would be permanent and disabling.

This case is presented to illustrate two special types of issues: It is typical of many cases involving "mild head injuries in which neurological and radiological evidence fails to show evidence of brain damage"; these are the cases in which neuropsychologists are most often called to testify. Because the patient is a highly educated person, it also illustrates the importance of applying the demographic corrections supplied by Heaton et al. (1991).

Additional tests administered were: The Wechsler Memory Scale-Revised (WMS-R) on which his scores were: Verbal Memory Index, 111; Visual Memory Index, 108; General Memory Index, 114; Attention/Concentration Index, 110; and Delayed Recall Index, 105.

HRB NORMS PROGRAM
Raw Score Transformations

Name: Case7   Sex: M
Age: 35   Years of Educ: 20
Date: 02/26/93   File Name: CASE7
Handedness: Right

Measure	Abbreviation	Raw Scores	Scaled Scores	T Scores
HALSTEAD REITAN BATTERY SCORES				
Halstead Impairment Index	HII	0.3	10	36#
Average Impairment Rating	AIR			
Category Test	CAT ERROR	19	12	46
Trail Making Test-A (secs)	TRAIL A	17	14	58
Trail Making Test-B (secs)	TRAIL B	41	14	57
Tact Perf Test-Time (min/blk)	TPT TIME	.306	12	52
Tact Perf Test-Memory (correct)	TPT MEM	8	11	44
Tact Perf Test-Location (correct)	TPT LOC	3	9	36#
Seashore Rhythm (correct)	SSHOR RHYM	22	6	28#
Speech Perception (errors)	SPCH PERC	1	15	57
Aphasia Screening (errors)	APHAS SCRN	0	13	57
Spatial Relations (rating)	SPAT REL			
Sensory-Perceptual Total (errors)	SP TOTAL	2	11	47
LATERALIZED SENSORIMOTOR/ PSYCHOMOTOR INDICES				
Finger Tapping-Dom (taps)	TAP DH	50.6	10	41
Finger Tapping-Non-dom (taps)	TAP NDH	47.8	11	44
Hand Dynamometer-Dom (kgs)	GRIP DH	59.33	14	56
Hand Dynamometer-Non-dom (kgs)	GRIP NDH	53.67	13	55
Grooved Pegboard-Dom (secs)	PEG DH			
Grooved Pegboard-Non-dom (secs)	PEG NDH			
Tact Perf Test-Dom (min/blk)	TPT DH	.363	13	59
Tact Perf Test-Non-dom (min/blk)	TPT NDH	.402	10	43L
Tact Perf Test-Both Hands (min/blk)	TPT BOTH	.155	13	56
Sensory-Perceptual-Right (errors)	SP R	1	12	49
Sensory-Perceptual-Left (errors)	SP L	1	10	51
Tactile Form Recog-Right (secs)	TFR R	5.5	17	68
Tactile Form Recog-Left (secs)	TFR L	5.5	16	65

# = Impaired
L = Right-left difference, with possible lateralizing significance

Figure 9. Case 7.

HRB NORMS PROGRAM
Raw Score Transformations

Page 2

Name: Case7   Sex: M
Age: 35   Years of Educ: 20
Date: 02/26/93   File Name: CASE7
Handedness: Right

Measure	Abbreviation	Raw Scores	Scaled Scores	T Scores
ADDITIONAL TEST SCORES				
Thurstone Word Fluency (correct)	WORD FLUEN	107	18	71
Boston Naming (correct)	BSTN NAME			
BDAE Complex Material (correct)	BDAE COMP			
WCST Perseverative Responses	WCST PSVR			
Seashore Tonal Memory (correct)	SSHOR TONAL			
Digit Vigilance Time (sec)	DIGIT TIME			
Digit Vigilance Errors	DIGIT ERROR			
Story Learning (points/trials)	STORY LEARN			
Story Memory (% loss)	STORY LOSS			
Figure Learning (points/trial)	FIGUR LEARN			
Figure Memory (% loss)	FIGUR LOSS			
PIAT Reading Recog (percentile)	PIAT RECOG			
PIAT Reading Comp (percentile)	PIAT COMP			
PIAT Spelling (percentile)	PIAT SPELL			

= Impaired

Figure 9. Case 7 (continued).

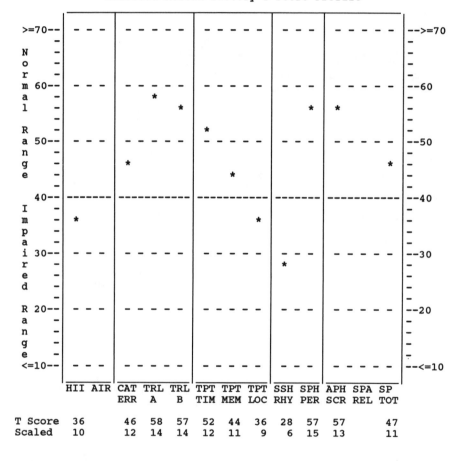

Name: Case7   Sex: M
Age: 35   Years of Educ: 20
Date: 02/26/93   File Name: CASE7
Handedness: Right

Figure 9. Case 7 (continued).

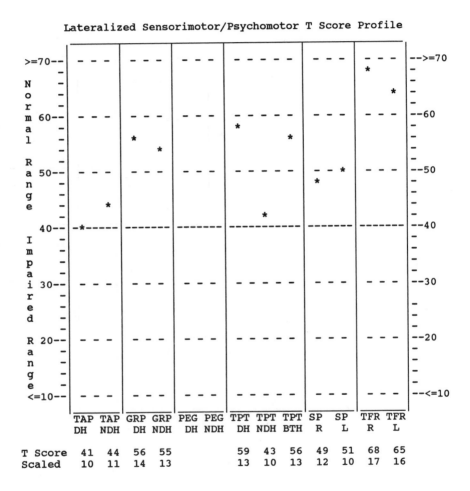

Page 4

Name:	Case7		Sex:	M
Age:	35		Yrs of Educ:	20
Date:	02/26/93		File Name:	CASE7
Handedness:	Right			

Lateralized Sensorimotor/Psychomotor T Score Profile

	TAP DH	TAP NDH	GRP DH	GRP NDH	PEG DH	PEG NDH	TPT DH	TPT NDH	TPT BTH	SP R	SP L	TFR R	TFR L
T Score	41	44	56	55			59	43	56	49	51	68	65
Scaled	10	11	14	13			13	10	13	12	10	17	16

Figure 9. Case 7 (continued).

Page 5

Name: Case7   Sex: M
Age: 35   Yrs of Educ: 20
Date: 02/26/93   File Name: CASE7
Handedness: Right

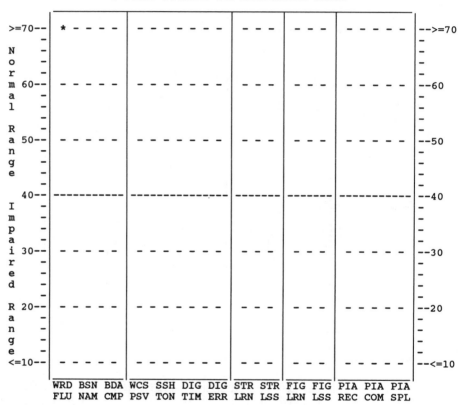

T Score Profile for Additional Tests

T Score   71
Scaled   18

Figure 9. Case 7 (continued).

SENSORY—PERCEPTUAL EXAMINATION

Case 7

Indicate Instance in which stimulus is not perceived or is incorrectly perceived.

Error Totals

Tactile:

Right Hand/Left Hand — RH [ ] LH [ ] Both: RH [ ] LH [ ] RH _0_ LH _0_

Right Hand/Left Face — RH [ ] LF [ ] Both: RH [ ] LF [ ] RH _0_ LF _0_

Left Hand/Right Face — LH [ ] RF [ ] Both: LH [ ] RF [ ] RF _0_ LH _0_

Auditory:

Right Ear/Left Ear — RE [ ] LE [ ] Both: RE [ ] LE [ ] RE _0_ LE _0_

Visual:

Above eye level
Eye level { RV [ ] LV [ ] Both: RV [ ] LV [ ] RV _0_ LV _0_
Below eye level

Finger Agnosia:

Right: 1 [ ] 2 [ ] 3 [ ] 4 [ ] 5 [ ] R _0/_
Left: 1 [ ] 2 [ ] 3 [ ] 4 [ ] 5 [4] L _1/_

Finger-tip Number Writing Perception:

Right: [4 6 3 5 / 5] [3 5 4 6] [6 5 4 3] [5 4 6 3] [6 3 5 4] R _1/_
Left: L _0/_

Astereognosis:

omitted

Right: [P N D]   Left: [D N P]   Both: Right: [N P D] Left: [ ] R ___
L ___

Tactile Form Recognition:

Errors: RH [○ □ △ ✚] LH [△ ✚ ○ □] RH [✚ ○ □ △] LH [□ △ ✚ ○] R _0_
Response Time: [1 .5 .5 1] [1 .5 .5 1] [.5 1 .5 .5] [.5 1 .5 .5] L _0_

Total Time: R _5.5_ L _5.5_

Visual Fields: WNL Left   Right

Figure 9. Case 7 (continued).

APHASIA SCREENING TEST   Case 7

Form for Adults and Older Children

Name: _____ Age: **35** Date: **2/6/93** Examiner: _____

1. Copy SQUARE	17. Repeat TRIANGLE
2. Name SQUARE	18. Repeat MASSACHUSETTS
3. Spell SQUARE	19. Repeat METHODIST EPISCOPAL
4. Copy CROSS	20. Write SQUARE
5. Name CROSS	21. Read SEVEN
6. Spell CROSS	22. Repeat SEVEN
7. Copy TRIANGLE	23. Repeat/Explain HE SHOUTED THE WARNING *A PERSON SHOUTED A CAUSE FOR OTHER PEOPLE TO* *LISTEN - (Q) ALERTING OTHER PEOPLE TO DANGER*
8. Name TRIANGLE	24. Write HE SHOUTED THE WARNING
9. Spell TRIANGLE	25. Compute 85 − 27 =
10. Name BABY	26. Compute 17 X 3 = *quickly done*
11. Write CLOCK	27. Name KEY
12. Name FORK	28. Demonstrate use of KEY
13. Read 7 SIX 2	29. Draw KEY
14. Read M G W	30. Read PLACE LEFT HAND TO RIGHT EAR.
15. Reading I	31. Place LEFT HAND TO RIGHT EAR
16. Reading II	32. Place LEFT HAND TO LEFT ELBOW *(laughs - appropriate response)*

Figure 9. Case 7 (continued).

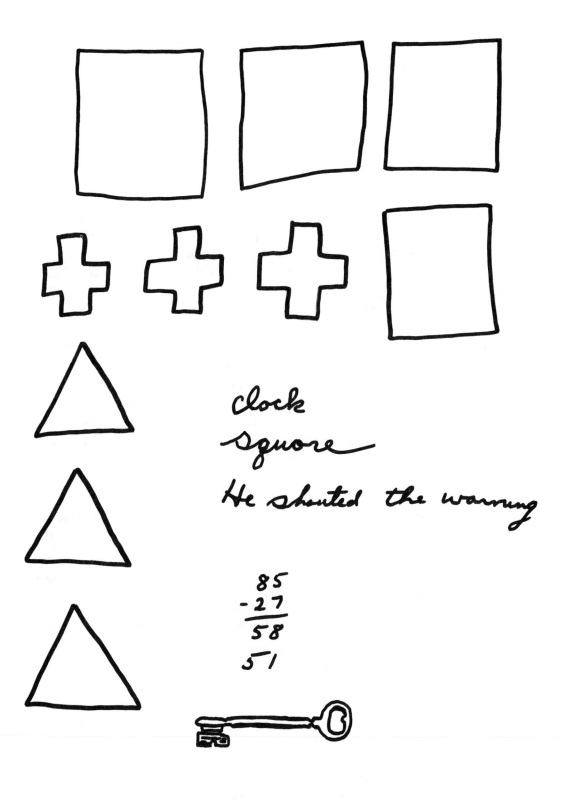

Figure 9. Case 7 (continued).

The Rey Auditory Verbal Learning Test (RAVLT) (Lezak, 1983) on which he learned a list of 15 unrelated words at a rate that was slightly more than one Standard Deviation below the Mean for a group of "professionals." More significantly, he showed a very significant interference effect when he was required to learn a new list of words after learning the first list; along with the five words he learned from the new list, he included four from the original list.

The Paced Auditory Serial Addition Test (PASAT), (Spreen & Strauss, 1991), which requires the ability to perform simple arithmetic calculations at a rapid pace, yielded a performance that was about one Standard Deviation below the Mean for his age.

The Stroop Neuropsychological Screening Test (SNST) (Trenerry, Crosson, Deboe, & Leben, 1989) requires the patient to name aloud, as rapidly as possible, the color of the ink in which color names are printed. This ink color is always different from the color name. (For example, the word red is never printed in red ink, but rather in a different color ink.) This requires the ability to provide rapid verbal responses in the face of competing or distracting stimuli. His performance on this test was at the sixth percentile for his age.

Because of the probability of future litigation in this case and the resulting potential for questions being raised about possible deception in such cases, particularly when they involve mild head injuries with no significant medical evidence of brain impairment, two of the special tests described in chapter 12 were administered. On the Rey Visual Memory Test (RVMT) (Lezak, 1983), he correctly reproduced all 15 stimuli. On the Portland Digit Recognition Test (PDRT) (Binder, 1992), which is a more complex test and more sensitive to attempted deception, his score was in the range that is characteristic of a group of subjects who had experienced head injuries and who had no motivation to obtain compensation.

1) Is There Cerebral Impairment?

Level of Performance: The Halstead Impairment Index is only .3, which is below the traditional cut-off for impairment, but the age and education corrected T score of 36 is impaired. The T score of 46 for the Category Test is not impaired, nor is the T score of 57 for part B of the Trail Making Test, but the TPT Location T score of 36 is. With two of the four most sensitive indicators being impaired, this method of inference lends a moderate degree of support for the presence of impairment.

Pattern of Performance: The VIQ/PIQ (132/125) and the Verbal/Visual Memory (111/108) relationships are normal, but the Aphasia/Spatial Relations (T scores of 57/47) relationship is a bit deviant, although neither is impaired. This method of inference lends virtually no support for the presence of cerebral impairment.

Right/Left Differences: The nondominant hand is slow in relation to the dominant hand on the TPT (T scores of 43 and 59), but the relationship is normal for all other motor and sensory tests. This method of inference lends only weak support for the presence of cerebral impairment.

Pathognomonic Signs: There were no pathognomonic signs.

Overall, there is fairly weak support for the presence of impairment.

2) What is the Severity of Cerebral Dysfunction?

Level of Performance: The level of performance is only mildly impaired.

Pattern of Performance: This method of inference does not contribute much to answering this question.

Right/Left Differences: This method of inference indicates at most mild impairment based on the deviant TPT relationship and the other normal relationships.

Pathognomonic Signs: There were no pathognomonic signs.

Overall, the evidence suggests that if there is any impairment, it is only mild.

3) Is the Lesion Progressive or Static?

Level of Performance: There is nothing to suggest a progressive lesion.

Pattern of Performance: There is nothing to suggest a progressive lesion.

Right/Left Differences: This method of inference does not contribute much to the answer of this question.

Pathognomonic Signs: There were no pathognomonic signs.

Overall, there is nothing to suggest that there is any progressive lesion.

4) Is the Lesion Diffuse or Lateralized?

Level of Performance: As usual, this method of inference does not contribute to the answer of this question.

Pattern of Performance: The relationships between the VIQ and PIQ and Verbal and Visual Memory are normal, while the Aphasia and Spatial Relations relationship provides at most very minimal support for right-hemisphere impairment. The fact that performance on Seashore Rhythm (*T* score of 28) is less adequate than performance on Speech Sounds Perception (*T* score of 57) also lends weak support for more right-hemisphere impairment. **(5-12)**

Right/Left Differences: The deviant TPT relationship suggests possible right-hemisphere impairment.

Pathognomonic Signs: There were no pathognomonic signs.

Overall, this appears to be a case of diffuse impairment, with only slight indications that the right hemisphere may be a bit more impaired than the left hemisphere. Note that the excellent *T* score of 71 on the Thurstone Word Fluency Test along with an Aphasia Screening Test performance within normal limits suggests a lack of impairment of the left hemisphere.

5) Is the Impairment in the Anterior or Posterior Part of the Cerebral Hemisphere?

Level of Performance: As usual, this method of inference does not contribute to the answer of this question.

Pattern of Performance: There is nothing in the pattern of performance which suggests any focal lesion.

Right/Left Differences: As usual, this method of inference does not contribute to the answer of this question.

Pathognomonic Signs: There were no pathognomonic signs.

Overall, there is no indication of any focal lesion.

6) What is the Most Likely Neuropathological Process?

This case is typical of many patients who have experienced mild closed head injuries. The impairment is mild and generally diffuse, although there may sometimes be evidence of slightly more focal impairment, particularly in the frontal and temporal regions. When there are disputes over claims for damages, questions about possible deception or exaggeration of deficits are frequently raised, and tests such as the RVMT and the PDRT should be added to the battery to assist in addressing them. In this case, performance on those two tests did not suggest any attempt at deception. The validity scales on the MMPI also reflected an honest approach to that test, and the profile on the clinical scales was normal.

7) What are the Implications for Everyday Functioning and Treatment?

This is a very bright man who is capable of understanding the implications of the test data, and the following description of them should be discussed with him directly in addition to sending a report of the evaluation to his physician and his attorney.

What he perceives as a memory problem is not so much a problem with memory as an impairment of attention and concentration when there are distractions present and a decrease in his ability to process information rapidly. The poor performance on Seashore Rhythm compared to Speech Sounds Perception illustrates the effect that a demand for rapid information processing has on his performance as does his impaired performance on the PASAT. Also significant is the fact that on the WMS-R, simple attention on Digit Span Forward and Visual Memory Span Forward, was significantly better than more complex attention or concentration on Digit Span Backward and Visual Memory Span Backward. Visual Memory Span Backward was only at the 36th percentile.

This suggests that he can compensate by reducing the demands for rapid information processing by requesting that information be provided to him in writing so that he can study it at his own pace instead of relying on his ability to comprehend verbal presentations.

His most impaired performance was on the SNST on which the competing stimuli coupled with the demand for rapid responses caused him a great deal of difficulty. The effect of interference was also seen in the number of intrusions from List A when he was required to learn List B on the RAVLT. This has two implications: He should be advised to keep his work environment as free from distractions as possible, which he can facilitate, for example, by establishing a specific time in his schedule when he will return phone calls and having his secretary screen calls and take messages for him. He should also arrange his schedule so that he allocates specific blocks of time to work on separate projects or sections of large projects and completes work on a project before he starts on another one.

He might also consider the use of electronic technology to assist in compensating for these deficits. Since his law firm makes extensive use of computer technology, he could take advantage of this by considering the addition of software, which facilitates functions such as scheduling and project planning. With project planning software, for example, he could identify all of the steps required to complete a project and rapidly determine the current status and the next action required on any project when he returns to work on it after an interruption. Small briefcase, or even pocket-size devices with the capacity to transfer data between them and his desktop computer are also available.

Probably the most important information that he should be given is the fact that he can expect a rapid recovery of functioning over the next 6 months or so. Periodic retesting with some of the tests used in this evaluation, such as the PASAT and the SNST, would document his progress and provide reassurance to him.

Case 8

This is a 44-year-old, white, left-handed woman with 12 years of education. She had reportedly worked successfully at a responsible secretarial job until about 2 years ago when she was hospitalized for the first time with a diagnosis of Schizophrenia, Undifferentiated Type. She was receiving neuroleptic medication at the time of testing. On the TPT, when she had failed to place a single block after 5 minutes, she removed the blindfold and refused to continue with that test.

1) Is There Cerebral Impairment?

Level of Performance: No Halstead Impairment Index was calculated because of her refusal to complete the TPT. The Category Test score was in the average range. Her *T* score of 36 on Part B of the Trail Making Test was in the impaired range, and her Digit Symbol Subtest score was in the impaired range and was the lowest of her WAIS-R subtest scores. This method of inference lends modest support for the presence of impairment.

Pattern of Performance: The VIQ/PIQ and the Aphasia/Spatial Relations relationships are normal, and this method of inference lends no support for the presence of cerebral impairment.

Right/Left Differences: The relationships between the two hands on Finger Tapping, Strength of Grip, and the Grooved Peg Board, all have possible lateralizing significance as indicated by the Ls next to them on the HRB Norms Transformation. This lends support for the presence of cerebral impairment. **(5-11)**

Pathognomonic Signs: There were no pathognomonic signs.

Overall, there is a rather modest level of support for the presence of impairment, although the fact that this woman reportedly has a schizophrenic disorder complicates the picture. A more detailed psychiatric history would be helpful in understanding the onset of her problems since a first schizophrenic episode at age 42 is unusual.

2) What is the Severity of Cerebral Dysfunction?

Level of Performance: The level of performance is generally only mildly impaired except for her performance on the Wisconsin Card Sorting Test, which was very severely impaired with 39 perseverative responses and not a single category achieved.

HRB NORMS PROGRAM
Raw Score Transformations

Name: Case8   Sex: F
Age: 44   Years of Educ: 12
Date: 02/26/93   File Name: CASE8
Handedness: Left

Measure	Abbreviation	Raw Scores	Scaled Scores	T Scores
HALSTEAD REITAN BATTERY SCORES				
Halstead Impairment Index	HII			
Average Impairment Rating	AIR			
Category Test	CAT ERROR	54	8	43
Trail Making Test-A (secs)	TRAIL A	42	6	35#
Trail Making Test-B (secs)	TRAIL B	104	7	38#
Tact Perf Test-Time (min/blk)	TPT TIME			
Tact Perf Test-Memory (correct)	TPT MEM			
Tact Perf Test-Location (correct)	TPT LOC			
Seashore Rhythm (correct)	SSHOR RHYM	29	14	61
Speech Perception (errors)	SPCH PERC	6	9	46
Aphasia Screening (errors)	APHAS SCRN	0	13	64
Spatial Relations (rating)	SPAT REL	2	11	58
Sensory-Perceptual Total (errors)	SP TOTAL	5	9	42
LATERALIZED SENSORIMOTOR/ PSYCHOMOTOR INDICES				
Finger Tapping-Dom (taps)	TAP DH	33.4	4	34#L
Finger Tapping-Non-dom (taps)	TAP NDH	37.8	7	46
Hand Dynamometer-Dom (kgs)	GRIP DH	18.3	4	33#L
Hand Dynamometer-Non-dom (kgs)	GRIP NDH	23.0	7	48
Grooved Pegboard-Dom (secs)	PEG DH	79	7	33#
Grooved Pegboard-Non-dom (secs)	PEG NDH	101	5	27#L
Tact Perf Test-Dom (min/blk)	TPT DH			
Tact Perf Test-Non-dom (min/blk)	TPT NDH			
Tact Perf Test-Both Hands (min/blk)	TPT BOTH			
Sensory-Perceptual-Right (errors)	SP R	3	9	41
Sensory-Perceptual-Left (errors)	SP L	2	8	43
Tactile Form Recog-Right (secs)	TFR R	8	13	65
Tactile Form Recog-Left (secs)	TFR L	11	10	53L

\# = Impaired
L = Right-left difference, with possible lateralizing significance

Figure 10. Case 8.

HRB NORMS PROGRAM
Raw Score Transformations

Page 2

Name:	Case8		Sex:	F
Age:	44		Years of Educ:	12
Date:	02/26/93		File Name:	CASE8
Handedness:	Left			

Measure	Abbreviation	Raw Scores	Scaled Scores	T Scores
ADDITIONAL TEST SCORES				
Thurstone Word Fluency (correct)	WORD FLUEN			
Boston Naming (correct)	BSTN NAME			
BDAE Complex Material (correct)	BDAE COMP			
WCST Perseverative Responses	WCST PSVR	39	6	34#
Seashore Tonal Memory (correct)	SSHOR TONAL			
Digit Vigilance Time (sec)	DIGIT TIME			
Digit Vigilance Errors	DIGIT ERROR			
Story Learning (points/trials)	STORY LEARN			
Story Memory (% loss)	STORY LOSS			
Figure Learning (points/trial)	FIGUR LEARN			
Figure Memory (% loss)	FIGUR LOSS			
PIAT Reading Recog (percentile)	PIAT RECOG			
PIAT Reading Comp (percentile)	PIAT COMP			
PIAT Spelling (percentile)	PIAT SPELL			
WAIS-R SCORES				
Verbal IQ (VIQ)	VIQ	100	10	50
Performance IQ (PIQ)	PIQ	88	8	42
Full Scale IQ (FSIQ)	FSIQ	95	9	46
Information	INFO	9	9	49
Digit Span	DIGIT SPAN	10	11	51
Vocabulary	VOCAB	9	9	48
Arithmetic	ARITH	13	13	65
Comprehension	COMP	10	10	51
Similarities	SIMIL	10	10	53
Picture Completion	PICT COMP	9	9	50
Picture Arrangement	PICT ARR	7	7	43
Block Design	BLOCK DESGN	7	7	42
Object Assembly	OBJ ASSMB	8	8	46
Digit Symbol	DIGIT SYMB	6	6	36#

= Impaired

Figure 10. Case 8 (continued).

Name: Case8   Sex: F
Age: 44   Years of Educ: 12
Date: 02/26/93   File Name: CASE8
Handedness: Left

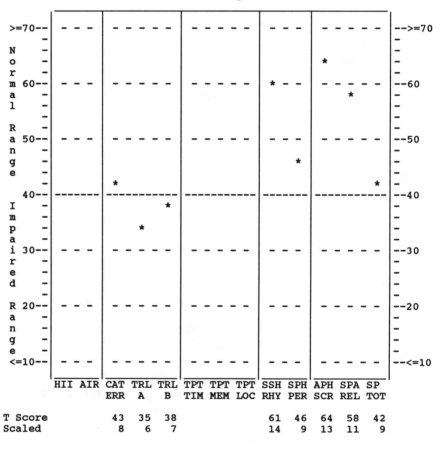

Figure 10. Case 8 (continued).

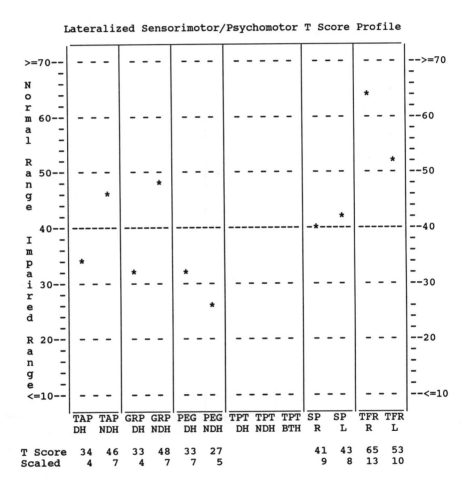

Figure 10. Case 8 (continued).

Page 5

Name: Case8   Sex: F
Age: 44   Yrs of Educ: 12
Date: 02/26/93   File Name: CASE8
Handedness: Left

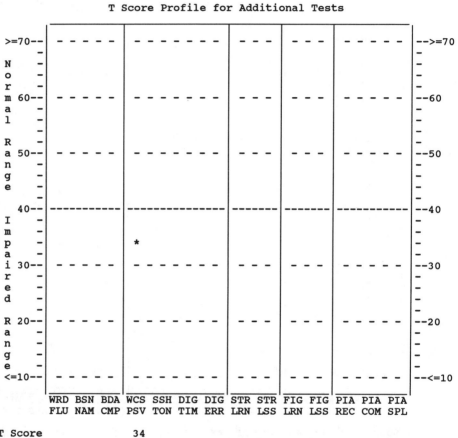

Figure 10. Case 8 (continued).

Page 6

Name: Case8   Sex: F
Age: 44   Yrs of Educ: 12
Date: 02/26/93   File Name: CASE8
Handedness: Left

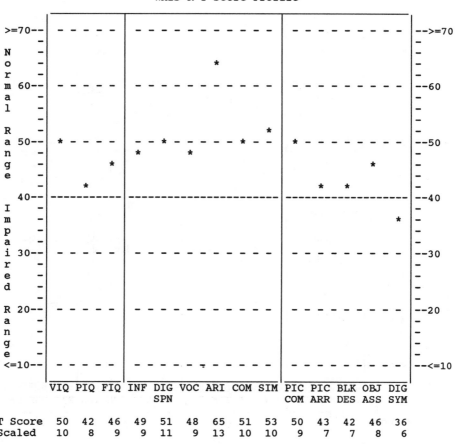

WAIS-R T Score Profile

	VIQ	PIQ	FIQ	INF	DIG SPN	VOC	ARI	COM	SIM	PIC COM	PIC ARR	BLK DES	OBJ ASS	DIG SYM
T Score	50	42	46	49	51	48	65	51	53	50	43	42	46	36
Scaled	10	8	9	9	11	9	13	10	10	9	7	7	8	6

Figure 10. Case 8 (continued).

SENSORY—PERCEPTUAL EXAMINATION   Case 8

Indicate Instance in which stimulus is not perceived or is incorrectly perceived.

Error Totals

Tactile:

Right Hand/Left Hand — RH ☐☐☐☐ LH ☐☐☐☐   Both: RH ☐☐☐☐ LH ☐☐☐☐   RH _0_ LH _0_

Right Hand/Left Face — RH ☐☐☐☐ LF ☐☐☐☐   Both: RH ☐☐☐☐ LF ☐☐☐☐   RH _0_ LF _0_

Left Hand/Right Face — LH ☐☐☐☐ RF ☐☐☐☐   Both: LH ☐☐☐☐ RF ☐☐☐☐   RF _0_ LH _0_

Auditory:

Right Ear/Left Ear — RE LE ☐☐☐☐   Both: ☐☐☐☐   RE LE ☐☐☐☐   RE ☐☐☐☐   LE _0_   _0_

Visual:

Above eye level
Eye level   { RV ▦ LV ▦   Both: RV ▦   LV ▦   RV _0_ LV _0_
Below eye level

Finger Agnosia:

Right: 1 ▦   2 ▦   3 ▦   4 ▦   5 |4|4| R _2/_
Left: 1 ▦   2 ▦   3 ▦   4 ▦   5 ▦   L _0/_

Finger-tip Number Writing Perception:

Right: |4|6|3|5| OK |3|5|4|6| |6|5|4|3| |5|4|6|3| |6|3|5|4| R _1/_
Left: |5| OK   L _2/_

Astereognosis:

Right: |P|N|D| Left: |D|N|P| D   Both: Right: N|P|D P|D   R _2_
                                               Left: D   L _1_

Tactile Form Recognition:

Errors: RH ○□△✛   LH △✛○□   RH ✛○□△   LH □△✛○   R _0_
Response Time: |1|1|1|1| |1|1|4|1| |1|1|1|1| |1|1|1|1| L _0_

                                    Total Time: R _8_   L _11_

Visual Fields: Left   Right

WNL ⊕   ⊕

Figure 10. Case 8 (continued).

Name: _____ Age: __44__ Date: __1/18/90__ Examiner: _____

1. Copy SQUARE	17. Repeat TRIANGLE
2. Name SQUARE	18. Repeat MASSACHUSETTS
3. Spell SQUARE	19. Repeat METHODIST EPISCOPAL
4. Copy CROSS	20. Write SQUARE
5. Name CROSS	21. Read SEVEN
6. Spell CROSS	22. Repeat SEVEN
7. Copy TRIANGLE	23. Repeat/Explain HE SHOUTED THE WARNING. *I D.K. HE LET SOMEONE KNOW THAT THERE WAS A DISASTER OR THAT SOMETHING HAPPENED.*
8. Name TRIANGLE	24. Write HE SHOUTED THE WARNING.
9. Spell TRIANGLE	25. Compute 85 – 27 = *See*
10. Name BABY	26. Compute 17 X 3 = *(Very fast response)*
11. Write CLOCK *ANYWHERE ON THE PAPER?*	27. Name KEY
12. Name FORK	28. Demonstrate use of KEY
13. Read 7 SIX 2	29. Draw KEY *Even though I clearly said that it did not have to be drawn c̄ one line, she thought that was the case. When I told her again, she wanted to start over but again drew with only one line.*
14. Read M G W	30. Read PLACE LEFT HAND TO RIGHT EAR.
15. Reading I	31. Place LEFT HAND TO RIGHT EAR
16. Reading II	32. Place LEFT HAND TO LEFT ELBOW *LH to R, then RH to L - Then "LH TO LE! D.K. HOW TO DO THAT!*

Figure 10. Case 8 (continued).

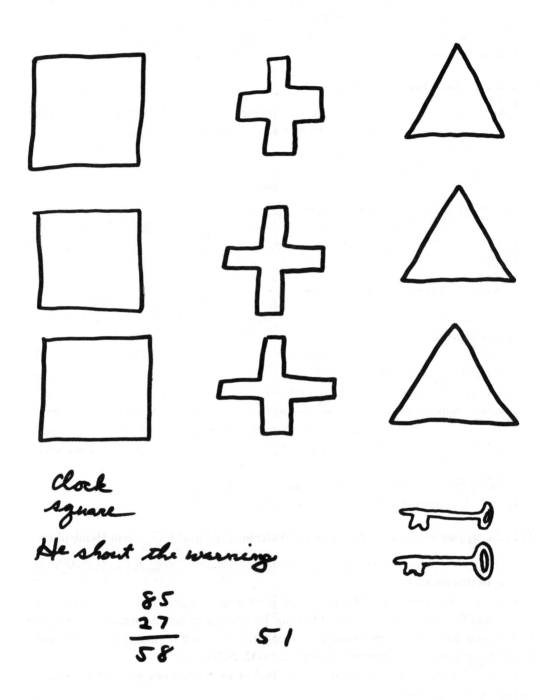

Figure 10. Case 8 (continued).

Pattern of Performance: This method of inference does not contribute much to answering this question.

Right/Left Differences: The deviant patterns noted on the motor tests are generally in the range 10 *T* score points of deviation, which suggests rather mild impairment.

Pathognomonic Signs: There were no pathognomonic signs.

Overall, the evidence suggests that the impairment is fairly mild.

3) Is the Lesion Progressive or Static?

Level of Performance: Her adequate performance on the Seashore Rhythm and Speech Sounds Perception Tests argues against a rapidly progressive lesion. **(6-11)**

Pattern of Performance: This method of inference does not usually contribute much to the answer of this question.

Right/Left Differences: This method of inference does not contribute much to the answer of this question.

Pathognomonic Signs: This method of inference does not contribute to the answer of this question in this case.

Overall, there is nothing to suggest that there is any progressive lesion.

4) Is the Lesion Diffuse or Lateralized?

Level of Performance: As usual, this method of inference does not contribute to the answer of this question.

Pattern of Performance: The relationships between the VIQ and PIQ and Aphasia and Spatial Relations are normal.

Right/Left Differences: The right/left relationships on finger tapping and strength of grip suggest impairment of the right hemisphere for this left-handed patient; the relationships on the grooved peg board and TFR time suggest impairment of the left hemisphere, although this is not as strong an indication. Overall, this looks like a pattern of bilateral impairment.

Pathognomonic Signs: There were no pathognomonic signs.

Overall, it appears that the impairment is bilateral.

5) Is the Impairment in the Anterior or Posterior Part of the Cerebral Hemisphere?

Level of Performance: As usual, this method of inference does not contribute to the answer of this question.

Pattern of Performance: The most significant data in regard to this question in this case is that from the Wisconsin Card Sorting Test, which indicates impairment of one or both frontal lobes. The impairment of motor functions, with normal sensory perceptual functions, also suggests anterior impairment. **(5-32, 5-37)**

Right/Left Differences: As usual, this method of inference does not contribute to the answer of this question.

Pathognomonic Signs: There were no pathognomonic signs.

Overall, there appears to be bilateral impairment of the frontal lobes.

6) What is the Most Likely Neuropathological Process?

The limitation of impairment to the frontal lobes makes a closed head injury unlikely; impairment is usually more diffuse in such cases. On the other hand, it is too widespread for a penetrating head injury. The mild level of impairment and the lack of any suggestion of a progressive lesion make a tumor unlikely. Similarly, the mild level of impairment coupled with the lack of impairment beyond the frontal lobes makes a vascular disorder unlikely.

A neurological consultation resulted in a report of "subtle, bifrontal upper motor neuron findings," and a CT scan revealed "enlarged frontal sulci." These studies did not shed any more light on the nature of the pathological process than did the neuropsychological evaluation.

7) What are the Implications for Everyday Functioning and Treatment?

The severity of this woman's deficits in problem-solving abilities makes it clear that she is unable to function independently. Any treatment planning is complicated by the lack of understanding of the neuropathological process underlying her cognitive deficits. Additional information about the nature of the onset of her problems might be helpful. Finally, repeat testing to monitor the progress of her condition is indicated.

Case No. 9

This is a 46-year-old, white, right-handed woman with 9 years of education. She had reportedly shown a steady decline in self-care skills, memory, and other cognitive functions over the past 2 or 3 years. Just prior to this evaluation, she had begun to show evidence of delusions and severe depression, which resulted in her first psychiatric hospitalization.

Her gait was normal, and she did not have any tremors, but gross movements of her arms were uncoordinated at times. Her speech was difficult to understand at times because of it's staccato nature. She refused to attempt the TPT and could not cooperate with the Sensory Perceptual Examination.

She showed evidence of dyspraxia on the Object Assembly subtest of the WAIS-R in that she recognized what some of the objects were, but said she couldn't "get them to go together right." On the Aphasia Screening Test, she made errors of dysnomia, constructional dyspraxia, spelling, and calculation.

Additional tests administered were: The Wechsler Memory Scale-Revised (WMS-R) on which her scores were: Verbal Memory Index, 65; Visual Memory Index, 55; General Memory Index, 50; Attention/Concentration Index, 68; and Delayed Recall Index, < 50.

The Rey Auditory Verbal Learning Test (RAVLT) (Lezak, 1983) on which she only learned two words on the first trial, learned eight words by the third trial, dropped to six and seven words on trials four and five, learned only one word on List B, and was unable to remember any words from List A on the final trial. This is a very severely impaired performance.

HRB NORMS PROGRAM
Raw Score Transformations

Name:	Case9	Sex:	F
Age:	46	Years of Educ:	9
Date:	02/26/93	File Name:	CASE9
Handedness:	Right		

Measure	Abbreviation	Raw Scores	Scaled Scores	T Scores
HALSTEAD REITAN **BATTERY SCORES**				
Halstead Impairment Index	HII	1.0	1	14#
Average Impairment Rating	AIR			
Category Test	CAT ERROR	138	0	16#
Trail Making Test-A (secs)	TRAIL A	104	1	18#
Trail Making Test-B (secs)	TRAIL B	750	1	17#
Tact Perf Test-Time (min/blk)	TPT TIME			
Tact Perf Test-Memory (correct)	TPT MEM			
Tact Perf Test-Location (correct)	TPT LOC			
Seashore Rhythm (correct)	SSHOR RHYM	15	3	30#
Speech Perception (errors)	SPCH PERC	25	3	29#
Aphasia Screening (errors)	APHAS SCRN	16	4	29#
Spatial Relations (rating)	SPAT REL	5	5	25#
Sensory-Perceptual Total (errors)	SP TOTAL			
LATERALIZED SENSORIMOTOR/ **PSYCHOMOTOR INDICES**				
Finger Tapping-Dom (taps)	TAP DH	20.8	1	24#
Finger Tapping-Non-dom (taps)	TAP NDH	16.2	0	20#L
Hand Dynamometer-Dom (kgs)	GRIP DH	22.3	5	39#
Hand Dynamometer-Non-dom (kgs)	GRIP NDH	19.0	5	39#
Grooved Pegboard-Dom (secs)	PEG DH	95	5	27#
Grooved Pegboard-Non-dom (secs)	PEG NDH	109	5	28#
Tact Perf Test-Dom (min/blk)	TPT DH			
Tact Perf Test-Non-dom (min/blk)	TPT NDH			
Tact Perf Test-Both Hands (min/blk)	TPT BOTH			
Sensory-Perceptual-Right (errors)	SP R			
Sensory-Perceptual-Left (errors)	SP L			
Tactile Form Recog-Right (secs)	TFR R	33	1	24#
Tactile Form Recog-Left (secs)	TFR L	35.5	1	24#L

\# = Impaired
L = Right-left difference, with possible lateralizing significance

Figure 11. Case 9.

HRB NORMS PROGRAM
Raw Score Transformations

Page 2

Name:	Case9		Sex:	F
Age:	46	Years of Educ:	9	
Date:	02/26/93	File Name:	CASE9	
Handedness:	Right			

Measure	Abbreviation	Raw Scores	Scaled Scores	T Scores
ADDITIONAL TEST SCORES				
Thurstone Word Fluency (correct)	WORD FLUEN			
Boston Naming (correct)	BSTN NAME			
BDAE Complex Material (correct)	BDAE COMP			
WCST Perseverative Responses	WCST PSVR	114	0	20#
Seashore Tonal Memory (correct)	SSHOR TONAL			
Digit Vigilance Time (sec)	DIGIT TIME			
Digit Vigilance Errors	DIGIT ERROR			
Story Learning (points/trials)	STORY LEARN			
Story Memory (% loss)	STORY LOSS			
Figure Learning (points/trial)	FIGUR LEARN			
Figure Memory (% loss)	FIGUR LOSS			
PIAT Reading Recog (percentile)	PIAT RECOG			
PIAT Reading Comp (percentile)	PIAT COMP			
PIAT Spelling (percentile)	PIAT SPELL			
WAIS-R SCORES				
Verbal IQ (VIQ)	VIQ	72	5	33#
Performance IQ (PIQ)	PIQ	68	4	30#
Full Scale IQ (FSIQ)	FSIQ	70	4	29#
Information	INFO	5	5	37#
Digit Span	DIGIT SPAN	4	5	33#
Vocabulary	VOCAB	5	5	36#
Arithmetic	ARITH	3	3	30#
Comprehension	COMP	5	5	37#
Similarities	SIMIL	5	5	39#
Picture Completion	PICT COMP	5	5	40
Picture Arrangement	PICT ARR	2	2	29#
Block Design	BLOCK DESGN	4	4	36#
Object Assembly	OBJ ASSMB	3	3	31#
Digit Symbol	DIGIT SYMB	2	2	28#

= Impaired

Figure 11. Case 9 (continued).

Name: Case9   Sex: F
Age: 46   Years of Educ: 9
Date: 02/26/93   File Name: CASE9
Handedness: Right

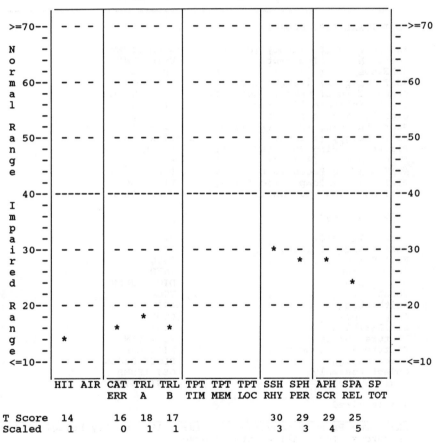

Halstead-Reitan Battery T Score Profile

		HII	AIR	CAT ERR	TRL A	TRL B	TPT TIM	TPT MEM	TPT LOC	SSH RHY	SPH PER	APH SCR	SPA REL	SP TOT
T Score		14		16	18	17				30	29	29	25	
Scaled		1		0	1	1				3	3	4	5	

Figure 11. Case 9 (continued).

Page 4

Name: Case9   Sex: F
Age: 46   Yrs of Educ: 9
Date: 02/26/93   File Name: CASE9
Handedness: Right

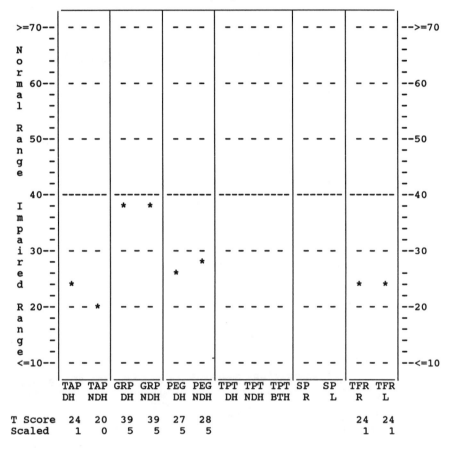

Figure 11. Case 9 (continued).

```
Name:        Case9                        Sex:        F
Age:         46                  Yrs of Educ:         9
Date:        02/26/93             File Name:          CASE9
Handedness: Right
```

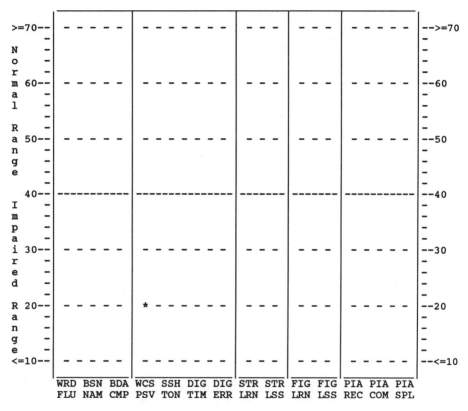

Figure 11. Case 9 (continued).

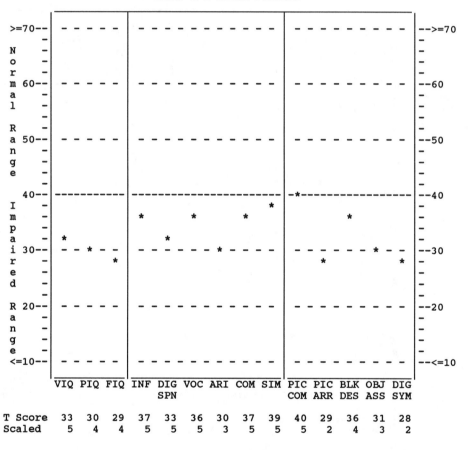

Page 6

Name: Case9   Sex: F
Age: 46   Yrs of Educ: 9
Date: 02/26/93   File Name: CASE9
Handedness: Right

WAIS-R T Score Profile

	VIQ	PIQ	FIQ	INF	DIG SPN	VOC	ARI	COM	SIM	PIC COM	PIC ARR	BLK DES	OBJ ASS	DIG SYM
T Score	33	30	29	37	33	36	30	37	39	40	29	36	31	28
Scaled	5	4	4	5	5	5	3	5	5	5	2	4	3	2

Figure 11. Case 9 (continued).

SENSORY—PERCEPTUAL EXAMINATION Case 9

Indicate Instance in which stimulus is not perceived or is incorrectly perceived.

Tactile: *Some confusion - Scattered - inconsistencies, suppressions, and "both" response when only one touched.* Error Totals

Right Hand/Left Hand — RH ☐☐☐ LH ☐☐☐ Both: RH ☐☐☐ LH ☐☐☐ RH _____ LH _____

Right Hand/Left Face — RH ☐☐☐ LF ☐☐☐ Both: RH ☐☐☐ LF ☐☐☐ RH _____ LF _____

Left Hand/Right Face — LH ☐☐☐ RF ☐☐☐ Both: LH ☐☐☐ RF ☐☐☐ RF _____ LH _____

Auditory:

Right Ear/Left Ear — RE ☐☐☐ LE ☐☐☐ Both: RE ☐☐☐ LE ☐☐☐ RE _0_ LE _0_

Visual: *Unable to focus - Has trouble c̄ eye contact.*

Above eye level
Eye level   { RV ☐☐☐ LV ☐☐☐ Both: RV ☐☐☐ LV ☐☐☐ RV _0_ LV _0_
Below eye level

Finger Agnosia: *Some confusion - unable to evaluate*

Right: 1 ☐☐ 2 ☐☐ 3 ☐☐ 4 ☐☐ 5 ☐☐ R _/_
Left: 1 ☐☐ 2 ☐☐ 3 ☐☐ 4 ☐☐ 5 ☐☐ L _/_

Finger-tip Number Writing Perception: *Unable to do*

Right: | 4 6 3 5 | | 3 5 4 6 | | 6 5 4 3 | | 5 4 6 3 | | 6 3 5 4 | R _/_
Left: L _/_

Astereognosis: *omitted*

Right: | P N D | Left: | D N P | Both: Right: | N P D / D | R _____
                                             Left: | D D | L _____

Tactile Form Recognition:

Errors: RH | ○ ☐ △ ✚ / △ | LH | △ ✚ ○ ☐ | RH | ✚ ○ ☐ △ | LH | ☐ △ ✚ ○ | R _1_
Response Time: | 1.5 5.0 4.0 4.0 | | 3.5 4 2 7 | | 5 2 9 2.5 | | 6 4.5 5 3.5 | L _0_

Difficult to evaluate.   Total Time: R _33.0_ L _35.5_

Visual Fields: Left   Right
WNL?

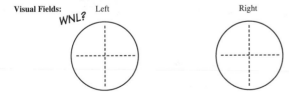

Figure 11. Case 9 (continued).

APHASIA SCREENING TEST   Case 9

Form for Adults and Older Children

Name: _____ Age: __46__ Date: __12/11/91__ Examiner: _____

1. Copy SQUARE	17. Repeat TRIANGLE
2. Name SQUARE *BOX (Q) TOY BOX (Q) PUT STUFF IN (E)*	18. Repeat MASSACHUSETTS
3. Spell SQUARE *S-Q-U-A-R*	19. Repeat METHODIST EPISCOPAL *EPISTOBAL*
4. Copy CROSS	20. Write SQUARE
5. Name CROSS *DK (Q) CROSS*	21. Read SEVEN
6. Spell CROSS *C-R-O-S-E*	22. Repeat SEVEN
7. Copy TRIANGLE	23. Repeat/Explain HE SHOUTED THE WARNING. *SOMEBODY'D GET HURT-IF THEY DIDN'T LISTEN*
8. Name TRIANGLE	24. Write HE SHOUTED THE WARNING.
9. Spell TRIANGLE *T-R-A-I-N-G-E-L*	25. Compute 85 − 27 = *74*
10. Name BABY	26. Compute 17 X 3 = *(Smiles-) Hm-Hm (5+8?)* *28* *(No response for >15* *seconds) 40*
11. Write CLOCK *CLOCK*	27. Name KEY
12. Name FORK *SS-FORK*	28. Demonstrate use of KEY *Put it in the door (show me)* *(Grabs book & says PUT IT IN THE KEY & TURN IT &* *OPEN THE DOOR*
13. Read 7 SIX 2 *7 SIX AND 2*	29. Draw KEY
14. Read M G W	30. Read PLACE LEFT HAND TO RIGHT EAR.
15. Reading I *"jerky" SEE THE BLACK (PAUSE) SEE THE BLACK* reading *DOG-*	31. Place LEFT HAND TO RIGHT EAR *(LH to L ear, then LH to R ear)*
16. Reading II *HE IS A FARMER-FAMOUS WINTER-WINNER* *OF THE DOG SHOW*	32. Place LEFT HAND TO LEFT ELBOW *(Makes several attempts, then YOU CAN'T* *DO THAT)*

Figure 11. Case 9 (continued).

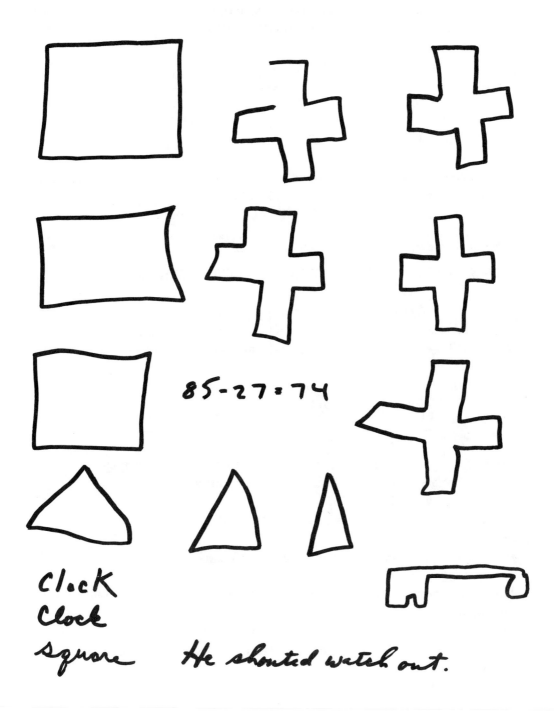

Figure 11. Case 9 (continued).

1) Is There Cerebral Impairment?

Level of Performance: *T* scores of 14 for the Halstead Impairment Index, 16 for the Category Test, and 17 for Part B of the Trail Making Test are all severely impaired. As indicated above, she refused to attempt the TPT. This method of inference lends strong support for the presence of impairment. **(4-1)**

Pattern of Performance: There are no unusual aspects of pattern seen, and this method of inference lends no support for the presence of cerebral impairment.

Right/Left Differences: None of the motor tests shows any lateralization, and sensory testing was not available, so this method of inference lends no support for the presence of cerebral impairment.

Pathognomonic Signs: The presence of the aphasia signs, particularly the significant dysnomia, supports the presence of impairment. **(4-56)**

Overall, there is a strong level of support for the presence of impairment.

2) What is the Severity of Cerebral Dysfunction?

Level of Performance: The level of performance is severely impaired on nearly all tests.

Pattern of Performance: This method of inference does not contribute much to answering this question.

Right/Left Differences: This method of inference does not contribute much to answering this question.

Pathognomonic Signs: The significant dysnomia suggests severe impairment.

Overall, the evidence suggests that the impairment is quite severe.

3) Is the Lesion Progressive or Static?

Level of Performance: Her poor performance on the Seashore Rhythm and Speech Sounds Perception Tests along with an apparent drop in her IQ makes a progressive condition a possibility. **(6-11)**

Pattern of Performance: This method of inference does not usually contribute much to the answer of this question.

Right/Left Differences: This method of inference does not contribute much to the answer of this question.

Pathognomonic Signs: This method of inference does not contribute to the answer of this question in this case.

Overall, there is a real possibility of a progressive condition based on the test data. Her history of a steady decline in level of functioning over the past several years confirms this.

4) Is the Lesion Diffuse or Lateralized?

Level of Performance: As usual, this method of inference does not contribute to the answer of this question.

Pattern of Performance: This method of inference does not suggest any lateralization.

Right/Left Differences: This method of inference does not suggest any lateralization.

Pathognomonic Signs: The aphasia signs point mainly to left-hemisphere impairment.
(4-56)

Overall, it appears that the impairment is diffuse.

5) Is the Impairment in the Anterior or Posterior Part of the Cerebral Hemisphere?

Level of Performance: As usual, this method of inference does not contribute to the answer of this question.

Pattern of Performance: This method of inference does not suggest any focal lesion.

Right/Left Differences: As usual, this method of inference does not contribute to the answer of this question.

Pathognomonic Signs: The aphasia signs point to impairment of the left frontal, temporal regions, but the pervasiveness of the overall impairment makes it clear that this is simply part of a diffuse process.

Overall, there is diffuse impairment.

6) What is the Most Likely Neuropathological Process?

This woman has a progressive, diffuse impairment that is generally quite severe. She has a progressive dementia, which apparently began at around age 44, with psychiatric symptoms becoming apparent about 2 years later. She does not have the tremor or gait disturbance which would be characteristic of Parkinson's disease, nor does she have the ataxic gait or incontinence, which are common with normal pressure hydrocephalus. The uncoordinated arm movements are suggestive of beginning choreiform movements, which are characteristic of Huntington's disease. In that disease atrophy of the caudate nucleus is revealed by a characteristic butterfly-shaped enlargement of the lateral ventricles, but this woman refused to have a CT scan.

In a case like this a family history is essential. Her family eventually revealed that there was a history of Huntington's disease in the family, which was well documented in the case of the patient's brother. The combination of dementia and psychiatric symptoms beginning at age 44, possible beginning choreiform movements, and the family history makes it virtually certain that this patient has Huntington's disease.

7) What are the Implications for Everyday Functioning and Treatment?

Unfortunately, there is no treatment for this disease. Both the dementia and the involuntary movements will get progressively worse. Death at an early age is expected. It may be helpful to other members of the family to refer them to the Huntington's Disease Association for counseling.

Case 10

This is a 48-year-old, white, right-handed woman with 12 years of education. She had reportedly shown a significant depression and decline in memory over the past several months following the death of her husband from complications of chronic alcohol abuse.

Additional tests administered were: The Russell Revision of the Wechsler Memory Scale (RRWMS) on which her verbal memory for both immediate and delayed recall was moderately impaired, and her visual memory for both immediate and delayed recall was severely impaired. On the Associate Learning subtest, she learned all six easy pairs on the first trial, retained them on the second and third trials, and learned all four hard pairs by the third trial.

On the MMPI, her F-K = –16, indicating a strong tendency to present herself in an unrealistically good light, and she had highly elevated scores on scales 4 and 9 reflecting significant antisocial tendencies.

On the Benton Judgment of Line Orientation Test (JOLO), her score was in the mildly impaired range.

1) Is There Cerebral Impairment?

Level of Performance: The Halstead Impairment Index, the Category Test, Part B of the Trail Making Test, and the Location score on the TPT are all impaired. This method of inference lends strong support for the presence of impairment. **(4-1)**

Pattern of Performance: The relationship between VIQ and PIQ is normal, but visual memory is more impaired than verbal memory. This method of inference lends only modest support for the presence of cerebral impairment.

Right/Left Differences: Although only the Finger Tapping and Grooved Pegboard scores show enough difference between the two hands to result in an L on page 1 of the Norms printout, note that Grip and TPT show a similar, but nonsignificant relationship on the page 4 profile. This method of inference also lends only modest support for the presence of cerebral impairment.

Pathognomonic Signs: There are no definite pathognomonic signs, but there was some mild dysnomia.

Overall, there is a fairly strong level of support for the presence of impairment.

2) What is the Severity of Cerebral Dysfunction?

Level of Performance: The level of performance is moderately to severely impaired on nearly all tests.

Pattern of Performance: This method of inference does not contribute much to answering this question.

Right/Left Differences: This method of inference does not contribute much to answering this question.

Pathognomonic Signs: The mild dysnomia does not suggest severe impairment.

Overall, the evidence suggests that the impairment is moderately severe.

3) Is the Lesion Progressive or Static?

Level of Performance: Her Speech Sounds Perception score is impaired, but her Seashore Rhythm score is in the average range. This makes a rapidly progressive condition rather unlikely. **(6-11)**

HRB NORMS PROGRAM
Raw Score Transformations

Name: Case10   Sex: F
Age: 48   Years of Educ: 12
Date: 02/26/93   File Name: CASE10
Handedness: Right

Measure	Abbreviation	Raw Scores	Scaled Scores	T Scores
HALSTEAD REITAN BATTERY SCORES				
Halstead Impairment Index	HII	0.9	4	26#
Average Impairment Rating	AIR			
Category Test	CAT ERROR	96	4	29#
Trail Making Test-A (secs)	TRAIL A	48	6	37#
Trail Making Test-B (secs)	TRAIL B	135	5	31#
Tact Perf Test-Time (min/blk)	TPT TIME	1.286	4	29#
Tact Perf Test-Memory (correct)	TPT MEM	7	9	44
Tact Perf Test-Location (correct)	TPT LOC	0	5	32#
Seashore Rhythm (correct)	SSHOR RHYM	24	8	43
Speech Perception (errors)	SPCH PERC	13	5	33#
Aphasia Screening (errors)	APHAS SCRN	9	6	34#
Spatial Relations (rating)	SPAT REL	3	9	46
Sensory-Perceptual Total (errors)	SP TOTAL	4	9	43
LATERALIZED SENSORIMOTOR/ PSYCHOMOTOR INDICES				
Finger Tapping-Dom (taps)	TAP DH	34.4	5	39#L
Finger Tapping-Non-dom (taps)	TAP NDH	36.2	7	47
Hand Dynamometer-Dom (kgs)	GRIP DH	23.7	5	39#
Hand Dynamometer-Non-dom (kgs)	GRIP NDH	22	6	44
Grooved Pegboard-Dom (secs)	PEG DH	93	5	26#L
Grooved Pegboard-Non-dom (secs)	PEG NDH	90	6	33#
Tact Perf Test-Dom (min/blk)	TPT DH	2.0	4	29#
Tact Perf Test-Non-dom (min/blk)	TPT NDH	1.25	5	32#
Tact Perf Test-Both Hands (min/blk)	TPT BOTH	.96	4	29#
Sensory-Perceptual-Right (errors)	SP R	1	12	51
Sensory-Perceptual-Left (errors)	SP L	3	7	39#
Tactile Form Recog-Right (secs)	TFR R	10	11	57
Tactile Form Recog-Left (secs)	TFR L	8	12	60

\# = Impaired
L = Right-left difference, with possible lateralizing significance

Figure 12. Case 10.

HRB NORMS PROGRAM
Raw Score Transformations

Page 2

Name:	Case10	Sex:	F
Age:	48	Years of Educ:	12
Date:	02/26/93	File Name:	CASE10
Handedness: Right			

Measure	Abbreviation	Raw Scores	Scaled Scores	T Scores
WAIS-R SCORES				
Verbal IQ (VIQ)	VIQ	86	8	40
Performance IQ (PIQ)	PIQ	81	6	33#
Full Scale IQ (FSIQ)	FSIQ	83	7	36#
Information	INFO	6	6	35#
Digit Span	DIGIT SPAN	8	10	47
Vocabulary	VOCAB	8	8	42
Arithmetic	ARITH	6	6	37#
Comprehension	COMP	9	9	47
Similarities	SIMIL	6	6	38#
Picture Completion	PICT COMP	5	5	37#
Picture Arrangement	PICT ARR	7	7	45
Block Design	BLOCK DESGN	5	5	36#
Object Assembly	OBJ ASSMB	5	5	36#
Digit Symbol	DIGIT SYMB	5	5	35#

\# = Impaired

Figure 12. Case 10 (continued).

Name: Case10   Sex: F
Age: 48   Years of Educ: 12
Date: 02/26/93   File Name: CASE10
Handedness: Right

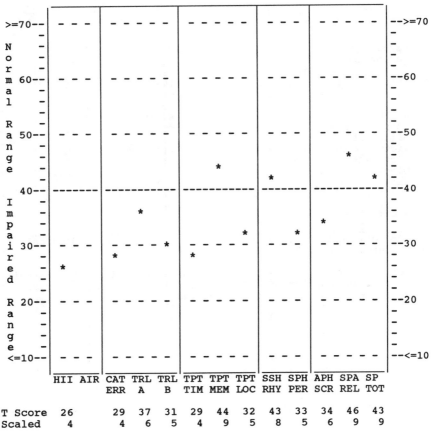

Figure 12. Case 10 (continued).

Page 4

```
Name:        Case10                              Sex:        F
Age:         48                        Yrs of Educ:          12
Date:        02/26/93                    File Name:          CASE10
Handedness:  Right
```

Lateralized Sensorimotor/Psychomotor T Score Profile

```
                TAP TAP  GRP GRP  PEG PEG  TPT TPT TPT  SP  SP  TFR TFR
                DH  NDH  DH  NDH  DH  NDH  DH  NDH BTH  R   L   R   L

T Score         39  47   39  44   26  33   29  32  29   51  39  57  60
Scaled           5   7    5   6    5   6    4   5   4   12   7  11  12
```

Figure 12. Case 10 (continued).

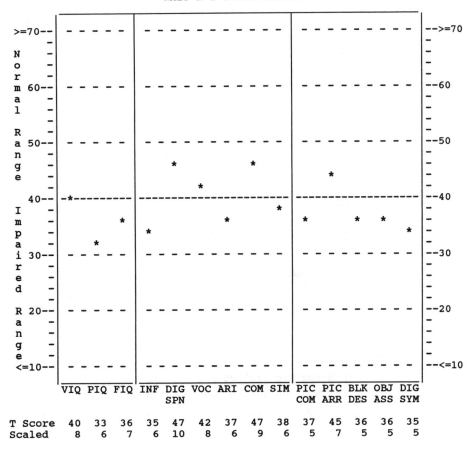

Page 5

Name: Case10   Sex: F
Age: 48   Yrs of Educ: 12
Date: 02/26/93   File Name: CASE10
Handedness: Right

WAIS-R T Score Profile

	VIQ	PIQ	FIQ	INF	DIG SPN	VOC	ARI	COM	SIM	PIC COM	PIC ARR	BLK DES	OBJ ASS	DIG SYM
T Score	40	33	36	35	47	42	37	47	38	37	45	36	36	35
Scaled	8	6	7	6	10	8	6	9	6	5	7	5	5	5

Figure 12. Case 10 (continued).

SENSORY—PERCEPTUAL EXAMINATION   Case 10

Indicate Instance in which stimulus is not perceived or is incorrectly perceived.

Tactile: **Error Totals**

Right Hand/Left Hand — RH [ ]   LH [ ]   Both: RH [ ]   LH [ ]   RH _0_ LH _0_

Right Hand/Left Face — RH [ ]   LF [ ]   Both: RH [X]   LF [ ]   RH _1_ LF _0_

Left Hand/Right Face — LH [ ]   RF [ ]   Both: LH [ ]   RF [ ]   RF _0_ LH _0_

Auditory: *Became confused - Required slightly louder stimuli than most patients we tested.*

Right Ear/Left Ear — RE [ ]   LE [ ]   Both: RE [ ]   LE [ ]   RE _−_ LE _−_

Visual: *Unable to do - confused.*

Above eye level
Eye level   { RV [ ]   LV [ ]   Both: RV [ ]   LV [ ]   RV _−_ LV _−_
Below eye level

Finger Agnosia: *Toward the end of the RH trials she became confused (although she had been following instructions correctly up until then)*

Right: 1 [ ]   2 [ ]   3 [3]   4 [5]   5 [ ]   R _2/_
Left: 1 [ ]   2 [ ]   3 [ ]   4 [ ]   5 [ ]   L _0/_

& said "I didn't ask you - do you want (me to lift) the exact finger or the whole hand?

Finger-tip Number Writing Perception: *"Oh, I'm blank"*

Right: [4 6 3 5 / A 4]   [3 5 4 6 / DK]   [6 5 4 3]   [5 4 6 3 / T]   [6 3 5 4 / O - no #s!]   R **X**
Left: [O]   [↑]   L **X**

↑"no #'s - I can't visualize it" "#'s-I can't keep that in my mind"

Astereognosis: *Persisted in responding with letters, although she reminded herself that she was to respond c̄ #'s.*

not attempted

Right: [P N D]   Left: [D N P]   Both: Right: [N P D / D] Left: [D D]   R **X**   L **X**

"I thought I already did that one (smiles) - I get carried away - I don't always make sense."

Tactile Form Recognition: ↓

Errors: RH [○ □ △ ✚]   LH [△ ✚ ○ □]   RH [✚ ○ □ △]   LH [□ △ ✚ ○]   R _0_
Response Time: [4 4 4 3]   [8 2 2 3]   [3 2 10 3]   [2 4 2 2]   L _0_

Total Time: R _33_   L _25_

Visual Fields: Left   Right

Unable to assess - no obvious problem ⊕   ⊕   *Had great difficulty understanding directions, became confused. Forgot what she was doing.*

Figure 12. Case 10 (continued).

APHASIA SCREENING TEST   Case 10

Form for Adults and Older Children

Name: _____ Age: __48__ Date: __3/4/93__ Examiner: _____

1. Copy SQUARE *I DON'T GET THE POINT OF THIS – I KNOW I'M NOT SUPPOSED TO - WELL, THAT'S ALRIGHT...*	17. Repeat TRIANGLE
2. Name SQUARE	18. Repeat MASSACHUSETTS
3. Spell SQUARE	19. Repeat METHODIST EPISCOPAL
4. Copy CROSS *THIS IS NOT IN MY MIND AT ALL - THIS IS NOT GOOD FOR ME – NO-WELL, I JUST LIFTED THE PENCIL TO*	20. Write SQUARE *WRITE IT? - ooo (smiles) WRITE IT, YOU SAID - NOT PRINT IT (whispers spelling to herself)*
5. Name CROSS	21. Read SEVEN *READ IT? - TO YOU? - OUT LOUD?*
6. Spell CROSS	22. Repeat SEVEN
7. Copy TRIANGLE	23. Repeat/Explain HE SHOUTED THE WARNING. *FOR HELP!- I d.k. WHAT ELSE (shrugs– smiles)*
8. Name TRIANGLE	24. Write HE SHOUTED THE WARNING. *(Did not remember the sentence) (R) SHOUTED – S-H-O-C-K-E-D- THERE.*
9. Spell TRIANGLE *T-R-A - 0000 – I D.K. HOW TO SPELL IT - T-R-A - Triangle - T-R-A-A-N-G-L-E*	25. Compute 85 – 27 = *"85 minus 27 equals is what it says, but I d.k. What you want me to do with it (smiles) I'm not being snotty (E) and write it down? - I'm still a finger girl (counting on her fingers) (Cont.)*
10. Name BABY *THAT? - SWEET BABY*	26. Compute 17 X 3 = *"What? (E) 17x3. Now what do I do? - 85 minus 27 (E) Oh-17x3. Is that a minus one, too? (Q) y.k. 85-27. Is that a minus one, too? (E) Let's see 85-27-Is that it? (E) oh,times - I can't do*
11. Write CLOCK *JUST ANYWHERE? WRITE? (pause) - WRITE WHAT? WHAT THAT DO?*	27. Name KEY *that in my head. Now if I had paper–85-27–Is that what you said? (Cont.)*
12. Name FORK *TELL YOU?*	28. Demonstrate use of KEY *"You want me to do what?- Not draw it-Do what with it? I d.k. what you want me to do!" (reaches for booklet) That's a skeleton key-"I know that" (E) (Eventually, ok)*
13. Read 7 SIX 2 *READ IT? TO YOU? OUT LOUD?*	29. Draw KEY *"I d.k. what I'm doing here-I really don't!-Where was I here?-This one is not for me-I'm sorry, I know that looks like nothing-I never saw one so hard to do-"*
14. Read M G W	30. Read PLACE LEFT HAND TO RIGHT EAR.
15. Reading I	31. Place LEFT HAND TO RIGHT EAR *WHAT? DO WHAT?! (E repeats slowly) (Then OK, giving herself verbal instruction)*
16. Reading II *(Slow & halting, but correct)*	32. Place LEFT HAND TO LEFT ELBOW *(Pt. repeats as she looks @ LH. Looks @ L elbow) DO WHAT NOW? THAT WOULD BE PRETTY HARD TO DO WHAT YOU SAID.*

25. (cont.) – My Mama is too- I d.k. if that's what you want, but I thought that's...

26. (Cont.) Say it again (R) I just can't get it in my head–17 what? (E) I just can't.

Figure 12. Case 10 (continued).

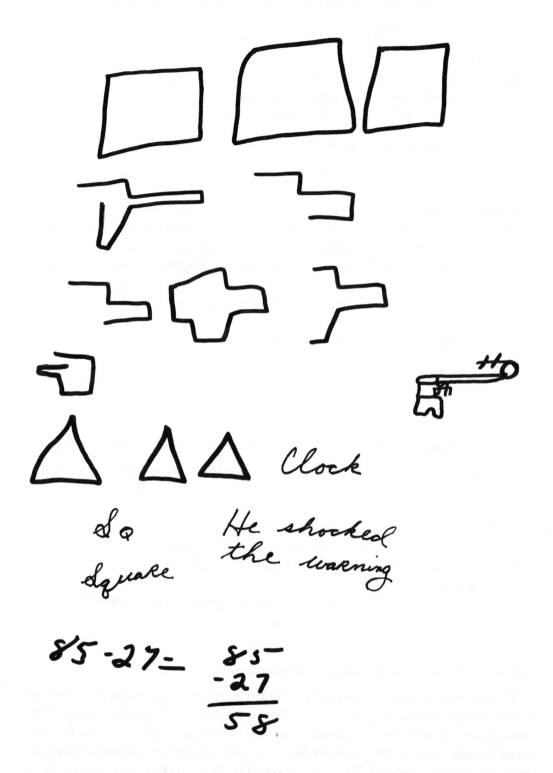

Figure 12. Case 10 (continued).

Pattern of Performance: This method of inference does not usually contribute much to the answer of this question.

Right/Left Differences: This method of inference does not contribute much to the answer of this question.

Pathognomonic Signs: This method of inference does not help answer this question.

Overall, a rapidly progressive condition is rather unlikely, but an adequate history would be needed to provide a more certain answer to this question.

4) Is the Lesion Diffuse or Lateralized?

Level of Performance: As usual, this method of inference does not contribute to the answer of this question.

Pattern of Performance: The greater impairment of visual memory than verbal memory suggests more right-hemisphere impairment, while the greater impairment on Aphasia (*T* score = 34) than Spatial Relations (*T* score = 46) and greater impairment on Speech Sounds Perception (*T* score = 33) than Seashore Rhythm (*T* score = 43) suggest more left-hemisphere impairment. This method of inference suggests impairment of both hemisphere, with the left hemisphere being more impaired. **(5-25, 5-12)**

Right/Left Differences: The right/left differences on motor tests noted above provide modest support for lateralization to the left hemisphere.

Pathognomonic Signs: The mild dysnomia suggests more left-hemisphere impairment. **(4-57)**

Overall, the left hemisphere appears more impaired, but the right hemisphere is not spared.

5) Is the Impairment in the Anterior or Posterior Part of the Cerebral Hemisphere?

Level of Performance: As usual, this method of inference does not contribute to the answer of this question.

Pattern of Performance: The greater impairment on TPT than on Tapping provides a suggestion of greater posterior impairment, but the lack of a significant number of sensory perceptual errors does not provide any further support for that. **(5-33)**

Right/Left Differences: As usual, this method of inference does not contribute to the answer of this question.

Pathognomonic Signs: The mild dysnomia does not provide much evidence for a focal lesion.

Overall, there is very little evidence of any focal lesion.

6) What is the Most Likely Neuropathological Process?

The significantly greater impairment of the left hemisphere with the right hemisphere not completely spared suggests the possibility of a left middle cerebral artery CVA, although one might expect the dysnomia and the verbal memory problems to be more severe in such a case. Furthermore, the history of slow, gradual deterioration of functioning is not consistent with a CVA. A tumor would be likely to show both more evidence of progression and greater severity. Imaging studies were not available, and the nature of the pathological process was uncertain.

7) What are the Implications for Everyday Functioning and Treatment?

The severity of this woman's cognitive deficits makes it unlikely that she can function adequately in an independent living situation. However, as might be expected from her MMPI, she refused placement in any type of assisted living situation, denying that she had any significant problems and contesting civil commitment. The court upheld her objections, and she returned to her apartment and refused any aftercare services.

Two years later, she was returned to the hospital after her apartment was badly damaged by a fire that probably resulted from careless smoking. She still denied that she had any problems and said she was certain that testing would confirm it.

A repeat neuropsychological evaluation was performed, and evidence of severe deterioration in all areas was found. She was unable to remember that she had had the TPT before and refused to continue after she could not place any blocks in nearly ten minutes. She could not understand the instructions for Part B of the Trail Making Test even after several repetitions and demonstrations. Her scores on all of the other tests had declined significantly. Both her verbal and visual memory were now very severely impaired on the RRWMS, and on the Associate Learning subtest she never learned more than four easy pairs and never learned a single hard pair in three trials. The severity of her impairment is perhaps best illustrated by the her performance on the Mental Control subtest, on which significant errors are unusual, even among impaired people: She made five errors in attempting to recite the alphabet, although she had been able to do so without error 2 years earlier, and was completely unable to count by threes.

A CT scan showed "ischemic changes in the frontal lobes, nothing acute." The most enlightening evidence of etiology was a cache of empty liquor bottles found in the disarray of her apartment by the social worker who visited it to get clothing for her after her readmission to the hospital. It seems most likely that this woman had an alcoholic dementia. An undisclosed history of past closed head injuries is not unusual in such cases, and that could account for some of the findings.

On this occasion, the court upheld a civil commitment, and the patient was placed in a nursing home.

This case illustrates some of the limitations of blind interpretation of test data, particularly when only a single evaluation is available. The clinical picture became much more clear after repeat testing, and the information provided by the social worker clarified the role of alcohol in this woman's deterioration.

Case 11

This is a 56-year-old, white, married, right-handed male chemical engineer who had demonstrated some mild decline in his work performance over the past 2 years, but who was still well respected and held an important position in his company. Three months prior to testing, this patient experienced acute medical distress involving visual disturbance and left-sided motor incoordination and severe weakness, as well as distortions in spatial problem-solving and memory. During testing, he appeared to understand all instructions, yet, at times, he had difficulty with attention and concentration. He was pleasant with the examiner, but showed clear frustration during more difficult test procedures.

1) Is There Cerebral Impairment?

Level of Performance: His Halstead Impairment Index of 0.9 (*T* score = 22), TPT total time of 24.6 minutes (.82 minutes per block) (*T* score = 38), Speech Sounds Perception Test score of 14 errors (*T* score = 30), Seashore Rhythm Test score of 13 correct (*T* score = 24), his poor scores on Finger Tapping (*T* scores = 16 and 7), Trails A and B (*T* scores = 15 and 14, respectively) and his many Sensory-Perceptual errors clearly indicate cerebral impairment. **(4-1)**

Pattern of Performance: There is considerable scatter in the *T* scores associated with this patient's Wechsler Intelligence Scale scores, as well as a significant variation between VIQ and PIQ (VIQ *T* score = 38; PIQ *T* score = 19). **(4-10)** These significant differences support the presence of cerebral impairment.

Right/Left Differences: Sensory and motor testing reveal bilateral deficits with severe impairment on the left side of the body on Finger Tapping, Strength of Grip, TPT, and the Sensory-Perceptual Examination. **(4-39)** The reader will notice that the administration of the TPT was unusual in the fact that the dominant hand was utilized for all three trials. This is consistent with the other data, which suggest that this patient could not use his left hand for any of the motor tasks, and the sensory-perceptual exam reflects lack of feeling on the left side of the body. These findings fully support the presence of cerebral impairment.

Pathognomonic Signs: The previously mentioned sensory and motor deficits are pathognomonic of cerebral impairment if we can rule out peripheral nerve and muscle damage, (which we can, by history, in this case). There were no indications of aphasic symptomatology on this examination; however, his drawing of the skeleton key was very poor in the constructional portion of the aphasia screening examination. Here again, we find strong support for cerebral impairment.

Overall, these four methods of inference clearly support the presence of cerebral impairment.

2) What is the Severity of Cerebral Dysfunction?

Level of Performance: This patient's Halstead Impairment Index itself indicates at least moderate to severe cerebral impairment. **(4-1)** This is further confirmed by the exceedingly poor Trails A and B, severely impaired PIQ (for a chemical engineer), and the significantly impaired Seashore Rhythm Test score.

Pattern of Performance: The VIQ *T* score differences (38 vs. 19) suggest moderate to severe impairment.

Right/Left Differences: The severe impairment of the left upper extremity on the TPT, Finger Tapping, Strength of Grip, and Sensory-Perceptual Examination all indicate moderate to severe cerebral dysfunction. **(4-39)**

Pathognomonic Signs: The constructional dyspraxia noted on the Aphasia Screening Examination suggest significant impairment.

In an overall sense, this patient must be considered to demonstrate at least moderate cerebral impairment.

HRB NORMS PROGRAM
Raw Score Transformations

Name:	Case11		Sex:	M
Age:	56	Years of Educ:		17
Date:	12/06/78	File Name:		CASE11
Handedness:	Right			

Measure	Abbreviation	Raw Scores	Scaled Scores	T Scores
HALSTEAD REITAN BATTERY SCORES				
Halstead Impairment Index	HII	0.9	4	22#
Average Impairment Rating	AIR			
Category Test	CAT ERROR	58	8	49
Trail Making Test-A (secs)	TRAIL A	233	1	15#
Trail Making Test-B (secs)	TRAIL B	427	1	14#
Tact Perf Test-Time (min/blk)	TPT TIME	.82	6	38#
Tact Perf Test-Memory (correct)	TPT MEM	7	9	45
Tact Perf Test-Location (correct)	TPT LOC	4	10	52
Seashore Rhythm (correct)	SSHOR RHYM	13	2	24#
Speech Perception (errors)	SPCH PERC	14	5	30#
Aphasia Screening (errors)	APHAS SCRN			
Spatial Relations (rating)	SPAT REL			
Sensory-Perceptual Total (errors)	SP TOTAL	60	1	26#
LATERALIZED SENSORIMOTOR/ PSYCHOMOTOR INDICES				
Finger Tapping-Dom (taps)	TAP DH	25	2	16#
Finger Tapping-Non-dom (taps)	TAP NDH	0	0	7#L
Hand Dynamometer-Dom (kgs)	GRIP DH	33	8	34#
Hand Dynamometer-Non-dom (kgs)	GRIP NDH	0	0	0#L
Grooved Pegboard-Dom (secs)	PEG DH			
Grooved Pegboard-Non-dom (secs)	PEG NDH			
Tact Perf Test-Dom (min/blk)	TPT DH	1.05	6	40
Tact Perf Test-Non-dom (min/blk)	TPT NDH	.93	6	38#
Tact Perf Test-Both Hands (min/blk)	TPT BOTH	.48	7	42
Sensory-Perceptual-Right (errors)	SP R	8	5	36#
Sensory-Perceptual-Left (errors)	SP L	52	2	21#L
Tactile Form Recog-Right (secs)	TFR R	0	19	77
Tactile Form Recog-Left (secs)	TFR L	99	1	15#L

\# = Impaired
L = Right-left difference, with possible lateralizing significance

Figure 13. Case 11.

HRB NORMS PROGRAM
Raw Score Transformations

Page 2

Name:	Case11	Sex:	M
Age:	56	Years of Educ:	17
Date:	12/06/78	File Name:	CASE11
Handedness: Right			

Measure	Abbreviation	Raw Scores	Scaled Scores	T Scores
WAIS SCORES				
Verbal IQ (VIQ)	VIQ	113	10	38#
Performance IQ (PIQ)	PIQ	85	3	19#
Full Scale IQ (FSIQ)	FSIQ	101	7	26#
Information	INFO	12	10	40
Digit Span	DIGIT SPAN	7	6	35#
Vocabulary	VOCAB	15	13	54
Arithmetic	ARITH	7	5	23#
Comprehension	COMP	15	12	52
Similarities	SIMIL	13	11	50
Picture Completion	PICT COMP	4	3	16#
Picture Arrangement	PICT ARR	6	6	38#
Block Design	BLOCK DESGN	8	7	35#
Object Assembly	OBJ ASSMB	4	3	28#
Digit Symbol	DIGIT SYMB	4	3	26#

= Impaired

Figure 13. Case 11 (continued).

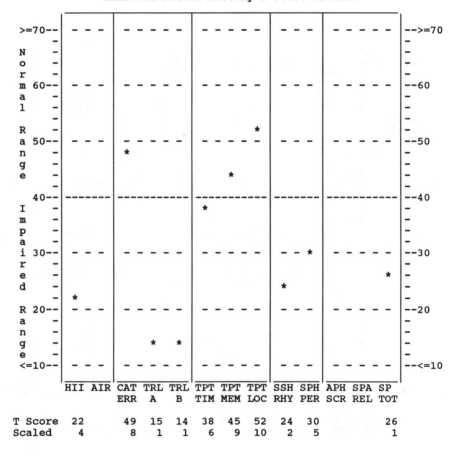

```
Name:        Case11                              Sex:       M
Age:         56                       Years of Educ:        17
Date:        12/06/78                     File Name:        CASE11
Handedness: Right
```

Halstead-Reitan Battery T Score Profile

	HII	AIR	CAT ERR	TRL A	TRL B	TPT TIM	TPT MEM	TPT LOC	SSH RHY	SPH PER	APH SCR	SPA REL	SP TOT
T Score	22		49	15	14	38	45	52	24	30			26
Scaled	4		8	1	1	6	9	10	2	5			1

Figure 13. Case 11 (continued).

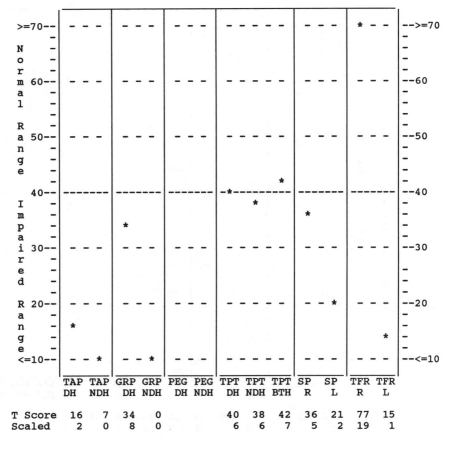

Page 4

Name: Case11
Age: 56
Date: 12/06/78
Handedness: Right

Sex: M
Yrs of Educ: 17
File Name: CASE11

Lateralized Sensorimotor/Psychomotor T Score Profile

	TAP DH	TAP NDH	GRP DH	GRP NDH	PEG DH	PEG NDH	TPT DH	TPT NDH	TPT BTH	SP R	SP L	TFR R	TFR L
T Score	16	7	34	0			40	38	42	36	21	77	15
Scaled	2	0	8	0			6	6	7	5	2	19	1

Figure 13. Case 11 (continued).

Name: Case11   Sex: M
Age: 56   Yrs of Educ: 17
Date: 12/06/78   File Name: CASE11
Handedness: Right

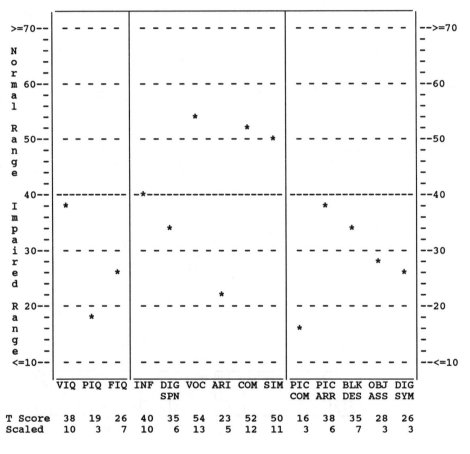

	VIQ	PIQ	FIQ	INF	DIG SPN	VOC	ARI	COM	SIM	PIC COM	PIC ARR	BLK DES	OBJ ASS	DIG SYM
T Score	38	19	26	40	35	54	23	52	50	16	38	35	28	26
Scaled	10	3	7	10	6	13	5	12	11	3	6	7	3	3

Figure 13. Case 11 (continued).

SENSORY—PERCEPTUAL EXAMINATION

Case 11

Indicate Instance in which stimulus is not perceived or is incorrectly perceived.

Error Totals

Tactile:

Right Hand/Left Hand — RH ☐☐☐ LH ☐☐☐ Both: RH ☐☐☐ LH ☐☐☐   RH _0_ LH _0_

Right Hand/Left Face — RH ☐☐☐ LF ☐☐☐ Both: RH ☐☐☐ LF ☐X☐X☐   RH _0_ LF _2_

Left Hand/Right Face — LH ☐☐☐ RF ☐☐☐ Both: LH ☐☐☐ RF ☐☐☐   RF _0_ LH _0_

Auditory:

Right Ear/Left Ear — RE ☐☐☐ LE ☐☐☐ Both: RE ☐☐☐ LE X☐X☐X☐X   RE _0_ LE _4_

Visual:

Above eye level / Eye level / Below eye level { RV ☐ LV ☐ Both: RV ☐ LV [XX/XX/XX]   RV _0_ LV _6_

Finger Agnosia:

Right: 1 ☐ 2 X☐X 3 X☐ 4 XX☐ 5 ☐X   R _6/20_
Left: 1 ☐ 2 ☐ 3 ☐ 4 ☐ 5 ☐   L _could not test_

Finger-tip Number Writing Perception:

Right: [4 6 3 5] [3 5 4 6 / 6] [6 5 4 3] [5 4 6 3 / 6] [6 3 5 4]   R _2/20_
Left: L _could not test_

Astereognosis:

Right: [P N D]   Left: [D N P]   Both: Right: [N P D] / Left: R _____
L _____

Tactile Form Recognition:

Errors: RH [○ □ △ ✛] LH [△ ✛ ○ □] RH [✛ ○ □ △] LH [□ △ ✛ ○]   R _0_
Response Time: [3 3 4 3] [ ] [3 2 3 3] [ ]   L _could not test_

Total Time: R _24"_ L _–_

Visual Fields: Left   Right

Figure 13. Case 11 (continued).

APHASIA SCREENING TEST   Case 11

Form for Adults and Older Children

Name: _____ Age: __*56*__ Date: __*12/6/78*__ Examiner: _____

1. Copy SQUARE	17. Repeat TRIANGLE
2. Name SQUARE	18. Repeat MASSACHUSETTS
3. Spell SQUARE	19. Repeat METHODIST EPISCOPAL
4. Copy CROSS	20. Write SQUARE
5. Name CROSS	21. Read SEVEN
6. Spell CROSS	22. Repeat SEVEN
7. Copy TRIANGLE	23. Repeat/Explain HE SHOUTED THE WARNING. *LOOK OUT FOR SOMETHING—DANGER?*
8. Name TRIANGLE	24. Write HE SHOUTED THE WARNING.
9. Spell TRIANGLE	25. Compute 85 – 27 =
10. Name BABY	26. Compute 17 X 3 =
11. Write CLOCK	27. Name KEY
12. Name FORK	28. Demonstrate use of KEY
13. Read 7 SIX 2	29. Draw KEY
14. Read M G W	30. Read PLACE LEFT HAND TO RIGHT EAR.
15. Reading I	31. Place LEFT HAND TO RIGHT EAR
16. Reading II	32. Place LEFT HAND TO LEFT ELBOW

Figure 13. Case 11 (continued).

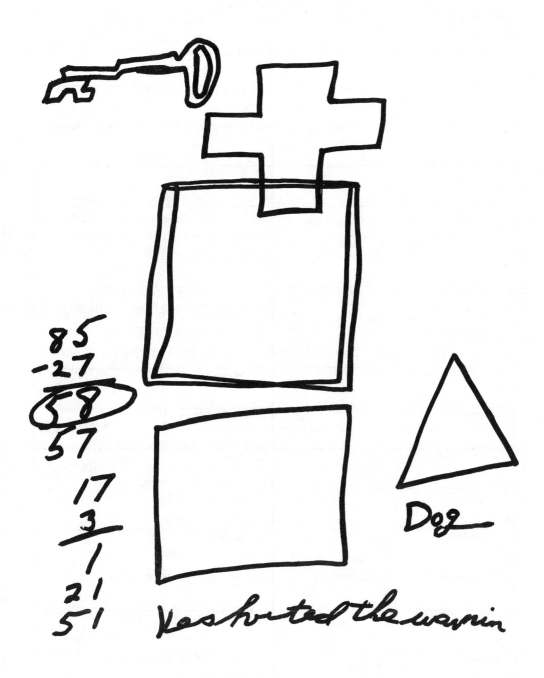

Figure 13. Case 11 (continued).

3) Is the Lesion Progressive or Static?

Level of Performance: The severely impaired Speech Sounds Perception and Seashore Rhythm test scores suggest an acute neurologic process and the possibility of a progressive lesion.

Pattern of Performance: This method of inference does not contribute to the answer of this question.

Right/Left Differences: The lack of left upper extremity motor and sensory-perceptual function, in relationship to better intact right upper extremity abilities suggest the possibility of an acute, vascular condition, which may have a slowly progressive nature, but will often show improvement from the acute disorder. **(7-20)**

Pathognomonic Signs: This method of inference does not contribute to the answer of this question.

Overall, these test data suggest the possibility of some progressive neurologic condition; however, a more probable hypothesis is that many of these data are indicative of an acute process, from which he may demonstrate some improvement over this short term. As usual, a complete history would be most helpful in answering this question.

4) Is the Lesion Diffuse or Lateralized?

Level of Performance: This method of inference does not contribute to the answer of this question.

Pattern of Performance: The differences between VIQ and PIQ on the Wechsler Intelligence Scale reveals lateralize deficits associated with the right-cerebral hemisphere. **(5-8)**

Right/Left Differences: This method of inference is very important in this case, since this patient has no use of his left upper extremity on the TPT, Finger Tapping, and Strength of Grip Test. He also demonstrates very severe left-sided sensory suppressions and sensory-perceptual impairment. These tests clearly indicate right-cerebral hemisphere impairment. **(5-11)** It should also be noted that scores associated with left-cerebral hemisphere functions on these same tests are at least mildly impaired.

Pathognomonic Signs: Constructional dyspraxia (poor drawing of the skeleton key) suggests impairment of right-cerebral hemisphere functions. **(5-22)**

Although there are indications of mild left-cerebral hemisphere dysfunction, severe deficits are noted in functions subserved by the right-cerebral hemisphere.

5) Is the Impairment in the Anterior or Posterior Part of the Cerebral Hemisphere?

Level of Performance: This method of inference does not contribute to the answer of this question.

Pattern of Performance: Since there are both sensory and motor deficits, there is no clear indication of more impairment in the anterior or posterior areas of the right-cerebral hemisphere.

Right/Left Differences: This method of inference does not contribute to the answer of this question.

Pathognomonic Signs: Since there are no indications of receptive or expressive difficulties, this does not contribute to the answer of this question.

This right-hemisphere lesion appears to affect both anterior and posterior cerebral functions.

6) What is the Most Likely Neuropathological Process?

Given this man's age of 56, the acuteness of this stage of his neuropathological condition, his severely impaired PIQ (for a chemical engineer), and his lack of use of and sensation in the left upper extremity, a cerebrovascular accident is the most likely condition. This total left upper extremity motor dysfunction and sensory deficits are also pathognomonic of such an accident. **(7-20)** Neuroimaging studies revealed a right middle cerebral artery occlusion.

7) What are the Implications for Everyday Functioning and Treatment?

The natural recovery curve for cerebrovascular accidents can be as short as 3 months or as long as 1 year depending on the severity of the hemorrhaging or occlusion and the availability of collateral blood supply. The fact that some cognitive functions remain intact or are mildly impaired in this particular patient suggests that some recovery will take place in this case. Given his total paralysis on the left side, return to completely normal function is not expected. Physical therapy and cognitive retraining, particularly in his visuospatial problem-solving skills, will be important, as will intervention with an occupational therapist. Return to his engineering duties may be impossible, and some alternative work in the engineering field where he can utilize his more intact verbal skills should be explored, as well as the possibility of an early retirement program.

Case 12

This 49-year-old white male with over 16 years of education recently retired from his position as an electrical engineer, due to increasingly impaired work performance over the past 2 years. This voluntary retirement was prompted by his family, which was concerned regarding his ability to handle activities of daily living successfully.

During the test session, he had considerable difficulty understanding instructions for most of the tests, and his memory and attentional functions were clearly impaired. He was persistent in attempting to carry out all assessment tasks, yet he demonstrated great fatigue during the administration of the TPT. At times, he appeared to confabulate when confronted with history and mental status questions for which he clearly had no answer.

1) Is there Cerebral Impairment?

Level of Performance: The Impairment Index of 1.0 (T score = 4), Category Test Score of 99 (T score = 23), Trail Making B of 135 (T score = 29), and TPT Localization of 1 (T score = 32) all indicate considerable cerebral impairment. **(4-1)** Other Halstead-Reitan test scores such as Seashore Rhythm, Speech Sounds Perception, Dominant Hand Tapping, and Grip Strength, as well as Sensory-Perceptual errors all indicate significant cerebral deficits.

HRB NORMS PROGRAM
Raw Score Transformations

Name:	Case12	Sex:	M
Age:	49	Years of Educ:	16
Date:	11/19/75	File Name:	CASE12
Handedness:	Right		

Measure	Abbreviation	Raw Scores	Scaled Scores	T Scores
HALSTEAD REITAN BATTERY SCORES				
Halstead Impairment Index	HII	1.0	1	4#
Average Impairment Rating	AIR			
Category Test	CAT ERROR	99	4	23#
Trail Making Test-A (secs)	TRAIL A	56	5	30#
Trail Making Test-B (secs)	TRAIL B	135	5	29#
Tact Perf Test-Time (min/blk)	TPT TIME	.98	5	32#
Tact Perf Test-Memory (correct)	TPT MEM	4	5	29#
Tact Perf Test-Location (correct)	TPT LOC	1	6	32#
Seashore Rhythm (correct)	SSHOR RHYM	15	3	25#
Speech Perception (errors)	SPCH PERC	13	5	29#
Aphasia Screening (errors)	APHAS SCRN			
Spatial Relations (rating)	SPAT REL			
Sensory-Perceptual Total (errors)	SP TOTAL	45	2	23#
LATERALIZED SENSORIMOTOR/ PSYCHOMOTOR INDICES				
Finger Tapping-Dom (taps)	TAP DH	13	0	7#L
Finger Tapping-Non-dom (taps)	TAP NDH	38	7	34#
Hand Dynamometer-Dom (kgs)	GRIP DH	22	5	13#L
Hand Dynamometer-Non-dom (kgs)	GRIP NDH	55	14	64
Grooved Pegboard-Dom (secs)	PEG DH			
Grooved Pegboard-Non-dom (secs)	PEG NDH			
Tact Perf Test-Dom (min/blk)	TPT DH	1.2	6	37#
Tact Perf Test-Non-dom (min/blk)	TPT NDH	1.08	6	35#
Tact Perf Test-Both Hands (min/blk)	TPT BOTH	.78	5	31#
Sensory-Perceptual-Right (errors)	SP R	28	1	21#
Sensory-Perceptual-Left (errors)	SP L	17	3	21#
Tactile Form Recog-Right (secs)	TFR R	0	19	78
Tactile Form Recog-Left (secs)	TFR L	0	19	78

# = Impaired
L = Right-left difference, with possible lateralizing significance

Figure 14. Case 12.

HRB NORMS PROGRAM
Raw Score Transformations

Page 2

Name:	Case12		Sex:	M
Age:	49		Years of Educ:	16
Date:	11/19/75		File Name:	CASE12
Handedness:	Right			

Measure	Abbreviation	Raw Scores	Scaled Scores	T Scores
WAIS SCORES				
Verbal IQ (VIQ)	VIQ	96	7	28#
Performance IQ (PIQ)	PIQ	97	6	24#
Full Scale IQ (FSIQ)	FSIQ	96	6	21#
Information	INFO	13	11	47
Digit Span	DIGIT SPAN	4	3	25#
Vocabulary	VOCAB	12	10	43
Arithmetic	ARITH	6	4	21#
Comprehension	COMP	9	6	32#
Similarities	SIMIL	10	8	38#
Picture Completion	PICT COMP	5	4	21#
Picture Arrangement	PICT ARR	9	9	46
Block Design	BLOCK DESGN	11	10	43
Object Assembly	OBJ ASSMB	9	8	38#
Digit Symbol	DIGIT SYMB	5	4	26#

= Impaired

Figure 14. Case 12 (continued).

```
Name:        Case12                                Sex:      M
Age:         49                         Years of Educ:       16
Date:        11/19/75                      File Name:      CASE12
Handedness: Right
```

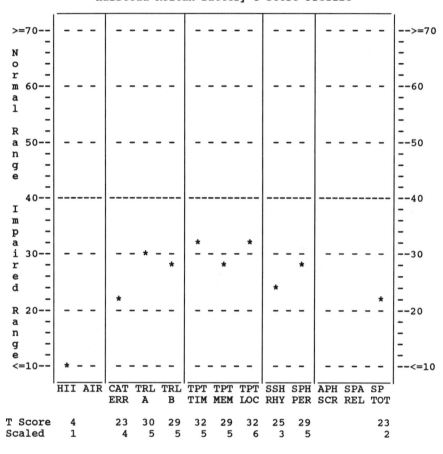

Figure 14. Case 12 (continued).

Page 4

Name:	Case12		Sex:	M
Age:	49		Yrs of Educ:	16
Date:	11/19/75		File Name:	CASE12
Handedness:	Right			

Lateralized Sensorimotor/Psychomotor T Score Profile

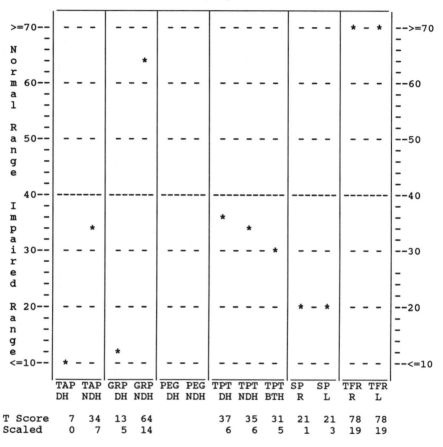

		TAP DH	TAP NDH	GRP DH	GRP NDH	PEG DH	PEG NDH	TPT DH	TPT NDH	TPT BTH	SP R	SP L	TFR R	TFR L
T Score		7	34	13	64			37	35	31	21	21	78	78
Scaled		0	7	5	14			6	6	5	1	3	19	19

Figure 14. Case 12 (continued).

Page 5

Name: Case12
Age: 49
Date: 11/19/75
Handedness: Right

Sex: M
Yrs of Educ: 16
File Name: CASE12

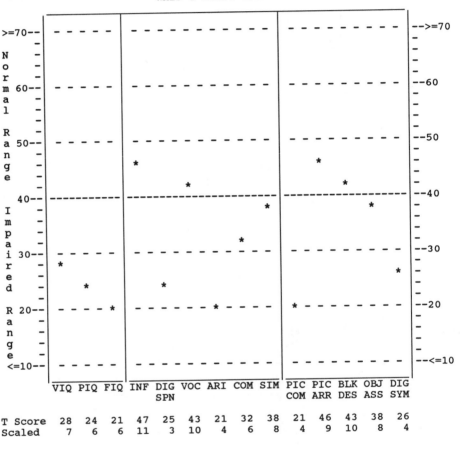

WAIS T Score Profile

	VIQ	PIQ	FIQ	INF	DIG SPN	VOC	ARI	COM	SIM	PIC COM	PIC ARR	BLK DES	OBJ ASS	DIG SYM
T Score	28	24	21	47	25	43	21	32	38	21	46	43	38	26
Scaled	7	6	6	11	3	10	4	6	8	4	9	10	8	4

Figure 14. Case 12 (continued).

SENSORY—PERCEPTUAL EXAMINATION

Case 12

Indicate Instance in which stimulus is not perceived or is incorrectly perceived.

Error Totals

Tactile:

Right Hand/Left Hand — RH ☐☐☐ LH ☐☐☐ Both: RH ☐☐☐ LH ☐☐☐ RH _0_ LH _0_

Right Hand/Left Face — RH ☐☐☐ LF ☐☐☐ Both: RH XXXX LF ☐☐☐ RH _4_ LF _0_

Left Hand/Right Face — LH ☐☐☐ RF ☐☐☐ Both: LH XXXX RF ☐☐☐ RF _0_ LH _4_

Auditory:

Right Ear/Left Ear — RE ☐☐☐ LE ☐☐☐ Both: RE XXXX LE ☐☐☐ RE _4_ LE _0_

Visual:

Above eye level / Eye level / Below eye level { RV ☐ LV ☐ Both: RV ☐ LV ☐ RV _0_ LV _0_

Finger Agnosia:

Right: 1 ☐ 2 ☐ 3 X 4 XXX 5 ☐ R _5/20_
Left: 1 ☐ 2 X 3 X 4 ☐ 5 ☐ L _1/20_

Finger-tip Number Writing Perception:

Right: | 4 6 3 5 | 3 5 4 6 | 6 5 4 3 | 5 4 6 3 | 6 3 5 4 | R _15/20_
DKDKDKDK / 6DKDK / DK6 6 / DK 3 6 / DK8
Left: DK 4 DK / 6 / 3 4 DK / 3 3 6 / 6 4 L _12/20_

Astereognosis:

Right: | P | N | D | Left: | D | N | P | Both: Right/Left: | N | P | D | R ____ L ____

Tactile Form Recognition:

Errors: RH | ○ □ △ ✚ | LH | △ ✚ ○ □ | RH | ✚ ○ □ △ | LH | □ △ ✚ ○ | R _0_ L _0_
Response Time: | 10 12 4 10 | 5 4 3 5 | 14 5 5 6 | 5 5 5 2 |

Total Time: R _66"_ L _34"_

Visual Fields: Left   Right

WNL

Figure 14. Case 12 (continued).

APHASIA SCREENING TEST   Case 12

Form for Adults and Older Children

Name: _____ Age: __49__ Date: _11/19/75_____ Examiner: _____

1. Copy SQUARE	17. Repeat TRIANGLE
2. Name SQUARE	18. Repeat MASSACHUSETTS
3. Spell SQUARE	19. Repeat METHODIST EPISCOPAL
4. Copy CROSS	20. Write SQUARE
5. Name CROSS	21. Read SEVEN **SERVE**
6. Spell CROSS	22. Repeat SEVEN
7. Copy TRIANGLE	23. Repeat/Explain HE SHOUTED THE WARNING. **Pt. refused to say anything.**
8. Name TRIANGLE	24. Write HE SHOUTED THE WARNING.
9. Spell TRIANGLE **T-R-A-I-N-G-L-E**	25. Compute 85 – 27 = **68**
10. Name BABY	26. Compute 17 X 3 = **31**
11. Write CLOCK	27. Name KEY
12. Name FORK	28. Demonstrate use of KEY
13. Read 7 SIX 2	29. Draw KEY
14. Read M G W	30. Read PLACE LEFT HAND TO RIGHT EAR.
15. Reading I	31. Place LEFT HAND TO RIGHT EAR
16. Reading II	32. Place LEFT HAND TO LEFT ELBOW

Figure 14. Case 12 (continued).

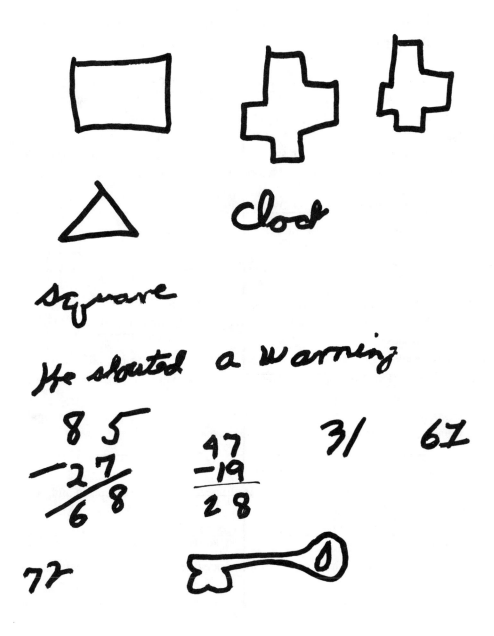

Figure 14. Case 12 (continued).

Pattern of Performance: Although the VIQ of 96 and PIQ of 97 are not significantly different, these overall IQ values are considerably lower then one would expect from an individual of his age, education, and vocation. These test scores (including subtest scores), support the presence of cerebral impairment.

Right/Left Differences: Right upper extremity deficits are noted on the TPT, Finger Tapping, and Strength of Grip tests, and the Sensory-Perceptual evaluation also indicates more right-sided impairment than that on the left. Such right/left differences support the presence of cerebral impairment. **(4-49)**

Pathognomonic Signs: A total of eight tactile and four auditory suppressions were noted on the Sensory-Perceptual Examination. In addition, on the Aphasia Screening Examination he spelled triangle as "traingle" and read the word seven as "serve." He had difficulty with mental calculations. He wrote "he shouted the warning" as "he shouted a warning," and some constructional dyspraxia (disproportional crosses and a skeleton key with no detail) was noted. All of these factors suggest cerebral impairment. **(4-56, 4-72)**

2) What is the Severity of Cerebral Dysfunction?

Level of Performance: As noted earlier, his poor performance on all subtests from the Halstead-Reitan Neuropsychological Test Battery and his average Wechsler Intelligence Scales scores in the presence of a high level of education and demanding vocation all suggest moderate to severe cerebral impairment.

Pattern of Performance: As above, his paucity of intact cognitive functions, in any areas other than information, vocabulary and picture arrangement, and block design suggest severe impairment.

Right/Left Differences: He has very severe right upper extremity deficits, with some indication of left-sided problems on motor and sensory examination, which supports the possibility of moderate to severe impairment.

Pathognomonic Signs: His spelling dyspraxia, dyscalculia, and constructional dyspraxia all indicate a severe level of cerebral impairment.

3) Is the Lesion Progressive or Static?

Level of Performance: The severely impaired Speech Sounds Perception and Seashore Rhythm Test scores, in combination with his probable decreased IQ scores suggest the possibility of a progressive condition. This, of course, is best answered by reviewing the history and through serial testing.

Pattern of Performance: This method of inference does not contribute to the answer of this questions.

Right/Left Differences: This method of inference does not contribute to the answer of this question.

Pathognomonic Signs: The history of decline over the past 2 years suggests that this condition is progressive.

4) Is the Lesion Diffuse or Lateralized?

Level of Performance: This method of inference does not contribute to the answer of this question.

Pattern of Performance: Since there is no significant difference between VIQ and PIQ, this condition may be diffuse or bilateral. **(5-2)**

Right/Left Differences: Although there are deficits on both sides of the body in motor and sensory assessment, there is clearly more impairment on the right side of the body, which would implicate left-cerebral hemisphere dysfunction.

Pathognomonic Signs: On the Aphasia Screening Examination, there are mixed lateralizing signs (verbal and constructional).

In an overall sense, there appears to be diffuse impairment, with more specifically lateralized deficits on the right side of the body (left-cerebral hemisphere).

5) Is the Impairment in the Anterior or Posterior Part of the Cerebral Hemisphere?

Level of Performance: This method of inference does not contribute to the answer of this question.

Pattern of Performance: Since there are both sensory and motor deficits, suppositions regarding anterior versus posterior impairment cannot be made.

Right/Left Differences: This method of inference does not contribute to the answer of this question.

Pathognomonic Signs: On the Aphasia Screening Examination and interview, this patient demonstrates both receptive and expressive difficulties, which, when coupled with his constructional dyspraxia, may indicate a more diffuse process.

6) What is the Most Likely Neuropathological Process?

This patient is suffering from a moderate to severe diffuse cerebral condition, with more lateralization to the left-cerebral hemisphere than the right. **(7-25)** It appears to be progressive, since he has demonstrated some decline for the past 2 years. Even though at 49 this man is not considered elderly, a degenerative condition such as Alzheimer's disease appears to be the most likely neuropathological condition. CT scan and later pathologist's report confirmed Alzheimer's disease.

7) What are the Implications for Everyday Functioning and Treatment?

Virtually every area of cognitive function, with the exception of overlearned verbal abilities, was impaired in this individual. His retirement from his electrical engineering work was appropriate, and counseling was initiated with the patient and his family with regard to maintaining a static, unchanging environment and assisting with future planning for his medical and the family's emotional needs.

Case 13

This 32-year-old black male with 12 years of education worked as an industrial plant manager. During one of his inspection rounds, he slipped and fell, hitting his head on a set of concrete steps. Although he only briefly lost consciousness, he was taken to the emergency room where standard neuroimaging was initiated and he was kept for observation. Three months later, neuropsychological assessment was initiated due to slow recovery and some difficulties on the job. He was friendly and cooperative throughout testing and appeared to understand all instructions. His test results were considered to be an accurate reflection of his current cognitive-behavioral functioning.

1) Is There Cerebral Impairment?

Level of Performance: The Halstead Impairment Index of 0.1 (*T* score = 56), Category Test Score of 40 (*T* score = 43), Trail Making B of 89 (*T* score = 41), and TPT Localization of 9 (*T* score = 75) all suggest no significant cerebral impairment. Scores that could be considered in an abnormal range are those for the dominant hand on the TPT, total time for the TPT, Trail Making A, Dominant Hand Grip Strength, and Fingertip Number Writing errors on the Sensory-Perceptual Examination.

Pattern of Performance: The difference between VIQ and PIQ scores of 18 points (18 *T* score points) is suggestive of some cerebral impairment. **(4-10)**

Right/Left Differences: Dominant hand performance on the TPT and Strength of Grip Test scores both indicate cerebral impairment. There are also bilateral fingertip number writing errors, which support this hypothesis.

Pathognomonic Signs: On the Aphasia Screening Examination, this patient had difficulty spelling the word triangle and called a fork a spoon (later changing his answer to fork). **(4-57)** No constructional dyspraxia was noted.

Overall, there is some support for cerebral dysfunction.

2) What is the Severity of Cerebral Dysfunction?

Level of Performance: With a low Halstead Impairment Index, good Category Test score, intact TPT Localization and Memory, Speech Sounds Perception, and Seashore Rhythm Test scores within normal limits, and a good Trail Making B score, overall cerebral impairment should be considered mild.

Pattern of Performance: The difference between VIQ and PIQ, as well as the low digit symbol score and overall variability between subtest scores on the Wechsler Intelligence Scale, indicate mild cerebral dysfunction.

Right/Left Differences: TPT dominant hand score and deficits in dominant hand Strength of Grip suggest at least mild impairment. **(4-35)**

Pathognomonic Signs: The previously mentioned pathognomonic signs on the Aphasia Screening Examination suggest mild to moderate cerebral dysfunction. **(4-57)**

3) Is the Lesion Progressive or Static?

Level of Performance: The overall intact scores on Speech Sounds Perception and Seashore Rhythm, as well as a good Category score and low Halstead Impairment Index suggest that this is not a progressive lesion. **(6-10, 6-11)**

Pattern of Performance: This method of inference does not contribute to the answer of this question.

Right/Left Differences: This method of inference does not contribute to the answer of this question.

HRB NORMS PROGRAM
Raw Score Transformations

Name:	Case13		Sex:	M
Age:	32		Years of Educ:	12
Date:	02/12/76		File Name:	CASE13
Handedness:	Right			

Measure	Abbreviation	Raw Scores	Scaled Scores	T Scores
HALSTEAD REITAN **BATTERY SCORES**				
Halstead Impairment Index	HII	.1	12	56
Average Impairment Rating	AIR			
Category Test	CAT ERROR	40	9	43
Trail Making Test-A (secs)	TRAIL A	36	7	35#
Trail Making Test-B (secs)	TRAIL B	89	8	41
Tact Perf Test-Time (min/blk)	TPT TIME	1.49	4	23#
Tact Perf Test-Memory (correct)	TPT MEM	9	14	60
Tact Perf Test-Location (correct)	TPT LOC	9	18	75
Seashore Rhythm (correct)	SSHOR RHYM	30	19	75
Speech Perception (errors)	SPCH PERC	2	13	58
Aphasia Screening (errors)	APHAS SCRN			
Spatial Relations (rating)	SPAT REL			
Sensory-Perceptual Total (errors)	SP TOTAL	10	6	35#
LATERALIZED SENSORIMOTOR/ **PSYCHOMOTOR INDICES**				
Finger Tapping-Dom (taps)	TAP DH	51	10	44
Finger Tapping-Non-dom (taps)	TAP NDH	46	10	44
Hand Dynamometer-Dom (kgs)	GRIP DH	35	9	34#L
Hand Dynamometer-Non-dom (kgs)	GRIP NDH	52	13	55
Grooved Pegboard-Dom (secs)	PEG DH			
Grooved Pegboard-Non-dom (secs)	PEG NDH			
Tact Perf Test-Dom (min/blk)	TPT DH	1.02	6	32#L
Tact Perf Test-Non-dom (min/blk)	TPT NDH	.28	12	55
Tact Perf Test-Both Hands (min/blk)	TPT BOTH	.19	11	52
Sensory-Perceptual-Right (errors)	SP R	7	6	36#
Sensory-Perceptual-Left (errors)	SP L	3	7	39#
Tactile Form Recog-Right (secs)	TFR R	0	19	81
Tactile Form Recog-Left (secs)	TFR L	0	19	80

# = Impaired
L = Right-left difference, with possible lateralizing significance

Figure 15. Case 13.

```
                    HRB NORMS PROGRAM
                 Raw Score Transformations

                          Page 2

Name:        Case13                    Sex:       M
Age:         32              Years of Educ:       12
Date:        02/12/76           File Name:        CASE13
Handedness:  Right
```

| | | Raw | Scaled | T |
Measure	Abbreviation	Scores	Scores	Scores
WAIS SCORES				
Verbal IQ (VIQ)	VIQ	126	13	68
Performance IQ (PIQ)	PIQ	108	9	50
Full Scale IQ (FSIQ)	FSIQ	119	11	60
Information	INFO	11	9	47
Digit Span	DIGIT SPAN	19	18	76
Vocabulary	VOCAB	13	11	57
Arithmetic	ARITH	15	13	63
Comprehension	COMP	17	14	69
Similarities	SIMIL	12	10	52
Picture Completion	PICT COMP	11	10	51
Picture Arrangement	PICT ARR	10	10	49
Block Design	BLOCK DESGN	14	13	60
Object Assembly	OBJ ASSMB	13	12	59
Digit Symbol	DIGIT SYMB	8	7	38#

```
# = Impaired
```

Figure 15. Case 13 (continued).

Name: Case13   Sex: M
Age: 32   Years of Educ: 12
Date: 02/12/76   File Name: CASE13
Handedness: Right

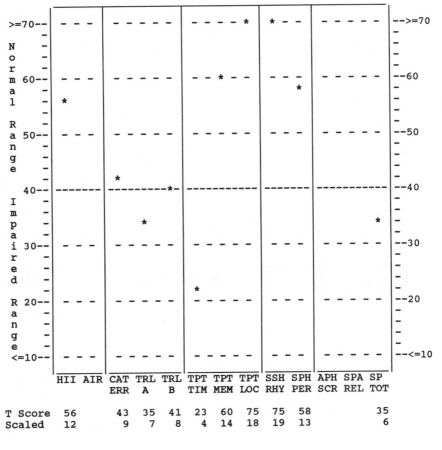

Halstead-Reitan Battery T Score Profile

	HII	AIR	CAT ERR	TRL A	TRL B	TPT TIM	TPT MEM	TPT LOC	SSH RHY	SPH PER	APH SCR	SPA REL	SP TOT
T Score	56		43	35	41	23	60	75	75	58			35
Scaled	12		9	7	8	4	14	18	19	13			6

Figure 15. Case 13 (continued).

Page 4

Name: Case13   Sex: M
Age: 32   Yrs of Educ: 12
Date: 02/12/76   File Name: CASE13
Handedness: Right

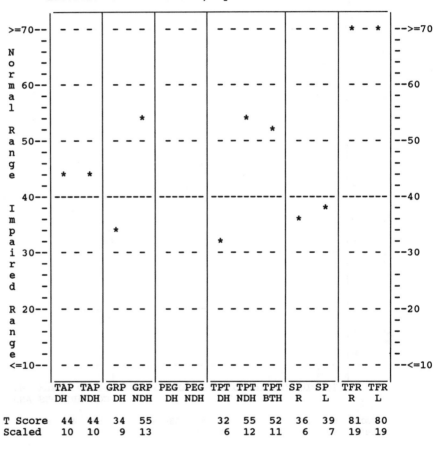

Lateralized Sensorimotor/Psychomotor T Score Profile

	TAP DH	TAP NDH	GRP DH	GRP NDH	PEG DH	PEG NDH	TPT DH	TPT NDH	TPT BTH	SP R	SP L	TFR R	TFR L
T Score	44	44	34	55			32	55	52	36	39	81	80
Scaled	10	10	9	13			6	12	11	6	7	19	19

Figure 15. Case 13 (continued).

Page 5

Name: Case13   Sex: M
Age: 32   Yrs of Educ: 12
Date: 02/12/76   File Name: CASE13
Handedness: Right

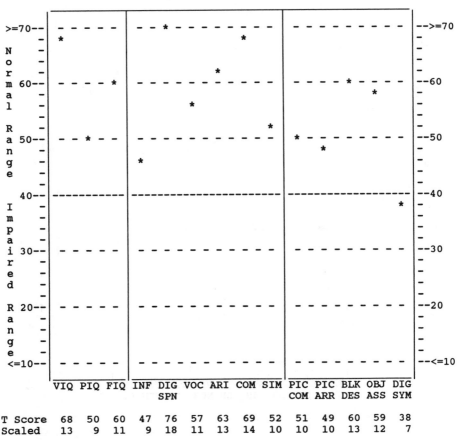

WAIS T Score Profile

	VIQ	PIQ	FIQ	INF	DIG SPN	VOC	ARI	COM	SIM	PIC COM	PIC ARR	BLK DES	OBJ ASS	DIG SYM
T Score	68	50	60	47	76	57	63	69	52	51	49	60	59	38
Scaled	13	9	11	9	18	11	13	14	10	10	10	13	12	7

Figure 15. Case 13 (continued).

SENSORY—PERCEPTUAL EXAMINATION Case 13

Indicate Instance in which stimulus is not perceived or is incorrectly perceived.

Figure 15. Case 13 (continued).

APHASIA SCREENING TEST

Case 13

Form for Adults and Older Children

Name: _____ Age: **32** Date: **2/12/76** Examiner: _____

1. Copy SQUARE	17. Repeat TRIANGLE
2. Name SQUARE	18. Repeat MASSACHUSETTS
3. Spell SQUARE	19. Repeat METHODIST EPISCOPAL
4. Copy CROSS	20. Write SQUARE
5. Name CROSS	21. Read SEVEN
6. Spell CROSS *S-C-R-O-S-S*	22. Repeat SEVEN
7. Copy TRIANGLE	23. Repeat/Explain HE SHOUTED THE WARNING. *SOMEONE SHOUTED A WARNING TO SOMEONE ELSE.*
8. Name TRIANGLE	24. Write HE SHOUTED THE WARNING.
9. Spell TRIANGLE *T-R-I-N . . . T-R-I-A-N-G-K-E*	25. Compute 85 − 27 =
10. Name BABY	26. Compute 17 X 3 =
11. Write CLOCK	27. Name KEY
12. Name FORK *SPOON . . . FORK*	28. Demonstrate use of KEY
13. Read 7 SIX 2	29. Draw KEY
14. Read M G W	30. Read PLACE LEFT HAND TO RIGHT EAR.
15. Reading I	31. Place LEFT HAND TO RIGHT EAR
16. Reading II	32. Place LEFT HAND TO LEFT ELBOW

Figure 15. Case 13 (continued).

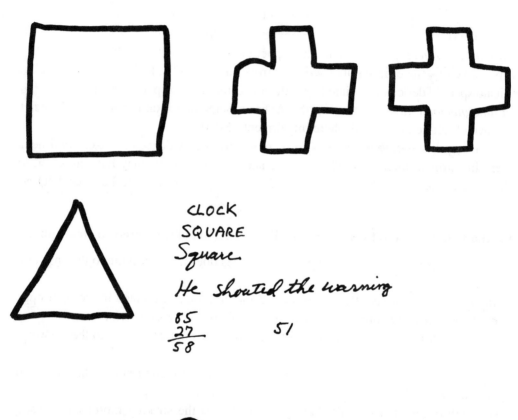

CLOCK
SQUARE
Square
He shouted the warning

85
27
58

51

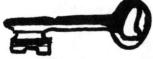

Figure 15. Case 13 (continued).

Pathognomonic Signs: This method of inference does not contribute to the answer of this question.

The lack of general impairment demonstrated by this patient, and the many areas of strength argue against a progressive neuropathological condition.

4) Is the Lesion Diffuse or Lateralized?

Level of Performance: This method of inference does not contribute to the answer of this question.

Pattern of Performance: The 18-point difference between VIQ and PIQ scores suggests some right-cerebral hemisphere impairment. **(5-8)**

Right/Left Differences: The dominant upper extremity deficits on TPT and Strength of Grip, as well as fingertip number writing errors on the right side as opposed to the left, indicate specific deficits associated with the left-cerebral hemisphere. **(5-11)**

Pathognomonic Signs: Errors on the Aphasia Screening Examination add further to evidence of left-cerebral hemisphere impairment. **(5-13)**

In an overall sense, there appears to be more striking evidence of left-cerebral hemisphere impairment than right. These motor and sensory deficits may have impaired his PIQ subtest scores, which could account for the 18-point difference between VIQ and PIQ.

5) Is the Impairment in the Anterior or Posterior Part of the Cerebral Hemisphere?

Level of Performance: This method of inferences does not contribute to the answer of this questions.

Pattern of Performance: Both sensory and motor deficits are noted in the right upper extremity, which affects our ability to determine anterior versus posterior lesion site.

Right/Left Differences: This method of inference does not contribute to the answer of this questions.

Pathognomonic Signs: This method of inference does not contribute to the answer of this question.

Although this lesion is undoubtedly focal, due to the striking motor and sensory deficits, there is nothing to indicate that it is clearly anterior or posterior.

6) What is the Most Likely Neuropathological Process?

The neurocognitive deficits revealed by this examination are generally mild **(7-2)** and lateralized to the left-cerebral hemisphere. **(7-20)** Since there is some sensory-perceptual deficit and motor impairment, the lesion is likely in the distribution of the left middle cerebral artery. Given the history of reported head injury, the most likely diagnosis is hemorrhage in the left-cerebral hemisphere. Head CT scan revealed a left subdural hematoma extending over portions of the frontal, temporal, and parietal lobes.

7) What are the Implications for Everyday Functioning and Treatment?

This slow hemorrhage was evacuated neurosurgically, and with short convalescence and physical therapy intervention, this patient returned to normal everyday functioning.

Case 14

This case involves a 36-year-old black female with 12 years of education, who worked in an textile plant. She was involved in a motor vehicle accident that resulted in loss of consciousness for 4 days, approximately 24 hours of retrograde amnesia, and a posttraumatic amnesia of almost 2 weeks. She was assessed approximately 3 months postinjury, while she was being evaluated for rehabilitation intervention. She was cooperative with all test procedures; however, her attention and concentration and ability to understand test instructions on first presentation were impaired.

1) Is There Cerebral Impairment?

Level of Performance: Her Halstead Impairment Index of 1.0 (*T* score = 4), Category Test score of 64 (*T* score = 36), Trail Making B score of 94 (*T* score = 35), and TPT Localization of 1 (*T* score = 31) all indicate significant cerebral impairment. **(4-1)** Other test scores such as the Speech Sounds Perception Test of 28 (*T* score = 25), Seashore Rhythm Test score of 15 (*T* score = 26), and numerous sensory and motor impairments add evidence to this cerebral impairment.

Pattern of Performance: Her VIQ and PIQ scores, as well as her subtest scaled scores on the Wechsler Intelligence Scale are generally below that which we would expect from a individual with her educational level (see *T* scores).

Right/Left Differences: There are considerable right/left differences on Finger Tapping, Strength of Grip, TPT, and Sensory-Perceptual Examination, which support the notion of cerebral impairment. **(4-39)**

Pathognomonic Signs: On the Aphasia Screening Examination, there was some indication of mild dysarthria and she perseverated and demonstrated confusion on several of the verbal tasks. Mild constructional dyspraxia was also noted, particularly in lack of detail on the skeleton key. All of these factors indicate cerebral impairment.

2) What is the Severity of Cerebral Dysfunction?

Level of Performance: As noted earlier, the Halstead Impairment Index of 1.0, poor Category Test score, TPT total time of 29.8 minutes (2.48 minutes per block and a *T* score of 16), as well as impaired scores on TPT Localization, Speech Sounds Perception, Seashore Rhythm, Trail Making A and B, the motor speed and strength test, and the sensory and perceptual examination suggest severe cerebral impairment. **(4-1)**

Pattern of Performance: Her Wechsler Intelligence Scale scores are generally depressed as are her neuropsychological test results, all of which suggest moderate to severe impairment.

Right/Left Differences: The dominant hand strength of grip score of 9 indicates a moderate to severe impairment on the right side of the body. **(4-53, 4-54)**

Pathognomonic Signs: The perseveration and confusion on the Aphasia Screening Examination also suggest moderate to severe impairment.

Moderate to severe overall dysfunction is indicated.

HRB NORMS PROGRAM
Raw Score Transformations

Name:	Case14		Sex:	F
Age:	36		Years of Educ:	12
Date:	04/03/75		File Name:	CASE14
Handedness:	Right			

Measure	Abbreviation	Raw Scores	Scaled Scores	T Scores
HALSTEAD REITAN BATTERY SCORES				
Halstead Impairment Index	HII	1.0	1	4#
Average Impairment Rating	AIR			
Category Test	CAT ERROR	64	7	36#
Trail Making Test-A (secs)	TRAIL A	54	5	28#
Trail Making Test-B (secs)	TRAIL B	94	7	35#
Tact Perf Test-Time (min/blk)	TPT TIME	2.48	2	16#
Tact Perf Test-Memory (correct)	TPT MEM	4	5	27#
Tact Perf Test-Location (correct)	TPT LOC	1	6	31#
Seashore Rhythm (correct)	SSHOR RHYM	15	3	26#
Speech Perception (errors)	SPCH PERC	28	3	25#
Aphasia Screening (errors)	APHAS SCRN			
Spatial Relations (rating)	SPAT REL			
Sensory-Perceptual Total (errors)	SP TOTAL	19	4	24#
LATERALIZED SENSORIMOTOR/ PSYCHOMOTOR INDICES				
Finger Tapping-Dom (taps)	TAP DH	24	2	24#L
Finger Tapping-Non-dom (taps)	TAP NDH	38	7	44
Hand Dynamometer-Dom (kgs)	GRIP DH	9	1	16#L
Hand Dynamometer-Non-dom (kgs)	GRIP NDH	31	9	57
Grooved Pegboard-Dom (secs)	PEG DH			
Grooved Pegboard-Non-dom (secs)	PEG NDH			
Tact Perf Test-Dom (min/blk)	TPT DH	1.44	5	29#
Tact Perf Test-Non-dom (min/blk)	TPT NDH	.88	6	31#
Tact Perf Test-Both Hands (min/blk)	TPT BOTH	.66	6	32#
Sensory-Perceptual-Right (errors)	SP R	13	4	25#
Sensory-Perceptual-Left (errors)	SP L	6	5	27#
Tactile Form Recog-Right (secs)	TFR R	1	19	86L
Tactile Form Recog-Left (secs)	TFR L	0	19	85

\# = Impaired
L = Right-left difference, with possible lateralizing significance

Figure 16. Case 14.

HRB NORMS PROGRAM
Raw Score Transformations

Page 2

Name: Case14   Sex: F
Age: 36   Years of Educ: 12
Date: 04/03/75   File Name: CASE14
Handedness: Right

Measure	Abbreviation	Raw Scores	Scaled Scores	T Scores
WAIS SCORES				
Verbal IQ (VIQ)	VIQ	87	4	29#
Performance IQ (PIQ)	PIQ	83	3	27#
Full Scale IQ (FSIQ)	FSIQ	84	3	25#
Information	INFO	6	4	27#
Digit Span	DIGIT SPAN	11	10	51
Vocabulary	VOCAB	7	5	30#
Arithmetic	ARITH	9	7	46
Comprehension	COMP	6	3	29#
Similarities	SIMIL	8	6	35#
Picture Completion	PICT COMP	7	6	36#
Picture Arrangement	PICT ARR	6	6	33#
Block Design	BLOCK DESGN	9	8	43
Object Assembly	OBJ ASSMB	6	5	31#
Digit Symbol	DIGIT SYMB	5	4	24#

= Impaired

Figure 16. Case 14 (continued).

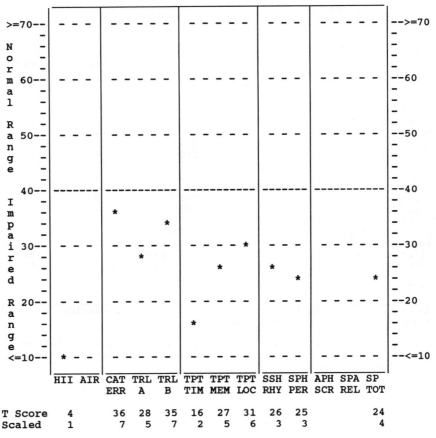

Figure 16. Case 14 (continued).

Name: Case14   Sex: F
Age: 36   Yrs of Educ: 12
Date: 04/03/75   File Name: CASE14
Handedness: Right

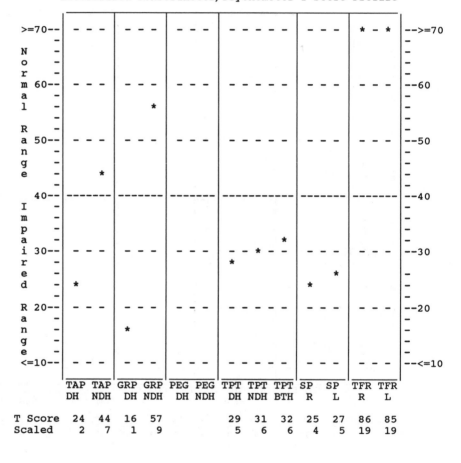

Figure 16. Case 14 (continued).

Page 5

Name: Case14   Sex: F
Age: 36   Yrs of Educ: 12
Date: 04/03/75   File Name: CASE14
Handedness: Right

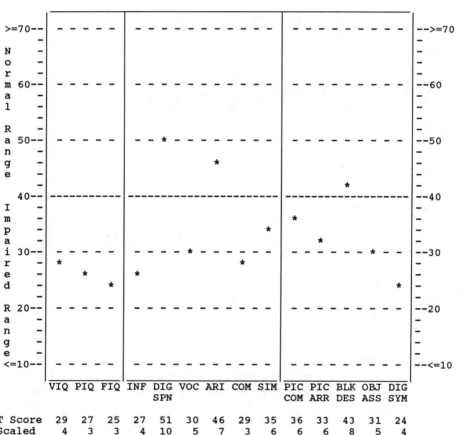

WAIS T Score Profile

	VIQ	PIQ	FIQ	INF	DIG SPN	VOC	ARI	COM	SIM	PIC COM	PIC ARR	BLK DES	OBJ ASS	DIG SYM
T Score	29	27	25	27	51	30	46	29	35	36	33	43	31	24
Scaled	4	3	3	4	10	5	7	3	6	6	6	8	5	4

Figure 16. Case 14 (continued).

SENSORY—PERCEPTUAL EXAMINATION Case 14

Indicate Instance in which stimulus is not perceived or is incorrectly perceived.

Error Totals

Tactile:

Right Hand/Left Hand — RH ☐☐☐ LH ☐☐☐ Both: RH ☐X☐ LH ☐☐☐   RH _1_ LH _0_

Right Hand/Left Face — RH ☐☐☐ LF ☐☐☐ Both: RH ☐☐☐ LF ☐☐☐   RH _0_ LF _0_

Left Hand/Right Face — LH ☐☐☐ RF ☐☐☐ Both: LH ☐☐☐ RF ☐☐☐   RF _0_ LH _0_

Auditory:

Right Ear/Left Ear — RE ☐☐☐ LE ☐☐☐ Both: RE X X X X LE ☐☐☐   RE _4_ LE _0_

Visual:

Above eye level
Eye level   { RV ☐☐☐ LV ☐☐☐ Both: RV ☐☐☐ LV ☐☐☐   RV _0_ LV _0_
Below eye level

Finger Agnosia:

Right: 1 ☐☐☐ 2 ☐X☐ 3 ☐☐☐ 4 ☐X☐ 5 ☐☐☐   R _2 /20_
Left: 1 ☐☐☐ 2 ☐☐☐ 3 ☐X☐ 4 ☐X☐ 5 ☐☐☐   L _2 /20_

Finger-tip Number Writing Perception:

	4 6 3 5	3 5 4 6	6 5 4 3	5 4 6 3	6 3 5 4	
Right:	36	5	6	6	3	R _6/20_
Left:		6 5	5	3		L _4/20_

Astereognosis:

Right: P N D   Left: D N P   Both: Right: | N P D | R _____
                                      Left: L _____

Tactile Form Recognition:

Errors: RH ○ □ △ ✛   LH △ ✛ ○ □   RH ✛ ○ □ △   LH □ △ ✛ ○   R _1_
Response Time: 3 4 3 3   3 4 3 4   4 3 2 3   3 4 3 2   L _0_

Total Time: R _25"_ L _26"_

Visual Fields: Left   Right

WNL ⊕   ⊕

Figure 16. Case 14 (continued).

APHASIA SCREENING TEST   Case 14

Form for Adults and Older Children

Name: _____ Age: __**36**__ Date: __**4/3/75**__ Examiner: _____

1. Copy SQUARE	17. Repeat TRIANGLE
2. Name SQUARE	18. Repeat MASSACHUSETTS **MASSACHUSES**
3. Spell SQUARE	19. Repeat METHODIST EPISCOPAL **" . . . CAPAL**
4. Copy CROSS	20. Write SQUARE
5. Name CROSS	21. Read SEVEN
6. Spell CROSS	22. Repeat SEVEN
7. Copy TRIANGLE	23. Repeat/Explain HE SHOUTED THE WARNING. **A POLICEMAN OR DOCTOR**
8. Name TRIANGLE	24. Write HE SHOUTED THE WARNING. **Note: explains words policeman . . . doctor**
9. Spell TRIANGLE	25. Compute 85 – 27 =
10. Name BABY	26. Compute 17 X 3 =
11. Write CLOCK	27. Name KEY
12. Name FORK	28. Demonstrate use of KEY
13. Read 7 SIX 2	29. Draw KEY
14. Read M G W	30. Read PLACE LEFT HAND TO RIGHT EAR.
15. Reading I	31. Place LEFT HAND TO RIGHT EAR
16. Reading II	32. Place LEFT HAND TO LEFT ELBOW

Figure 16. Case 14 (continued).

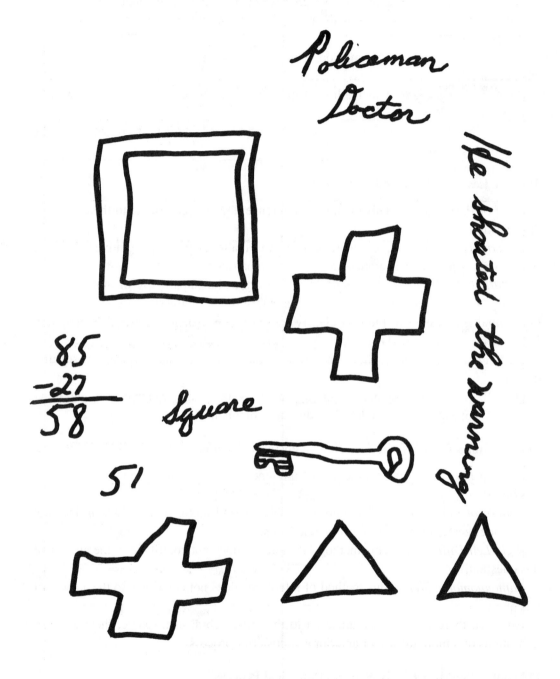

Figure 16. Case 14 (continued).

3) Is the Lesion Progressive or Static?

Level of Performance: The poor Speech Sounds Perception and Seashore Rhythm Test scores indicate an acute and possibly progressive neuropathological condition.

Pattern of Performance: This method of inference does not contribute to the answer of this question.

Right/Left Differences: This method of inference does not contribute to the answer of this question.

Pathognomonic Signs: This method of inference does not contribute to the answer of this question.

In an overall sense, the history and serial assessments will best contribute to the answer of this question.

4) Is the Lesion Diffuse or Lateralized?

Level of Performance: This method of inference does not contribute to the answer of this question.

Pattern of Performance: There are deficits in virtually all areas of cognitive/behavioral functioning, which suggest a bilateral or diffuse impairment.

Right/Left Differences: Although there appears to be impairment on both sides of the body demonstrated by the TPT, Finger Tapping, Strength of Grip, and Sensory-Perceptual Examination, there is clearly more evidence of left-cerebral hemisphere impairment than right. **(5-11)**

Pathognomonic Signs: There are both verbal and visuospatial problem-solving deficits.

Overall, the left-cerebral hemisphere appears to be more impaired than the right, however, there appears to be an underlying, diffuse component.

5) Is the Impairment in the Anterior or Posterior Part of the Cerebral Hemisphere?

Level of Performance: This method of inference does not contribute to the answer of this question.

Pattern of Performance: There are both sensory and motor deficits, which does not allow for either anterior or posterior delineations.

Right/Left Differences: This method of inference does not contribute to the answer of this question.

Pathognomonic Signs: This method of inferences does not contribute to the answer of this question.

Although there is some lateralization to the left-cerebral hemisphere, there are also indications of a more diffuse or anterior and posterior process.

6) What is the Most Likely Neuropathological Process?

The history clearly indicates that this patient suffered a closed head injury and the neuropsychological test data suggest more impairment to the left-cerebral hemisphere than the right. Head CT scan revealed multiple sights of contrecoup injury resulting in contusions and hemorrhages in several locations, including white matter. Upon emergency room admission, there were indications of increased intracranial pressure, which was treated pharmacologically.

7) What are the Implications for Everyday Functioning and Treatment?

This patient's neurocognitive deficits are quite severe and will not allow her to return to her textile work at this time. She demonstrates cognitive impairment in virtually all areas and must undergo extensive rehabilitation treatment involving physical therapy, speech therapy, occupational therapy, cognitive retraining, and psychological intervention. Significant improvement will undoubtedly take place over the first 18 to 24 months, following the natural recovery curve from moderate to severe closed head injury. Neuropsychological reevaluation every 9 to 12 months is highly recommended in order to document improvements in her condition and to determine the best emphasis for rehabilitation efforts to remediate and help her to cope with and adapt to her deficits.

Case 15

This 65-year-old white, married male had 20 years of education and was a retired pharmacist. Approximately 18 months prior to this assessment he had begun to complain of double vision and significant memory problems, as well as some lower extremity motor weakness. At about that time, he had his first seizure and was hospitalized for a full neurologic workup. Later in the process of his treatment, the present neuropsychological assessment was completed. He was physically ill at the time of this evaluation, and many of the test measures had to be discontinued. Under these adverse conditions, he cooperated as best he could and attempted to complete all test procedures.

1) Is There Cerebral Impairment?

Level of Performance: The four most sensitive indicators of cerebral impairment (the Halstead Impairment Index, Category Test, TPT Localization, and Trail Making B) were all severely impaired and clearly indicate cerebral impairment. **(4-1)** All other Halstead-Reitan test scores were also in the impaired range (*T* scores range from 8 to 41).

Pattern of Performance: There is a 34-point difference between VIQ and PIQ, which is 16 *T* score points. **(4-10)** This significant difference supports the presence of cerebral impairment.

Right/Left Differences: Greater impairment on the left side of the body on Finger Tapping, Strength of Grip, and Sensory-Perceptual functions support the notion of cerebral impairment.

Pathognomonic Signs: Dysnomia, dyslexia, right/left confusion, dysgraphia, and constructional dyspraxia on the Aphasia Screening Examination suggest the presence of cerebral impairment. **(4-56, 4-57)**

Given the deficits in almost every area of neurocognitive function, there can be no doubt that this patient does demonstrate cerebral impairment.

HRB NORMS PROGRAM
Raw Score Transformations

Name: Case15   Sex: M
Age: 65   Years of Educ: 20
Date: 03/22/82   File Name: CASE15
Handedness: Right

Measure	Abbreviation	Raw Scores	Scaled Scores	T Scores
HALSTEAD REITAN BATTERY SCORES				
Halstead Impairment Index	HII	1.0	1	8#
Average Impairment Rating	AIR			
Category Test	CAT ERROR	124	2	25#
Trail Making Test-A (secs)	TRAIL A	122	1	16#
Trail Making Test-B (secs)	TRAIL B	300	2	18#
Tact Perf Test-Time (min/blk)	TPT TIME	7.8	0	17#
Tact Perf Test-Memory (correct)	TPT MEM	2	3	24#
Tact Perf Test-Location (correct)	TPT LOC	0	5	35#
Seashore Rhythm (correct)	SSHOR RHYM	0	1	21#
Speech Perception (errors)	SPCH PERC	60	1	14#
Aphasia Screening (errors)	APHAS SCRN			
Spatial Relations (rating)	SPAT REL			
Sensory-Perceptual Total (errors)	SP TOTAL	54	1	28#
LATERALIZED SENSORIMOTOR/ PSYCHOMOTOR INDICES				
Finger Tapping-Dom (taps)	TAP DH	44	8	40
Finger Tapping-Non-dom (taps)	TAP NDH	27	3	20#L
Hand Dynamometer-Dom (kgs)	GRIP DH	36	9	41
Hand Dynamometer-Non-dom (kgs)	GRIP NDH	21	6	26#L
Grooved Pegboard-Dom (secs)	PEG DH			
Grooved Pegboard-Non-dom (secs)	PEG NDH			
Tact Perf Test-Dom (min/blk)	TPT DH	4.5	2	28#
Tact Perf Test-Non-dom (min/blk)	TPT NDH	10.0	0	17#L
Tact Perf Test-Both Hands (min/blk)	TPT BOTH	10.0	1	18#
Sensory-Perceptual-Right (errors)	SP R	23	2	30#
Sensory-Perceptual-Left (errors)	SP L	31	2	22#
Tactile Form Recog-Right (secs)	TFR R	46	1	12#
Tactile Form Recog-Left (secs)	TFR L	158	1	13#L

# = Impaired
L = Right-left difference, with possible lateralizing significance

Figure 17. Case 15.

HRB NORMS PROGRAM
Raw Score Transformations

Page 2

Name:	Case15		Sex:	M
Age:	65		Years of Educ:	20
Date:	03/22/82		File Name:	CASE15
Handedness:	Right			

Measure	Abbreviation	Raw Scores	Scaled Scores	T Scores
WAIS SCORES				
Verbal IQ (VIQ)	VIQ	116	10	28#
Performance IQ (PIQ)	PIQ	82	3	12#
Full Scale IQ (FSIQ)	FSIQ	98	6	12#
Information	INFO	12	10	32#
Digit Span	DIGIT SPAN	9	8	39#
Vocabulary	VOCAB	14	12	43
Arithmetic	ARITH	7	5	18#
Comprehension	COMP	16	13	50
Similarities	SIMIL	12	10	41
Picture Completion	PICT COMP	4	3	14#
Picture Arrangement	PICT ARR	4	4	30#
Block Design	BLOCK DESGN	5	4	22#
Object Assembly	OBJ ASSMB	5	4	32#
Digit Symbol	DIGIT SYMB	3	2	22#

= Impaired

Figure 17. Case 15 (continued).

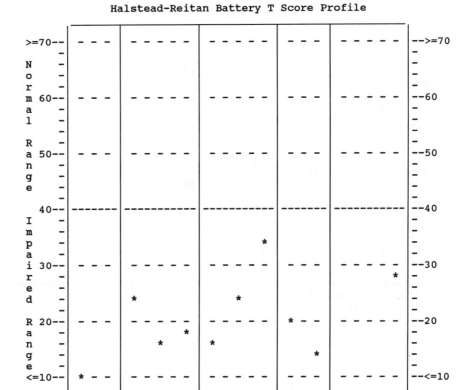

Figure 17. Case 15 (continued).

Name: Case15   Sex: M
Age: 65   Yrs of Educ: 20
Date: 03/22/82   File Name: CASE15
Handedness: Right

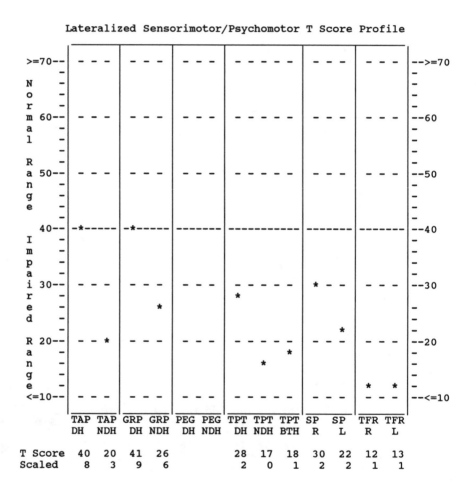

Figure 17. Case 15 (continued).

Page 5

Name: Case15   Sex: M
Age: 65   Yrs of Educ: 20
Date: 03/22/82   File Name: CASE15
Handedness: Right

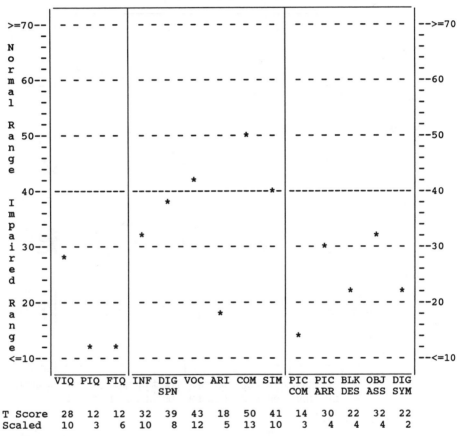

WAIS T Score Profile

	VIQ	PIQ	FIQ	INF	DIG SPN	VOC	ARI	COM	SIM	PIC COM	PIC ARR	BLK DES	OBJ ASS	DIG SYM
T Score	28	12	12	32	39	43	18	50	41	14	30	22	32	22
Scaled	10	3	6	10	8	12	5	13	10	3	4	4	4	2

Figure 17. Case 15 (continued).

SENSORY—PERCEPTUAL EXAMINATION   Case 15

Indicate Instance in which stimulus is not perceived or is incorrectly perceived.

Error Totals

Tactile:

Right Hand/Left Hand — RH [ ][ ][ ] LH [ ][ ][ ] Both: RH [ ][X][ ] LH [X][ ][X]   RH _1_ LH _2_

Right Hand/Left Face — RH [ ][ ][ ] LF [ ][ ][ ] Both: RH [X][ ][ ] LF [X][X]   RH _1_ LF _2_

Left Hand/Right Face — LH [ ][ ][ ] RF [ ][ ][ ] Both: LH [ ][ ][ ] RF [X][ ][ ]   RF _1_ LH _0_

Auditory:

Right Ear/Left Ear — RE [ ][ ][ ] LE [ ][ ][ ] Both: RE [ ][ ][ ] LE [ ][ ][ ]   RE _4_ LE _3_

Visual:

Above eye level
Eye level   { RV [grid] LV [grid] Both: RV [X grid] LV [X][ ][X]   RV _1_ LV _2_
Below eye level

Finger Agnosia:

Right: 1 [ ][X] 2 [ ][ ] 3 [X][ ] 4 [X][X] 5 [ ][X]   R _5 /20_
Left: 1 [X][ ] 2 [X][ ] 3 [X][X] 4 [X][ ][X] 5 [ ][X]   L _7 /20_

Finger-tip Number Writing Perception:

Right: | 4 6 3 5 | | 3 5 4 6 | | 6 5 4 3 | | 5 4 6 3 | | 6 3 5 4 | R _10/20_
       | 4 | | 6   8 | | 8   6 | | 586 | | 3 6 |
Left: | 5 3 8 | | 6 7 5 | | 3 7 5 | | 4 5   6 | | 8   4 5 | L _15/20_

Astereognosis:

Right: [P | N | D]   Left: [D | N | P]   Both: Right: [N | P | D] / Left: [ ]   R _____
                                                                                         L _____

Tactile Form Recognition:

Errors: RH [○][□][△][✚] LH [△][✚][○][□] RH [✚][○][□][△] / [△] LH [□][△][✚][○]   R _0_
Response Time: RH [ ]   LH [ ]   RH [ ]   LH [ ]   L _0_

Total Time: R _46"_   L _158"_

Visual Fields: Left   Right

WNL [circle with crosshairs]   [circle with crosshairs]

Figure 17. Case 15 (continued).

APHASIA SCREENING TEST   Case 15

Form for Adults and Older Children

Name: _____ Age: __65__ Date: __3/22/82__ Examiner: _____

1. Copy SQUARE	17. Repeat TRIANGLE
2. Name SQUARE	18. Repeat MASSACHUSETTS *"...sess*
3. Spell SQUARE	19. Repeat METHODIST EPISCOPAL
4. Copy CROSS	20. Write SQUARE
5. Name CROSS *A STAR...OR A RECTANGLE. INSIGNIA –* *NAZIS*	21. Read SEVEN
6. Spell CROSS	22. Repeat SEVEN
7. Copy TRIANGLE	23. Repeat/Explain HE SHOUTED THE WARNING. *THERE WAS A CERTAIN AMOUNT OF DANGER* *OR CONCERN THAT WAS TO BE EXPRESSED*
8. Name TRIANGLE	24. Write HE SHOUTED THE WARNING.
9. Spell TRIANGLE	25. Compute 85 – 27 =
10. Name BABY	26. Compute 17 X 3 =
11. Write CLOCK	27. Name KEY
12. Name FORK	28. Demonstrate use of KEY
13. Read 7 SIX 2	29. Draw KEY
14. Read M G W *M-G-M*	30. Read PLACE LEFT HAND TO RIGHT EAR.
15. Reading I	31. Place LEFT HAND TO RIGHT EAR *R - R looks confused*
16. Reading II	32. Place LEFT HAND TO LEFT ELBOW

Figure 17. Case 15 (continued).

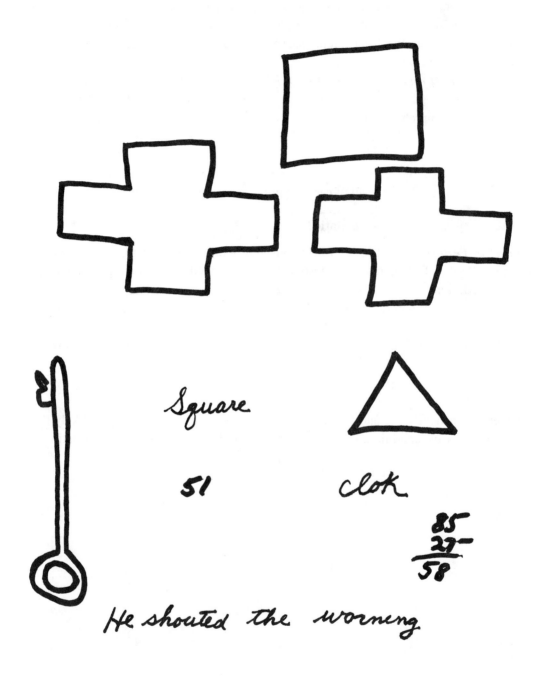

Figure 17. Case 15 (continued).

2) What is the Severity of Cerebral Dysfunction?

Level of Performance: All individual Halstead-Reitan test scores indicate severe cognitive disruption, particularly given his probable premorbid level of functioning given 20 years of education and his vocation as a pharmacist. His severe visuospatial problem-solving deficits on the Wechsler Intelligence Scales also suggest a significant decline and moderate to severe cerebral dysfunction.

Pattern of Performance: His VIQ-PIQ split of 34 points indicates severe cerebral impairment, as does his dramatic subtest scatter from a scaled score of 3 on Digit Symbol to a 16 on Comprehension.

Right/Left Differences: This method of inference does not contribute to the answer of this question.

Pathognomonic Signs: The previously mentioned aphasic errors and constructional dyspraxia indicate a severe level of cerebral impairment for this patient.

3) Is the Lesion Progressive or Static?

Level of Performance: The VIQ-PIQ split and poor Speech Sounds Perception and Seashore Rhythm Test scores (these tests were discontinued) suggest the possibility of a progressive lesion.

Pattern of Performance: This method of inference does not contribute to the answer of this question.

Right/Left Differences: This method of inference does not contribute to the answer of this question.

Pathognomonic Signs: This method of inference does not contribute to the answer of this question.

Given this patient's age and the severity of his overall deficits, it is highly likely that this is a progressive condition. Here again, history would provide valuable information.

4) Is the Lesion Diffuse or Lateralized?

Level of Performance: This method of inference does not contribute to the answer of this question.

Pattern of Performance: The 34-point difference between VIQ and PIQ suggests a right-cerebral hemisphere lesion. **(4-10)**

Right/Left Differences: Although he performed poorly on the Tactual Performance Test, and this measure was eventually discontinued, there are indications from the Finger Tapping and Strength of Grip tests that the left upper extremity is more impaired than the right (indicating right-cerebral hemisphere involvement). **(5-11)** The Sensory-Perceptual Examination demonstrates bilateral tactile, auditory, and visual suppressions, as well as bilateral finger and fingertip agnosia, and astereognosis. Here again, more deficits are associated with the right-cerebral hemisphere.

Pathognomonic Signs: On the Aphasia Screening Examination, there are indications of both right and left-cerebral hemisphere dysfunction.

This lesion appears lateralized to the right-cerebral hemisphere; however, it is also clear that there are deficits associated with the left-cerebral hemisphere. With the exception of some verbal functions, which have remained intact, there is generalized neurocognitive impairment.

5) Is the Impairment in the Anterior or Posterior Part of the Cerebral Hemisphere?

Level of Performance: This method of inference does not contribute to the answer of this question.

Pattern of Performance: Since there are both sensory and motor deficits, differentiation between anterior and posterior effects is not possible.

Right/Left Differences: This method of inference does not contribute to the answer of this question.

Pathognomonic Signs: This method of inference does not contribute to this answer of this question.

Anterior or posterior delineations are not possible in this case.

6) What is the Most Likely Neuropathological Process?

Given this patient's physical illness, Halstead Impairment Index of 1.0, extremely poor Category Test of 124, and the huge difference between his VIQ and PIQ scores, the most likely neopathological process is neuroplastic disease. **(7-10)** Head CT scan revealed a right frontal glioma, which was subsequently removed and regrew for a second and finally third time. The present neuropsychological assessment followed this third operation and delineated the severe neurocognitive deficits associated with this destructive tumor.

7) What are the Implications for Everyday Functioning and Treatment?

Unfortunately, this patient died 5 months after this assessment from medical complications associated with this tumor. Recovery from the effects of this neoplastic disease, if it had been controlled, would not likely have been complete, and rehabilitation efforts would have been necessary to restore some everyday functioning.

SECTION 2
CLINICAL APPLICATIONS

Chapter 10

Beyond the Test Data

Up to this point, the emphasis in this volume has been on understanding the implications of test data. In actual clinical evaluations the neuropsychologist must go beyond the test data to examine other sources of information. In even the simplest cases of referrals to answer diagnostic questions, test data must be viewed within the context of other information. Heaton et al. (1991), for example, have made it clear that performance on neuropsychological tests is affected by age, sex, and education. An IQ of 95, which is within the average range, has very different diagnostic implications for a person who dropped out of school in the ninth grade than it does for a person with 18 years of education and a graduate degree. Similarly, a score of 55 errors on the Category test has different implications for a 30-year-old person than it does for a 70-year-old. It is clear, then, that in every case one must consider basic demographic information in order to understand the implications of test data. In many cases, this information can be obtained simply by questioning the patient, but in certain situations this can yield inaccurate information and, consequently, incorrect inferences may be made.

When questions about everyday functioning and rehabilitation are to be considered, as is increasingly the case, one must consider still more information about the patient, particularly in forensic cases. One must understand what the person was like before the brain injury. What kind of child, parent, spouse, student, or worker was she or he? Then one must understand how this person views the changes in his/her life that the injury or disease has caused and how others perceive the changes. How have relationships with family, friends, and coworkers changed (Jarvis, 1988a)?

An understanding of these factors often requires additional sources of information. The testing that produces the test data also yields valuable observations of the patient's behavior during testing. Interviews with the patient, family members, teachers, employers, and others are often essential sources of information. Another source that is critical in some cases is information obtained from a variety of records: previous testing, medical, school, employment, and court records.

Observations During Testing

Everyone who has a neuropsychological evaluation comes to the experience with some perception of the purpose of the examination. This may be the same as the examiner's perception, or it may be quite different. It is not unusual for hospitalized patients to believe that the purpose of the evaluation is to determine, "whether I can ever go home."

This, of course, is almost always inaccurate. While one might assume that any patient who has this perception will put forth the best possible effort in order to be discharged from the hospital, this is not necessarily the case, since some patients may fear leaving a hospital for any of a variety of reasons. It is useful to give patients a simple explanation of the purpose of the evaluation before testing is started and to assess their reactions to it.

Similarly, some patients have inaccurate expectations about the nature of a neuropsychological evaluation, particularly if they have been recently subjected to a variety of medical procedures including unpleasant, invasive ones. Therefore, it is important to explain that this evaluation will not involve medical procedures, but will assess the differences in one's ability to perform different types of tasks. Once again, one should evaluate the patient's understanding of and reaction to this information.

Testing occurs within the context of an interpersonal relationship between the patient and the examiner. It is reasonable to assume that the patient's behavior within this situation is similar to his/her behavior in a variety of other important relationships. If, for example, a patient is hostile toward the examiner, the same behavior may characterize relationships with other "authority figures," for example. In some cases, the patient's behavior with the examiner may be quite different from the behavior reported or observed with other people. When this occurs, it is important to examine the characteristics of the examiner, such as gender and age, and the ways that the behavior of the examiner differs from those of people toward whom the patient responds differently. Finally, it is important for the examiner to examine his/her feelings about and reactions to the patient. Does one feel angry, protective, or hopeless about the patient? What is it that evokes these feelings? All of this information about the patient's way of relating to the examiner has implications for how the patient will relate to other people in everyday activities and in the rehabilitation process.

During testing, the patient's cooperation and effort should be assessed. If these are judged to be less than optimal, test results must be considered with caution. Other factors such as the patient's understanding of the English language; visual and auditory acuity; and, particularly for some tests like the MMPI, his/her reading ability should also be evaluated. One is not assessing the adequacy of brain functioning if the patient does not understand the test instructions or cannot hear the examiner or understand the language adequately.

Beyond that basic consideration, a patient's cooperation and effort may fluctuate from one test to another. A patient may produce a hasty, sloppy performance on a simple task such as copying a design because he/she considers it degrading to be asked to do such a basic thing. On tasks that are very difficult for them, patients may react in a variety of ways. Some, of course, may persist in attempting to complete the task. Others may give up and refuse to continue when they encounter difficulty. Still others may argue with the examiner, saying the test is flawed or the examiner is trying to "trick" them; and some may "just go through the motions" of the task, responding at random in a passive-aggressive manner. Each of these styles of dealing with tasks of differing levels of difficulty has implications for the way the patient will handle tasks of everyday living and respond to rehabilitation and treatment. Patients vary considerably in the amount and type of structure they require in order to complete testing. Some can complete testing in a single 4- or

5-hour session that requires 8 or 10 hours for other patients. Some can complete testing in 1 day that requires several half-day sessions for others. Some can perform tests readily with only the briefest of "standard" instructions, while others require considerable repetition and elaboration of instructions for some or all of the tests. At times, a patient will be unable to perform a test under anything resembling the standard conditions, but may be able to do so if certain requirements are changed, such as allowing a patient to respond by pointing to the answer rather than giving a verbal response. Any such modification should be made only after first attempting the standard procedure, all modifications should be fully described, and resulting data should be interpreted with caution. Patients also vary considerably in the type and frequency of reinforcement they require to produce their best possible performance. The types of support, encouragement, and structure that facilitate patient performance can provide clues to treatment strategies that may be effective. Information about all of these factors should be recorded and considered along with the test data in answering referral questions about diagnosis, everyday functioning, and rehabilitation planning.

Certain types of behavior have specific implications for neurologic or psychiatric disorders. Several types of abnormal movements may have diagnostic and treatment implications, including such common ones as Parkinsonian movements, the mouth and facial movements of tardive dyskinesia, and the restlessness of the patient with akisthisia.

There are many other aspects of patient behavior that may have implications for neurologic disorders. Speech patterns may show dysarthria, scanning speech, or word-finding difficulty. Intentional memory problems may be evidenced by failure to remember appointments, and incidental memory problems may be evidenced by failure to remember the examiner's name. Visual-spatial problems may be reflected in difficulty finding the way to the testing room or to nearby facilities such as the bathroom or cafeteria.

Hemineglect may be suspected when a patient appears clumsy and frequently bumps into objects on one side of the body. It was demonstrated dramatically by one patient who, when the triangle was placed in his hand on the Tactile Form Recognition Test, said, "Now you gave me one that's not on the board." (The triangle is the form at the far left side of the board.) Visual field testing verified that he had a homonomous hemianopsia, but it was his spontaneous comment that demonstrated how disabling this lesion might be in his everyday functioning.

Schizophrenic disorders may be suspected when one observes loose associations; use of neologisms; expression of delusions; evidence of hallucinations; and a distant, schizoid way of relating to the examiner. Depression may be reflected in giving up easily as task difficulty increases, statements derogating one's own performance, and other evidence of low self-esteem.

Finally, patients make some assessment of the adequacy of their own performance on tests. Frequently they indicate this by their spontaneous comments; sometimes it is useful to ask them how well they think they did. On some tests it is very difficult for anyone to estimate the adequacy of his/her own performance. Patients have no way of knowing how many errors on the Category Test signify an adequate performance, for example, without even considering the unlikely possibility that they will count their errors. On timed tests this difficulty is even greater, perhaps most extremely on the TPT on which the blindfold adds an additional disorienting impediment. On these types of tests, then, patients' judgments of the adequacy of their performance are, perhaps, less important in regard to their accuracy in comparison to test norms than they are in terms of their feelings about their own abilities and the effect those feelings have on their behavior.

On certain other tests it is much easier to judge the adequacy of one's own performance, either because the standard of performance is visible on tasks such as copying designs or because one may readily compare one's performance on the test to one's own past performance on tasks like defining words or solving arithmetic problems. On such tests it is not unusual for patients to make comments such as, "I used to know that," or "I used to be able to do that."

Patients who have the most accurate perceptions of their own abilities appear to have the best chance of functioning at their optimal levels in everyday activities and the best rehabilitation prognosis. Those who lack awareness of their deficits are likely to overextend themselves in some situations and may, at times, place themselves in dangerous situations. On the other hand, those who grossly overestimate their deficits may fail to function as well as they could and attempt to remain overly dependent on others. In either case, the discrepancy has significant implications for rehabilitation and discharge planning.

Interview Data

There are two general types of information one should gather from interviews: information about the patient's past, and information about his/her present circumstances. Information about past events often helps clarify diagnostic and etiological questions, as well as providing information about pre-injury functioning. Information about the patient's present circumstances is essential for prediction of everyday functioning and planning rehabilitation.

Some neuropsychologists rely on formal questionnaires that patients, and sometimes relatives, complete (e.g., Chelune & Moehle, 1986). While this may result in a saving of the examiner's time and may yield standard data for all patients, it suffers from one of the same limitations that sole reliance on test data suffers from: The examiner is largely deprived of information about *how* people behave in response to the questions. In contrast, in an interview some people will give self-assured, well-rehearsed answers to questions, while others will express uncertainty and vagueness. Furthermore, an interview may capture nuances that cannot be discerned from a questionnaire but that may have significant implications. Therefore, if a standardized questionnaire is used, it seems important to use it as a guide to an interview and not as the only source of information.

Medical History

A family medical history should be obtained. A few neurological diseases such as Huntington's disease are hereditary. In the case of Huntington's disease, a definitive diagnosis usually cannot be made until middle age, but each child of a parent who has the disease has a 50% chance of getting it. Early signs of cognitive losses in a person who is at risk can, therefore, have enormous significance. Much more commonly, a family history of conditions such as cardiovascular or respiratory disease may indicate risk factors that are relevant to a patient's brain functioning. A family history of one of the major psychiatric disorders may alert one to the possibility of the same disorder in cases in which there are indications of diffuse impairment of brain functioning with no clear etiology, and patients with such disorders may appear "brain damaged" on neuropsychological testing (Golden, 1977; Heaton & Crowley, 1981).

Although it is often difficult to obtain information about the prenatal period, particularly for adult patients, there are sometimes important events during this period that have adverse effects on brain functioning. These include things such as illness of the mother and medications, alcohol, and other drugs used during pregnancy. Problems during labor and delivery, including trauma and anoxia, may also have long-lasting effects.

The history of childhood development may reveal early indications of impaired brain functioning. Significant delays in learning to walk and talk may have such implications. Similarly, difficulty or delay in learning to read and write and hyperactivity or hypoactivity may be significant. Such problems are usually identified in early school years and may only be apparent later if school records indicate that the child was referred to special education classes.

An individual medical history is essential. High on any list of significant medical factors are head injuries and seizures. Whenever head injuries are identified, one should attempt to determine how long the person was unconscious and the duration of any retrograde amnesia and posttraumatic amnesia, since these factors are often predictors of outcome.

Information should be obtained about the details of seizures: their nature, precipitants if any, their frequency and severity, as well as medications taken to control them. These factors, particularly the frequency and severity, provide indications of the degree of impairment of brain functioning, and a description of the seizures may give some indication of the location of the causal lesion.

Multiple sclerosis (MS) is the most common neurological disease among young adults, with the modal age of onset in the mid-30s, but it can be notoriously difficult to diagnose. In the past there has often been a period of several years between the appearance of the first symptoms and a definite diagnosis, although the availability of MRI scans today is leading to more rapid diagnosis. Among the most common early symptoms are sensory disturbances in the limbs, disturbance of gait and balance, visual loss in one eye, double vision, and progressive weakness (Scheinberg & Smith, 1987). Since the symptoms of MS, particularly in the early stages, may remit spontaneously at times, they are sometimes mistakenly diagnosed as conversion symptoms, and futile attempts at psychiatric or psychological treatment may be made. Reports of this type of history should lead to referral for a neurological evaluation.

Infectious diseases that effect the central nervous system directly, such as encephalitis and meningitis, are obviously significant since they may result in residual impairment of brain functioning. In some cases patients and families may not know the specific diagnosis of such a disease. They may, however, be aware that there was a high fever associated with delirium or coma, and such events should be noted since they may be associated with neurologic impairment.

A history of cardiovascular or respiratory disease may be significant. Either of them may result in reduced supply of oxygen to the brain. A history of cardiovascular disease may involve cardiac arrest and may be associated with strokes. Respiratory diseases such as emphysema or chronic obstructive pulmonary disease (COPD) may result in hypoxia, and the severity of COPD is correlated with the severity of cognitive impairment (Prigatano et al., 1983).

There are a number of systemic diseases that can directly affect the brain. These include systemic lupus erythematosus (SLE), which is a disease of the connective tissues that effects many different parts of the body and can sometimes attack the brain, directly causing significant cognitive deficits.

The human immunodeficiency virus (HIV), which causes AIDS, can also affect the brain. In some cases this eventually leads to AIDS dementia, but cognitive impairment is sometimes seen long before that, even before a diagnosis of AIDS can be made in some cases. With the recent concern over AIDS, there may be a tendency to neglect the problems of "older" sexually transmitted diseases, but it is important to remember that syphilis, if not treated adequately, can attack the central nervous system in its tertiary stage.

Information about the use of alcohol and other drugs, both past and present, should be a part of every history. It is interesting to note that if one asks a large number of people in the general population (e.g., job applicants) how much they drink, most will say essentially, "not much." Of course, what is "not much" for one person will be an enormous amount for some others. Therefore, it is necessary to obtain specific information about the quantity and pattern of consumption.

Some people will report that they do not drink at all, and it is easy to assume that this is, therefore, not a potential problem area, which is sometimes correct. However, this should be explored further before dismissing it. Ask, "Nothing, you *never* drank at all?", and "When did you stop drinking, why did you stop?" The person who stopped "last week" or "last month" is often one who has had a serious problem with alcohol, and the reason for stopping, most recently, may indicate the nature of the functional impairments caused by it.

Chronic excessive use of alcohol may cause serious impairment of brain functioning. Both the length of time a person has been drinking and the quantity consumed may be relevant, with the person who has frequently consumed enough to cause withdrawal symptoms probably being at greatest risk.

In order to obtain a full picture of the potential effects of alcohol use/abuse it is necessary to find out what happens both while the person is drinking and after each drinking episode, "the morning after": "What is it like when you are drunk (or drinking)?" Loss of control of behavior may result in head injuries. Blackouts, defined in this context as the failure to remember, after sobering up, events and behavior that occurred while intoxicated, are very commonly associated with eventual cognitive impairment.

The morning-after events and behavior provide clues to withdrawal, and thus addiction, which has implications for cognitive impairment. Frequent hangovers, particularly when accompanied by nausea, anorexia, tremors or "the shakes," and resolutions (often quickly forgotten) to quit or reduce drinking are serious warning signs. Of still greater concern is drinking in the morning to relieve hangover symptoms and "get started" for the day. People who do this with any regularity are at risk to show eventual cognitive impairment (Parsons & Farr, 1987).

The use of certain recreational drugs has become relatively common in some segments of our society today, and some of them are used in combination with alcohol. The illegal status of such drugs creates an additional problem: Users may be reluctant to admit to the use of illegal drugs. At times, they may not have reliable information about the dosages they are consuming and, in fact, may not even be certain about what drugs they are using at times.

With these warnings in mind, many users tend to prefer certain drugs or general classes of drugs. Marijuana generally has a soporific effect. Chronic, heavy users are often listless and lacking in initiative and energy. There are a few people who experience acute psychotic, schizophrenic-like reactions to smoking marijuana. Cocaine is essentially a stimulant that produces brief, intense high levels of energy and activity. Following this is a period of depression, which gets more intense with repeated use. In chronic users serious paranoia with delusions and hallucinations may develop. Heroin and other natural and synthetic opiates and their derivatives have extremely sedating effects. Problems may include malnutrition secondary to effects of life style changes made to support the use with its potential for causing cognitive deficits. Stimulants such as "speed" have many of the same effects as cocaine, and psychedelic drugs such as LSD and other natural and synthetic drugs may cause acute psychotic reactions.

Regardless of the drugs used, it is important to identify the route of administration. Inquiry should always be made about intravenous or IV use. This is almost always associated with more serious patterns of use and addiction. Thus, all of the adverse effects associated with specific drugs are more likely to occur and to be more severe. In addition, needle sharing by IV drug users carries a high risk of AIDS transmission.

An adequate history requires identification of *all* medications, including nonprescription drugs that are being taken. If one inquires about the reasons why each drug is taken, a chronic medical problem that the patient forgot to mention otherwise because the medicine is "controlling" it may be identified. Next, it is important to recognize that many combinations of medications, including nonprescription drugs, produce adverse effects. Therefore, it is important to determine who has prescribed each of the drugs that are being used. When several different physicians are involved, none may be aware of all the drugs being used, and the potential for adverse interactions increases.

In some cases patients may be taking larger or more frequent doses than are prescribed. Be particularly alert to this problem when people have been taking medication to relieve pain, induce sleep, or relieve anxiety for long periods of time. The drugs used for these purposes are particularly subject to abuse. In such cases it is sometimes wise to "reconcile" prescriptions with actual use by checking how much medicine was obtained with the quantity in the patient's possession.

Finally, it is important to recognize that older people often have different reactions than younger people have to medications. They may require smaller doses to obtain therapeutic effects, and they may have more frequent and more severe adverse effects to some drugs alone or in combination with others. Furthermore, if they are experiencing memory problems, they are at greater risk for misuse of medications.

Educational History

As indicated earlier, education is one of the key variables affecting performance on neuropsychological tests. Other aspects of a patient's educational history in addition to the total number of years of formal education often have neuropsychological implications. The same number of years spent in special education classes and college preparatory classes obviously have different implications. Similarly, a person who "just made it through" high school has a different premorbid level of functioning than one who was an honor society member with a high grade point average. In other words, not only the number of years of education but also the level of performance during school years is important. The area of study is also important, particularly at the college and post-college levels. Different patterns of premorbid cognitive strengths should be expected from a person who has completed an engineering degree and one who has completed a theology degree, for example.

Work History

Although there are no normative data available for neuropsychological tests for different occupations, work history has implications that are similar to those of educational history. One would expect generally higher levels of performance from people with occupational histories that are more demanding than from people who had worked only at unskilled jobs. Different patterns of cognitive strengths would also be expected from people with histories of different types of jobs.

It is important to recognize that job titles often provide little real information about the demands of the work a person actually performs. To obtain this information one must determine precisely what duties a person performed and the type and amount of supervision that was received. Some carpenters, for example, do only "rough" work, while others do "finish" work or handle all aspects of a total building project guided only by plans and specifications. Similarly, not all attorneys argue cases in court, as the ones depicted on popular television shows do; some spend all of their time in offices, rarely interacting with other people.

One should also inquire about the pattern of the patient's jobs: What was the first job? How long did it last? Why did the person leave? What was the next job, and so on? Such a detailed chronology may be useful in planning rehabilitation efforts.

A patient's history of military experience should receive the same attention as other aspects of work history. Not only the branch of service but the specific assignments and duties should be determined. The highest rank attained and the pattern of promotions and demotions, as well as any disciplinary actions received, may be significant.

Current Living Situation and Activities

Just as important as a past history is a picture of a patient's current situation. At a very basic level are the source and amount of a patient's income and the type and location of his/her residence. In connection with the residence it is important to determine who, if anyone, shares the residence with the patient and what is the nature of the relationship between them. The key factor in the relationship is the division of responsibilities among the people involved and the type of support available to the patient. One may think of parent-child relationships, for example, as typically involving dominance and a greater share of responsibility by the parent, but these roles may be reversed. It is helpful to determine such information as who provides the income, who does the shopping and prepares meals, who does other household chores, who pays the bills, and so on. The most important information is often a picture of whether there have been any changes in these responsibilities and, if so, when and why.

One should also obtain a clear, detailed picture of the daily activities of the patient. This may be facilitated by taking the patient and/or a relative through the details of a typical day, perhaps the day before the interview. This may be done by inquiring about things such as what time the patient got up in the morning, whether he/she bathed and got dressed, ate breakfast, and so on. Then one can go through the day's activities in sequence, determining how much time is spent in each one and how independently the patient functions in each. Sleep patterns should be determined, focusing on the nature and pattern of any changes that have occurred.

Review of Records

Since at times the memories of patients and/or others are inadequate and there may be no one who knows the details of past education, work, or medical history available to interview, reviewing various types of records may be the only way to obtain important information. Review of records is essential in all cases in which there is any type of adversarial or legal proceeding involved. The prototype of this is litigation over personal injury, but it includes other situations such as worker's compensation claims, disability retirement actions, civil commitment proceedings, and some criminal cases. In many of these cases there is an assumption on the part of the party who is being asked to compensate the patient that both the patient and his/her relatives have an interest in maximizing the patient's deficits. If the neuropsychologist relies only on information obtained from them, all conclusions regarding the patient's deficits will be challenged. If conclusions are based on a review of relevant records along with other data, they will be easier to defend.

Medical Records

A review of past medical records may be helpful in several ways. In those cases in which neuropsychological test data suggest the presence of brain damage of unknown etiology, medical records may reveal the probable cause of the damage. In those cases in which there is an identified head trauma, medical records should be checked to determine the length of the resulting coma, the duration of retrograde and posttraumatic amnesia, the extent of hemorrhaging and edema, other complications, and the type of treatment rendered and the patient's response to it.

In other cases, records may reveal evidence of earlier brain-impairing events. Such information may lead to a better understanding of the effects of the most recent injury. It is clear that the effects of brain injuries are cumulative, and the effects of any single injury may be much more severe if it was preceded by earlier injuries (Gronwall & Wrightson, 1975; Saunders & Harbaugh, 1984). Medical records may also verify or provide additional details about any of the types of significant events discussed in the preceding section on the medical history.

Medical records may be difficult for a nonmedically trained person to understand. Some of the terminology may seem obscure, and the frequent use of abbreviations cryptic. The statement, "pt c/o sob," for example, is not a comment on the patient's ancestry. It translates to, "The patient complains of shortness of breath." The Glossary and List of Abbreviations contained in the Appendix are provided to assist with interpretation, but it is wise to consult a medical dictionary whenever additional unfamiliar terms are encountered.

School Records

The purpose of reviewing school records is to obtain detailed and accurate information similar to that obtained from reviewing the medical history. When this is done, discrepancies between reports by patients and relatives and the information in the records are sometimes found, particularly in cases involving claims for compensation.

In one case, for example, a patient who was involved in litigation over an injury and his wife both reported that he had graduated from high school with "average" grades. Review of his high school transcripts, however, revealed that he had received mostly failing grades before dropping out of school at age 17. Furthermore, review of his military records indicated that he had failed the GED test a year later. This information resulted in the interpretation of his test scores as showing little, if any, decline from his pre-injury level of functioning in contrast to the major decline that was claimed.

Matarazzo, in his APA presidential address (Bales, 1990), provided a similar example of a woman who was suing for damages resulting from toxic exposure. She had an IQ of 84 and reported that she had graduated from high school with a B average. This might have contributed to a substantial monetary award if an examination of her school records, which revealed that she had dropped out of school in the 10th grade after receiving mostly Ds and Fs, had not been conducted.

This is not to say that most people misrepresent their school records, but since the validity of evidence (sources of data) is usually a contested issue in cases involving compensation claims, it is important to rely on "primary sources." That is, one should obtain, or have the attorney involved in the case obtain, official transcripts of school records directly from the schools.

Employment Records

The purpose of reviewing employment records is to obtain the same type of information about a patient's work history that was described earlier. Employment files are generally less standardized than school records, and it is, therefore, important to know what type of records one should request. Useful ones include a chronological record of job appointment, promotions, transfers, and termination of employment; wage records; leave use records; job descriptions, at least for the highest level or most recent position; records of on-the-job and inservice training received; and performance evaluations.

Many people who have had military service have copies of their discharge papers available for examination. Such forms include information about the length of service; type of discharge; rank at the time of discharge; "time lost," which refers to the results of disciplinary actions; duties of the last position held, which is listed as military occupational specialty (MOS); and service schools attended. In many cases a review of this record is adequate. In some cases, however, copies of official and more detailed records sent directly to an attorney should be reviewed.

Employment records may be difficult to obtain, or may even be nonexistent, for some people. These include people who have been self-employed or employed by small businesses that do not keep detailed records, and some professionals. In compensation cases where the stakes are high, the level of success in self-employment may be verified through tax records. In cases of employment by a small business it may be possible to interview the employer or supervisor by telephone. And in cases of some professions and licensed occupations it is possible to verify, at least, the possession of a license. This can usually be done by a phone call to the appropriate regulatory agency. In the case of a patient who claimed that he was an attorney a call to the Bar Association not only verified that fact, but also produced the information that he had been suspended for nonpayment of renewal fees for the past 2 years, which shed additional light on the course of his illness.

To summarize, no clinical neuropsychological evaluation is adequate or complete if it is based only on test data. Information obtained from observing the patient's behavior and interviewing the patient and others must always be considered. In many cases, particularly those involving compensation claims, a variety of records must also be reviewed. If these things are not done, conclusions about diagnoses and implications for everyday functioning and rehabilitation are likely to be faulty.

Chapter 11

Neuropsychological Rehabilitation

Background

The purpose of this chapter is to provide an introduction to this rapidly developing new aspect of clinical neuropsychology. The history and background of these developments will be reviewed briefly. A framework for conceptualizing an approach to cognitive rehabilitation will be proposed, and the major areas of cognitive deficits that are frequently treated will be discussed. Some of the treatment tools that are frequently used today will be described, and two illustrative rehabilitation cases will be presented. An attempt at comprehensive coverage is not intended; the field has expanded and continues to change too much and too rapidly to allow that within the confines of a single chapter. It is, instead, intended to elucidate some principles that should prove to be enduring and to identify some techniques that appear to have promise in the rehabilitation of certain cognitive deficits.

While focusing on teaching a method for interpretation of neuropsychological data for diagnostic purposes Jarvis & Barth (1984) identified the importance of going beyond that to the identification of the implications for treatment and rehabilitation:

> ...the evaluation and description of neuropathology is one step in an extensive process aimed at delineating a patient's cognitive and behavioral strengths and weaknesses, so that appropriate treatment and rehabilitation may be initiated. (p. 2)

The implications for daily functioning and treatment, however, received meager treatment in Jarvis & Barth (1984, pp. 35-36), reflecting, in part at least, the state of the neuropsychological literature, if not the state of the art. This was fairly typical of the neuropsychological literature of that era. Golden's (1978) book, for example, while giving equal billing to diagnosis and rehabilitation in the title, devoted less than 18% of the text to the latter topic.

Since then, two major factors dictate more attention to this issue: Neurodiagnostic procedures, particularly the refinement and wide availability of Magnetic Resonance Imaging (MRI) (Council on Scientific Affairs, 1988) have changed so dramatically that neuropsychological *diagnostic* evaluations are much less essential, except perhaps in cases of mild head injuries and early dementia (Heinrichs, 1990).

Concurrently, there has been a major expansion in the neuropsychological literature emphasizing treatment and rehabilitation. The number of articles about treatment and rehabilitation of brain-injured patients in general psychological and neuropsychological journals has increased significantly, and new journals such as *Cognitive Rehabilitation* and *The Journal of Head Trauma Rehabilitation* have appeared. Major books such as *Neuropsychological Rehabilitation* (Meier, Benton, & Diller, 1987) and *Introduction to Cognitive Rehabilitation* (Sohlberg & Mateer, 1989) now make frequent appearances in publisher's catalogs.

Conceptualization of the Rehabilitation Process

The goal of rehabilitation is to return the patient to the highest level of independent functioning and the best quality of life that are possible. There are three different approaches to this: (1) The first choice of both therapists and patients is usually to *restore functioning* to its premorbid level. A model for this is the use of exercise to restore functioning following neuromuscular injuries. (2) When restoration is not possible, efforts may be directed toward teaching patients to use *alternate behaviors to compensate* for lost or damaged functions. Teaching manual sign language to deaf people is a common example of this approach. (3) The third approach is to provide *external aids or substitutes* for the lost or damaged part of the body. There are many common examples of this approach ranging from the use of prostheses to replace lost limbs to the use of corrective lenses to improve vision. As specific cognitive deficits and treatment tools are discussed in this chapter reference will be made to this system of classification.

There is widespread agreement that a comprehensive neuropsychological evaluation, which identifies cognitive assets as well as deficits, is an essential first step in planning for rehabilitation (e.g., Bennett, 1988; Gianutsos & Matheson, 1987; Goldstein, 1987; Jarvis, 1988; Lezak, 1987a; Reitan & Wolfson, 1988a). For example, Bennett (1988) has outlined detailed hypotheses regarding the relationships between performance on the Halstead-Reitan Battery and Wisconsin Card Sorting Test and the following functional areas: Sensory Input, Attention and Concentration, Learning and Memory, Language, and Executive Functions.

An assessment of other characteristics of the person's behavior and environment is also needed. Individual factors such as energy level, stamina, frustration tolerance, emotional lability, impulse control, initiative; and environmental factors such as amount of structure, demands for performance, and potential for constructive change in both physical and social factors should be considered. Jarvis and Barth (1979) and Jarvis and Vollman (1983) have identified the importance of identifying these types of psychosocial factors.

Following the neuropsychological evaluation, it is necessary to inform or educate patients and families about the findings and their implications. They may be unaware of some deficits that are responsible for significant behavioral deficiencies. O. M., who is described in Rehabilitation Case 2, was unaware that it was a severe visual field loss that interfered with his ability to read. In some cases an explanation of the nature of a deficit and simple advise about how to compensate for it are sufficient to produce satisfactory improvement in behavior as was the case with the patient R. D., described by Gianutsos and Matheson (1987). In other cases the deficits are less obvious or patients' and families' denial of losses is so great that more extensive education is required. Showing them the profile resulting from the neuropsychological evaluation, having the patient repeat tests that demonstrate specific deficits, and demonstrating how the deficits shown on tests are related to performance of important tasks may all be helpful. However it is accomplished, understanding of deficits and how rehabilitation tasks and everyday functioning are related to them will improve patients' participation in rehabilitation programs.

Few patients will have a single deficit; most will have many. It is futile to attempt a "shotgun approach" in which one attempts to address all of a patient's deficits at once. It is also useless to attempt to remediate higher-order deficits such as certain executive functions when more basic cognitive functions such as attention are so deficient that a patient cannot even attempt the tasks intended to treat the higher-order deficit. In addition, deficits in some basic skills such as perception and attention may result in *apparent* deficits in areas such as practic abilities and memory (Gianutsos & Matheson, 1987). Unless the deficits in basic skills are addressed first, treatment of the others will be unsuccessful or, at best, unnecessarily prolonged and difficult.

It is necessary to prioritize deficits in the order in which they need to be addressed. Reitan and Wolfson (1988a, 1988b) have suggested one simple model for doing this. Their model identifies the primacy of intact sensory input, which must lead to adequate attention, concentration, and memory. These are prerequisites for the use of language and other "practic" skills, which are in turn required for adequate concept formation, reasoning, and logical analysis. Bracy (1984) suggests a somewhat more detailed model that relies on a hierarchy of "twenty four basic cognitive abilities." The influence of Luria's concept of "functional systems" is apparent in many current approaches to such prioritization, and a familiarity with it (Luria, 1963, 1966, 1977) should assist therapists in developing individual rehabilitation plans. Approaches that have been used in attempts to treat some of the most common cognitive deficits are discussed in the next section.

Treatment of Specific Deficits

Disorders of Attention/Concentration

Although there are probably no "pure" tests of attention, a number of neuropsychologists (e.g., Bennett, 1988; Lezak, 1983; Reitan & Wolfson, 1988; Sohlberg & Mateer, 1989) have suggested that a variety of tests such as the Seashore Rhythm Test, the Speech Sounds Perception Test, and the Digit Span Subtest of the WAIS-R have a major attentional requirement. Since these tests all have differing requirements for attention, as well as requirements for other cognitive abilities, performance on them should be examined carefully to assess impairment of attention.

It is generally agreed that adequate attention and concentration are the foundation on which all other cognitive functions must rest (e.g., Bracy, 1984; Lezak, 1983; Posner & Rafal, 1987; Reitan & Wolfson, 1988a). Benedict (1989) reviewed the effectiveness of a wide range of cognitive remediation strategies. Although he notes a number of methodological problems with the studies he reviewed, he concludes that attention and speed of processing may be improved by repeated practice of appropriate training tasks.

Ben-Yishay et al. (1987) have described the Orientation Remediation Module (ORM) developed by the NYU group for treatment of attention disorders. This consists of five tasks arranged in a hierarchy to train patients to: (1) attend to and respond to environmental stimuli, (2) time responses to environmental cues, (3) be actively vigilant, (4) estimate time, and (5) synchronize responses with complex rhythms. They indicate that training on the ORM has led to improvement on psychological tests that have a significant attentional component and appears to generalize to other functional behaviors. They state that a computerized version of the ORM has been developed and point out the advantages of such a tool, although this version of the ORM does not appear to be widely available at this point. In its absence, the direct application of much of the work of the NYU group has been limited because the ORM relies on "tailor-designed electronic gadgets" (Ben-Yishay, et al., 1987, p. 166).

Benedict (1989) notes that performance feedback and reinforcement play significant roles in improving performance on attention tasks. Since computers are well suited to provide feedback and immediate reinforcement, it follows that the use of computer programs may be quite helpful in restoring adequate attention, and it is not surprising that most of the Computer Assisted Cognitive Retraining (CACR) programs include attention training modules (e.g., Bracy, 1989; Gianutsos & Klitzner, 1981; Sbordone, 1987).

Studies using the single case experimental design such as the ones reported by Gray and Robertson (1989) in which attention training with CACR programs resulted in improvement of specific attentional skills support this use of CACR. Sohlberg and Mateer (1989) report similar findings using a combination of computer programs from different sources and paper-and-pencil tasks along with specially designed audio tapes. Niemann, Ruff, and Baser (1990) report a study in which an experimental group received attention training using Sbordone's "Digit-Digit Attention Test" computer program (Sbordone, Seecof, & Hall, 1983) among other attention training tasks while a control group received compensatory memory training. The performance of the experimental group improved on post-training measures of both attention and memory while the control group, which had memory training, failed to show any improvement on post-test measures of attention. This lends support to the hypothesis that attentional skills are prerequisites for other skills such as memory. There is, therefore, considerable evidence that the area of attention is one in which restoration appears to be a reasonable goal for some patients.

Visual Perceptual Disorders

Visual perceptual disorders may be demonstrated on a variety of assembly tasks such as the Block Design, Object Assembly, and Picture Arrangement Subtests of the WAIS-R and design copying tasks such as those on the Aphasia Screening Test (Bennett, 1988; Gianutsos & Matheson, 1987; Reitan & Wolfson, 1988a; Sohlberg & Mateer, 1989). Since these tests all have a practic component to them, it is necessary to distinguish between it and the perceptual component. The Benton Judgment of Line Orientation Test (Benton, et al., 1978) is useful in this regard.

Gianutsos and Matheson (1987) have stressed the importance of the identification and treatment of the perceptual deficits underlying defective performance on a variety of tests that have practic components. A number of the computer programs developed by the Gianutsos group have been used successfully for both diagnosis and treatment (Gianutsos & Klitzner, 1981). Robertson, Gray, and McKenzie (1988) describe the treatment of visual neglect problems using some of these programs along with the self-instructional procedures described by Meichenbaum (Meichenbaum & Goodman, 1971).

Training in visual scanning using similar programs to compensate for a visual field loss, which made functional reading impossible, is described in Rehabilitation Case 2. This is an area where teaching compensatory skills seems to be the most reasonable goal.

Disturbance of Executive Functions

The executive functions involve formulating goals, planning activities to achieve the goals, carrying out the activities, and performing the activities effectively. The issue is one of *whether or not* a person will do something (on his/her own) and *how* it will be done, not what he/she *can* do. Disturbances in executive functions, which typically result from frontal lobe damage, may render a person incapable of functioning independently and, at the same time, alienate one from others due to the resulting loss of self-care and social skills (Lezak, 1983). "Neuropsychologically, these processes involve logical analysis, concept formation, flexibility of thinking, and the ability to benefit from past trial-and-error experiences" (Bennett, 1988, p. 20). Therefore, one may expect to see evidence of deficits in executive functions manifested in impaired performance on the Category Test, the Trail Making Test, and the Wisconsin Card Sorting Test.

Benedict (1989) concludes that deficits in self-regulation skills, which are usually included among the executive functions, seem to respond best to behavior modification approaches and that long-term reliance on externally provided reinforcement is often necessary.

Sohlberg and Mateer (1989) emphasize the importance of providing a high degree of *structure* for patients in the treatment of executive function deficits. They describe a treatment program in which patients are guided through a series of six increasingly complex activities:

1. *Listing the steps in an activity.* Patients are required to list the steps required to complete an activity such as grocery shopping, washing a car, or getting ready for bed without regard for the sequence of steps.

2. *Sequencing the steps.* Patients are required to put the steps required to perform the activities in Step 1 in the proper sequence.

3. *Initiating an activity.* Patients are required to practice initiating activities such as conversations. The therapist helps patients become aware of problems in initiation of activities and provides structure for them, such as clues to initiation.

4. *Completing an errand.* Patients are required to carry out an errand such as finding out the schedule of the cashier's office or getting a bus schedule.

5. *Planning a group activity*. Patients are required to plan and carry out an activity involving the participation of one or more additional people, such as planning a birthday party for another patient.

6. *Repairing a plan*. Patients are required to "repair" or revise a plan after the therapist adds a complication to the activity planned in Step 5 (adapted from Sohlberg & Mateer, 1989, pp. 246-247).

Retraining of executive functions is obviously more complicated than retraining of attention skills, for example, and there is less clear evidence regarding the outcome of such training. It seems likely that the use of video recording and feedback would be helpful in some aspects of executive skills training such as initiating conversations, as it appears to be in social skills training. There also appears to be little evidence regarding the generalization of training in this area from one content domain to another, for example, whether training in grocery shopping enhances one's ability to cook a meal. It may well be that domain-specific training will be required for some patients; this, of course, will require a detailed analysis of the patients' individual circumstances in order to select those domains for training that will have the greatest payoff in terms of enhancing independence of functioning and quality of life. A combination of restoration of function and teaching compensatory skills is appropriate in this area.

Disturbances of Memory

The Halstead-Reitan Battery provides only a limited assessment of memory functioning. The Memory and Localization components of the TPT and Subtest 7 of the Category Test require nonverbal incidental memory, but other aspects of memory are not assessed directly. Therefore, at least one supplemental memory test such as the Russell Revision of the Wechsler Memory Scale (Russell, 1975) or the Wechsler Memory Scale-Revised (Wechsler, 1987) should be added.

Since memory deficits are among the most common results of a variety of brain injuries and often among the most severely disabling ones in terms of independent and productive functioning, this is an area of great importance to the rehabilitation neuropsychologist. Wehman et al. (1989), for example, found that memory problems were among the most common impediments to productive employment.

The study of normal memory goes back, at least, to the early years of experimental psychology, and attempts to treat disturbances in memory probably have nearly as long a history. Most of those efforts, unfortunately, are of little value to rehabilitation neuropsychologists today. While there is considerable agreement on what does not work, there is little consensus on what does work.

There is no convincing evidence that repeated practice of memory exercises based on the "memory as muscle" model is of any value. Thus, the numerous computer-assisted cognitive rehabilitation (CACR) programs, which use this approach, seem to be exercises in futility. Approximately 100 hours of practice with several such programs over a 3-month period by one patient who had severe memory problems resulting from cerebral anoxia provided some verification of this. As O'Connor and Cermak (1987) put it, "To assume that the addition of computerization to our armament of failures will result in success is ludicrous" (p. 274). In spite of this, the notion that training with a computer can "improve memory" still persists among some neuropsychologists. Twenty-nine percent (9 of 31) of the programs described by Story and Sbordone (1988), for example, as "appropriate to computer-assisted treatment of impairments of the brain injured" (p. 45) are reputed to improve memory.

Benedict (1989) concludes that mnemonic techniques such as visual imagery and the PQRST (preview, question, read actively, and test) (Barth & Boll, 1981) seem to be helpful to some patients. However, these seem to have limited value for many brain-injured patients. The PQRST technique is limited to use in improving retention of material that one reads, and it might be of some value in helping people who have only mild deficits to improve study techniques if they are going to return to school. It is not likely to be useful to people with more severe deficits.

The effectiveness of visual imagery also seems to be limited to special situations. Wilson (1987) describes three conditions limiting its use: (1) It seems to be limited to the learning of material in the "paired associate model" such as learning pairs of words or pairing faces with names; (2) a high degree of patient motivation is required, although this is probably a requirement for success with any technique; and (3) names to be learned must be taught one at a time. In addition, it appears that visual imagery is most likely to be successful when a therapist supplies or suggests the images to the patient (Wilson, 1987). This, of course, limits the patient's independence.

O'Connor and Cermak's (1987) conclusion regarding the state of the art is cautious:

> At present, rehabilitative techniques have not successfully met the needs of the memory-impaired individual. Memory improvement strategies such as the use of imagery, mnemonic devices, and external memory aids provide limited relief for memory problems. They do not, however, effect dramatic or generalized changes in memory. (p. 276)

If general recovery of memory is not feasible, patients with memory deficits may become more independent and productive if they can learn to perform specific useful tasks. The work of Schacter and others on domain specific procedural learning shows considerable promise in this regard (Schacter & Glisky, 1986). In one series of experiments severely amnestic patients were taught procedures for using an Apple computer to perform a number of operating system commands and write programs using commands such as HOME, PRINT, SAVE, LIST, and CATALOG.

Procedural learning, as implemented by Schacter, utilizes the method of vanishing cues:

> The method of vanishing cues requires the completion of a fragment on each learning trial, with the fragment cue being *reduced* gradually across trials. For example, on Trial 1 patients are exposed to a definition of a computer-related term (e.g., to store a program), and are then provided with the target word in a letter-by-letter manner until they identify it (e.g., S _ _ _; SA _ _; SAV_; SAVE). (Schacter & Glisky, 1986, p. 268)

On subsequent trials patients are able to identify the word with fewer letter cues until they can produce it without any cue, thus the "method of vanishing cues."

According to Schacter and Glisky (1986) these techniques can be used to teach patients skills in a wide range of domains including adaptive skills such as learning the names of staff in the rehabilitation setting and performing productive tasks such as household duties. Glisky and Schacter (1989) reported using this method to train a severely amnestic patient in computer data entry procedures to a level at which she was able to obtain employment. The method of vanishing cues has also been used to teach patients to remember their daily schedules in a rehabilitation program (E. Dells-Cotgageorge, personal communication, 1991). Those readers who are interested in the theoretical issues regarding procedural learning and its relationship to other memory phenomena are referred to Roediger (1990) for a recent review of the field.

It seems, in general, that the efforts of therapists and patients are better invested in developing compensatory techniques and external aids than in attempting to restore memory functioning. It is important to remember, however, that complaints of memory problems may, in some cases, actually be a result of attention deficits. Several promising approaches to teaching compensation for memory deficits are described in a subsequent section.

Behavioral/Personality Deficits

The MMPI, or MMPI-II, is often included as part of a comprehensive neuropsychological evaluation in order to assess the effects of brain injury on personality. It is also important to gather data about behavioral or emotional dysfunction from direct observation of patients in the hospital or rehabilitation center or their own home, school, or work settings. Family members often provide the best source of information about both the present and past behavior of patients in this regard (Jarvis, 1988a).

Sometimes medical specialists give brain-injured patients a "clean bill of health" when, following a brain injury, there are no longer abnormal findings on neurological examination or imaging studies such as CT or MRI scans even though the patients, and more often their families, report significant behavioral or "personality" problems. Case 2 in chapter 13 illustrates such a case. Mooney (1988) and Lezak (1987b) have indicated that personality changes may be more important than cognitive changes in determining the severity of disability.

Kreutzer, Leininger, Sherron, and Groah (1990) have described some of the common psychosocial dysfunctions resulting from brain injuries: depression, aggressive behavior, dysfunctional family systems, impaired self-awareness, and substance abuse. For each of them they list factors that lead to a high risk of occurrence, which may assist in anticipating problems during the early stages of planning for rehabilitation. They also describe the symptoms of each, which should be particularly helpful to rehabilitation workers who have limited experience with psychiatric populations, and they identify treatment considerations for each type of dysfunction.

Since some "personality problems" or psychosocial dysfunctions appear much like deficits in social skills or executive functions, it is far from clear whether it is better to approach them from a cognitive or an interpersonal perspective. Until there is evidence supporting one approach over the other, it appears wise to be aware of both approaches and to consider using them in combination.

Dunn (1987) describes an approach to social skills training that is characteristic of many such endeavors. Social skills training groups often are led by a pair of therapists so that they can model behavior for patients. Groups are usually highly structured with "lessons" prepared in advance by the therapists. They typically consist of doing things rather than talking about them, and there is an emphasis on providing feedback to people about their performance. Video recording and playback is a useful tool to enhance this. Braunling-McMorrow, Lloyd, and Fralish (1986) describe a social skills training program for brain-injured patients in which they used the table game "Sorry" as one of the tools. They reported that patients' social skills improved during the 16 sessions of treatment and generalized to other activities in the rehabilitation setting.

In addition to specialized skill training groups, more general group therapy is often believed to be beneficial for brain-injured patients. Sbordone (1990) has offered suggestions for specific techniques for each stage of recovery that appear useful in psychotherapy with brain-injured people.

Sohlberg and Mateer (1989) have listed several apparent advantages to using such groups: support, modeling, generalization, accurate self-perception, and economic therapy ratio. Just as it is in social skills training groups, a high degree of structure is important in more general therapy groups with brain-injured patients. Therapists often plan topics for discussion and provide more frequent advice and suggestions than in groups for some other types of patients. Since many brain-injured patients have attentional problems that make it difficult to follow group interactions and processes, therapists need to intervene frequently to clarify these issues. Similarly, memory problems result in a defective sense of continuity from one session to another. Because of this, it is important for therapists to begin each session with a statement of the purpose of the group, a summary of important events from past sessions, and a review of the expectations for group participation. At the end of each session the therapists should help the patients to summarize the session, highlighting what was learned and how participants can use it outside of the group. Many of these techniques are similar to those used by Yalom (1983) in his "focus groups."

Individual psychotherapy may also be helpful to some brain-injured patients, and it, too, usually needs to be highly structured and directive. For the most severely impaired patients behavioral techniques such as contingency contracting may be needed to increase the frequency of adaptive behaviors. Social skills, for example, may be improved in this way. Grief work to assist in coping with losses resulting from brain injury may be helpful to some patients. While psychodynamically oriented therapy is probably not helpful for most brain-injured patients, cognitive behavioral approaches can be helpful for some less severely impaired patients.

Family therapy is an important part of the treatment of brain-injured patients. If it is not provided, many patients will not be able to readjust to living outside of the hospital or rehabilitation center, and many families will needlessly disintegrate. A primary need of families is information. Just as brain-injured patients need education about the effects of their injuries, their families need it, perhaps even more than the patients themselves. Without accurate information families may show one of two extreme attitudes toward the injured family member. Some, especially when the patient has no obvious physical deficits, may assume that nothing is wrong with the him/her and believe he/she is just lazy, obstinate, or looking for sympathy. Others may assume that the patient is unable to do anything independently, and foster a high degree of dependency. Eisner and Kreutzer (1989) have described a number of useful sources of information for families that can assist them in making a constructive adjustment to the brain injury of a family member.

Just as some brain-injured patients need help with grief over the loss of functions, grief over the loss of the person who was father, mother, child, or spouse is an issue for many families. The former parent, child, or spouse is gone, and a different person has been sent to them by the hospital. Similarly, they may now be unable to meet the requirements of the earlier role and, instead, now end up in a more dependent role. When this happens, the whole family needs help in exploring the feelings about this and reintegrating into a new family with meaningful new roles for everyone.

Family intervention is often best accomplished in multiple-family groups, which may be available in rehabilitation centers that treat a number of brain-injured patients. For the therapist who is not working in such a center, referral of families to support groups provided by local chapters of the National Head Injury Foundation, National Multiple Sclerosis Society, Parkinson's Disease Foundation, and others may accomplish some of the same goals.

Most of the approaches used in treating personality problems and behavioral deficits involve teaching compensatory skills, although some restoration of functioning may be possible.

Rehabilitation Tools

The preceding section mentioned several different types of tools that have been used in the treatment of different cognitive deficits. In this section a sample of the ones that may be most useful and available to the neuropsychologist will be described in more detail. Techniques that require highly specialized, expensive, or custom-made equipment are not described.

Computer-Assisted Cognitive Rehabilitation (CACR)

The most recent addition to cognitive rehabilitation tools has been the microcomputer. This has allowed widespread dissemination of specific rehabilitation procedures (computer programs) among different rehabilitation programs. It also makes replication of research findings more feasible in comparison to the specialized, custom-made tools used in some programs. Unfortunately, this research development has not yet occurred to the extent one might have hoped for. Many programs described as useful in CACR have been marketed widely without any research data to support their clinical use.

In any event, the microcomputer is very much a part of cognitive rehabilitation today. It may have arrived when Lynch (1983a) made the "discovery" in 1978 that his head-injured patients seemed to receive cognitive benefits from recreational use of Atari video games. Since then, CACR has become a growth industry within the field of rehabilitation. The early history of this, reviewed by Bracy, Lynch, Sbordone, and Berrol (1985), shows a close tie to academic psychology and neuropsychology in the early work of

Rosamond Gianutsos who extended her early use of computers to evaluate visual functioning into cognitive retraining (Gianutsos & Matheson, 1987).

There are many different sources of software for therapists who want to explore the use of CACR as a rehabilitation tool. One of the factors to consider in selecting CACR software is whether or not one wants to rely on a single "package," which is said to provide a comprehensive training program or system or to select individual programs from different sources to train patients in specific areas. In addition to comprehensive CACR systems, there are programs that address broad areas such as language problems, and there are a number of sources of individual programs, each aimed at specific deficits.

It is not possible in this overview to provide more than a broad picture of the many types of programs that have been proposed for use in CACR because they are changing so rapidly, but some of the more widely used ones have been described by Bracy (1989), Gianutsos and Matheson (1987), Sbordone (1987), and Smith (1984). Lynch (1983b) has also described the use of general purpose programs such as word processing programs and speed reading programs in cognitive rehabilitation. Finally, there are thousands of video games and educational programs in the public domain, but most of them need to be modified for use in CACR since they are lacking in the user friendliness that is essential for CACR clients. Jarvis (1990) has described some of the problems this lack causes for patients and suggested ways of correcting them. Several important features of some of the widely used programs are listed in Table 5.

Unfortunately, there is no adequate catalog or directory of CACR software. Kreutzer, Hill, and Morrison (1987) prepared a guide to CACR software, but it was far from complete at the time of publication, and it is now out of print.

If CACR stands the test of time and rigorous outcome research, a comprehensive, periodically updated directory of available software will be a necessary tool for therapists. The (Buros) Mental Measurement Yearbook (Conoley & Kramer, 1989) with it's reviews of psychological tests by independent reviewers might serve as a useful model. It would seem most useful if it were published by an organization that does not have potentially conflicting interests in marketing software. Considering the content of such a directory, publication in the form of a computer data base file might be particularly effective.

Although microcomputers will undoubtedly prove to be useful tools in rehabilitation of brain-injured patients, it is important to view this in a realistic context. Their use in education provides one possible perspective. A few years ago some radical computer advocates suggested that the roles of classroom teachers would soon be drastically curtailed. While some teachers use computers today in creative ways to improve the education they provide, that revolution has not come about. It seems possible, in fact, that a backlash against the radical proposals has limited to some extent the changes that have occurred. This, if it happened, represents a loss, but it is clear that computers cannot replace the human element that teachers provide in education. Similarly, neuropsychologists and other rehabilitation professionals must recognize that computers, by themselves, will not rehabilitate brain-injured patients. Their use in CACR can provide a tool that may be a useful part of the overall rehabilitation program.

Table 5
Features of Selected CACR Software

Author/ Source	Program Coverage	Content Areas	User Modifiable?	Color/ Sound?	User Instructions?	Research Base
Bracy	CP	Attention, visual/spatial, memory, problem solving, conceptual	No	Yes	Yes	Limited
Gianutsos	SD	Visual/spatial, scanning, attention, memory	Some are	No/ Yes	Yes	More adequate than most
J. Smith	SD	Wide variety of language skills	Includes authoring program**	No/ Yes	Yes	Limited
Sbordone	SD	Attention, problem solving	No	Yes	Yes	Limited
Various General Purpose	IT	Speed reading, word processing, etc.	No	Varies	Not for use in CACR	None
Public Domain	IT	Educational and video games	Yes (Most require major modification)	Varies	Not for use in CACR	None

CP   Described as providing a Comprehensive CACR Program.

SD   Described as providing training for Specific Deficits.

IT   Specific use must be identified by each therapist.

**   The Authoring Program allows therapists to "write" specific lessons for individual patients.

The Functions of the Computer and the Therapist

One useful way of conceptualizing the computer-therapist relationship in CACR is to visualize the computer's functions from an operant behavioral perspective and the therapist's functions from a cognitive behavioral perspective. From this point of view the Operant Computer presents stimuli to the patient, records the patient's responses, provides immediate feedback regarding the accuracy of responses and appropriate reinforcement, and stores and summarizes data about patient performance. The advantages provided by computers in performing these functions are significant. Stimuli can be presented with complete consistency in whatever pattern the therapist, or programer, specifies and for as many repetitions as are required. Provision of feedback and reinforcement is completely consistent and reliable. Similarly, the storage and summarization of data are automatic and reliable while the human therapist is free to concentrate on other functions. Finally, in comparison to some of the rehabilitation tasks, which have used custom-built electrical/mechanical devices, tasks presented on microcomputers can be transported on disks from one laboratory or rehabilitation center to another with ease and accuracy.

Human therapists, free of many of the repetitive tasks performed by the computer, can perform other functions. First, they must select the specific software that will elicit the desired response behavior from the patient and shape it in the desired manner. They must observe patients' behavior, make judgements about factors such as motivation and fatigue, and intervene appropriately with social reinforcement for example. It is also clear that teaching of self-instructional techniques (Meichenbaum & Goodman, 1971) by therapists enhances learning with CACR. Therapists also need to look for patterns in patients' behavior such as their responses to their errors. They should then explore with the patients the meaning of the behavior and assist them in identifying and implementing more adaptive ways of accomplishing the rehabilitation tasks. Finally, they need to help patients generalize the skills they learn in using the computer to other "real world" tasks.

Other Electronic Tools

The ready availability of microcomputers led to the development of CACR programs to assist in restoring some cognitive functions and helping to compensate for deficits in others. Similarly, the current proliferation of pocket-sized and smaller electronic devices, which include programable data bases, now opens the way for their use as compensatory memory tools. There are devices that will allow storage of a variety of types of information including names, addresses, phone numbers, and schedules. Some also include programable alarm clocks to provide reminders to check the schedule, take medications, and so forth. Costs range from about $10 to several hundred dollars depending on the versatility of the products and the rapidly changing market. As new, more sophisticated products are developed, older ones rapidly decline in price. Parente and Anderson-Parente (1990) have described a number of potentially useful electronic tools and provide information about sources for some of them. Because of the rapidly changing technology, the best advice one can give therapists about selection in this situation may be to study current advertising and shop the discount stores. Even some of the relatively simple, inexpensive devices can be adapted to the needs of many patients, especially if they are used in conjunction with that rehabilitation therapist's old standby, a pocket notebook that includes a calendar, schedule, and section for listing other information.

A major problem with the use of some of these devices as rehabilitation tools is the complexity of the procedures required to store and retrieve information, or to program them. Bracy et al. (1990) attempts to address this problem by developing the "Computer Assisted Memory (CAM) System." This uses a multisection notebook in which a variety of information is recorded in conjunction with a credit card size device, which includes a programable database and alarm clock. As is often the case with the smallest devices, the programing of it is complicated. Consequently, the CAM System includes a series of 30 detailed lessons for the patient and an Instructor's Manual. A description of treatment outcome research with the CAM System would have enhanced its usefulness.

Therapists who want to explore this approach might consider designing their own "system" based on a simple programable alarm and a notebook, which contains sections that indicate what should be done each time the alarm sounds, and lists of important information such as names, addresses, and phone numbers. The information provided could be tailored to specific patient needs, and procedures for using the system could be taught using the method of vanishing cues. The effectiveness of this should then, of course, be evaluated using the single case experiment method (e.g., Gianutsos & Gianutsos, 1987). Sohlberg and Mateer (1989) have described a "Memory Notebook" that can be customized for individual patients and a method for teaching the use of it. An individual notebook might contain sections for (a) personal data, (b) calendar and schedule, (c) maps and directions, (d) names and identifying information, and (e) instructions for performing important tasks. The utility of such a system might be enhanced through the addition of an inexpensive electronic device with a programable alarm and/or database. Such electronic tools are clearly external aids and do not take the place of thoughtful therapeutic intervention.

Other Non-Electronic Tools

Although the lure of electronic technology is seductive, it is important to recognize that some rehabilitation tasks can be presented more simply, less expensively, and sometimes more effectively using more "primitive" tools.

One of the simplest techniques is to modify the environment so that external cues are always available. The possibilities are limited only by the creativity of the therapist who takes the time to observe patients in their natural environments and identifies the problems that are created by the interaction of the patients' deficits and features of the environment. Examples include creating environmental features such as a prominently placed bulletin board, which contains schedules and messages, rearranging and labeling shelves, using painted outlines of tools on a board where they will be hung, and posting step-by-step instructions for the use of appliances such as a washing machine or dishwasher on the wall next to each appliance.

Kreutzer, Wehman, Morton, and Stonnington (1988) describe a process for the development of compensatory tools to be used in vocational settings. The three steps in the process are: (1) a neuropsychological evaluation to identify cognitive deficits and strengths, (2) an analysis of the tasks to be performed by the client, and (3) development of a series of detailed instructions or materials that will assist in accomplishing the tasks. This process can obviously be used to assist people in carrying out a variety of self-care and independent living tasks as well as vocational ones.

A specific problem that some people who have right-cerebral hemisphere lesions have in finding their way around (Vogenthaler, 1987) provides another example of a problem that may be better treated by using less exotic, nonelectronic methods. Wilson (1987) reports her attempts to teach F. D. (who had suffered a right posterior CVA) several commonly traveled routes within the hospital using four procedures during 6 weeks of training: extra rehearsal, essentially traveling the routes repeatedly; a "fading procedure," following a chalk line, which was gradually rubbed out; a "letter sequencing cue," in which he was to go from A to B, and so forth, which were letters chalked on the wall along the route; and a "letter-word mnemonic strategy," in which he was supposed to use the aid "**ReaL** **E**mergency" (with the letters R, L, and E highlighted) to help him remember to turn right, then left, and then to go through the "Emergency Exit." Wilson apparently considered this attempt at training to be a failure: "He was never able to go straight to any destination without reading signs, responding to cues, or looking in his notebook for directions" (Wilson, 1987, p. 141).

This apparent failure may be instructive. First, it appears that Wilson attempted to teach F. D. several different routes simultaneously. This may have been too much information for him to learn at once, and there may have been interference effects. It appears to be more effective if a brain-injured patient is taught one task at a time, and additional tasks are only introduced after earlier ones have been learned thoroughly. Second, instead of considering behavior such as responding to cues and using a notebook for directions to be a sign of failure, perhaps patients should be *taught* to do these things. If they learn to follow a route using these aids, they may eventually be able to "fade" or drop them. This is, in fact, what people who have not had brain injuries often do in learning new complicated routes, consult a map the first few times the route is traveled, and then refer to it less frequently, but keep it handy in case they forget part of the route.

Georgemiller and Hassan (1986) suggest that people with route-learning deficits due to right-hemisphere lesions may be assisted by the use of sequential verbal instructions as opposed to visual maps. This led to the development of the "Verbal Map" tool by Jarvis and Hamlin (1991), which has been described in the following 12 steps:

1. Choose a common route that is troublesome for the patient (e.g., from the patient's bedroom to the dining room or occupational therapy area).

2. Walk through the route with the patient, identifying the starting point, all choice points such as turns, and the end point or destination.

3. At the starting point, all choice points, and destination ask the patient to stop, look around, and identify a visible "marker," which he/she can label (e.g., a phone booth or a fire extinguisher on the wall), and the instructions to be executed at that point (e.g., turn right).

4. Each time the patient is to turn, have him/her pat the appropriate thigh while verbalizing the instructions. Model this, "Turn right," while patting your right thigh.

5. Print the "verbal map" as a series of instructions that will direct the patient from one visual marker to the next until the destination is reached. "When you see x, do y." For example, A. Go to the door of your room and find the phone booth. B. Walk to the phone booth. C. When you get there, pat your left thigh and turn left. D. Walk to the Exit sign, and so forth.

6. Walk through the route behind the patient, listening to make certain that the "verbal map" is complete and accurate and that the patient vocalizes the instructions and gives the appropriate motor cues, thigh pats, at each turn correctly. (It is important for the therapist to be aware that those of us without perceptual-spatial deficits may have difficulty conceptualizing the task of getting from Point A to Point B without using perceptual-spatial cues.)

7. Have the patient travel the route regularly using the "verbal map" as a guide and evaluate the ability to do this accurately.

8. Once the patient is able to do this accurately and efficiently, begin to wean him/her from the use of the printed "verbal map" and rely on the memory of it in order to increase independence of functioning.

9. Teach the patient how to reverse the map to get back to the original starting point. Some patients may be able to learn this fairly easily; for others it may be necessary to repeat the first eight steps in the reverse direction. This is important to give a sense of "spatial security."

10. Repeat the first nine steps to teach the patient how to travel a different, more complex route to a different destination.

11. After the patient has learned how to use "verbal maps" well, teach the patient and family members how to *create* new ones, using steps 1 through 9, so that the technique can be used in a variety of different situations after the patient leaves the rehabilitation center.

12. Follow up with the patient and family to see whether they need any assistance in adapting the technique to their unique circumstances. (pp. 51-52)

Any attempt to use this technique should be preceded by a thorough neuropsychological evaluation that identifies the patient's strengths as well as deficits. For patients with adequate left-hemisphere dependent cognitive functions such as verbal memory the steps described above may be adequate. O. M., whose treatment is described in Rehabilitation Case 2, and who had suffered a right posterior CVA and had a pattern of deficits similar to Wilson's (1987) patient F. D., learned to use this technique quite effectively as it is described. For patients with additional problems it may be helpful to add tactile and kinesthetic cues by adding the use of a three-dimensional model for the patient to practice tracing the route by hand between Steps 2 and 3.

Reitan has developed a unique system called the Reitan Evaluation of Hemispheric Abilities and Brain Improvement Training (REHABIT) System, which is said to provide a comprehensive rehabilitation "package" (Reitan & Wolfson, 1988a, 1988b). Following a neuropsychological evaluation with the Halstead Reitan Neuropsychological Battery, patients are retrained with the more than 250 training items of REHABIT, which are organized in five "Tracks" that cover areas such as language skills, abstract reasoning, organization, planning, visual-spatial, sequential, and manipulatory skills. Reports of research on REHABIT (Reitan & Wolfson, 1988b; Sena, 1985, 1986; Sena & Sena, 1986a, 1986b), while less comprehensive than those of the NYU group's reports on the ORM, for example, are more extensive than research reported on many of the computer-assisted techniques.

The tools described in this section are either ones that teach compensatory skills or provide external aids, although REHABIT is claimed to provide some restoration of function.

Comprehensive Rehabilitation Programs

Many of the tools described can be used by neuropsychologists with patients who are seen in general clinical settings such as mental health centers, psychiatric or general hospitals, or even private offices (Sbordone, 1987). In recent years, however, there has been an increasing recognition that some brain-injured patients are treated most effectively in specialized rehabilitation programs staffed with multidisciplinary teams of rehabilitation professionals. Treatment in such settings may have several advantages: (a) the specialized expertise of many different rehabilitation professionals can be focused on the patients' needs, (b) individual rehabilitation programs may be developed to meet each patient's unique needs, and (c) patients with similar experiences and problems may be helpful to each other in terms of confronting destructive denial and supporting each other in their struggles in rehabilitation.

The brain injury rehabilitation program at New York University Medical Center Institute of Rehabilitation was one of the earliest and most innovative programs. Barth and Boll (1981) indicate that the NYU group includes a "behaviorally oriented engineer" who designs the rehabilitation tasks and the devices that patients use to execute them. In addition to numerous paper-and-pencil tasks these include various electrical and mechanical devices such as timers and an electronic adaptation of the Purdue Peg Board (Ben-Yishay et al., 1978). The work of this group has been extremely influential in shaping both research and theory about cognitive rehabilitation. It has probably not, however, seen a great deal of direct application in the everyday practice of the majority of clinical neuropsychologists because many of the rehabilitation tasks require highly specialized equipment, which has not been marketed by the NYU group.

Kreutzer et al. (1988) and Wehman and Kreutzer (1990) have described a comprehensive rehabilitation program that focuses specifically on returning brain-injured people to productive employment. An important feature of their program is "supported employment" in which a "job coach" selects appropriate jobs; develops necessary modifications of tasks and compensatory techniques; and works with the patient, supervisors, and peers on the job to assist in integrating the patient into the job setting. It appears that this approach could also be adapted to assist brain-injured people to resume constructive roles in their family homes or in group living settings.

There have been many recent descriptions of other comprehensive rehabilitation programs for brain-injured patients. Caplan (1987) and Meier et al. (1987), for example, include descriptions of several exemplary ones. These programs are typically multidisciplinary in nature. The core disciplines include the medical specialties of neurology and physiatry (rehabilitation medicine, physical therapy, occupational therapy, speech therapy, social work, and psychology, including neuropsychology and behavioral psychology). Others that may be included, depending on both the nature of patient needs and program directors' biases, are psychiatry, education, recreational therapy, vocational rehabilitation or therapy, and optometry or opthalmology.

The medical director of a program may be either a neurologist or a physiatrist. When the program treats mainly patients who are in the acute stage following brain injury a neurologist's diagnostic skills may be most important. Somewhat later in the recovery process a physiatrist's diagnosis of functional physical deficits and strengths and prescribed interventions play greater roles.

Many people who have experienced brain injuries suffer from physical disabilities, either as a result of injury to the motor component of the central nervous system or from direct injury to other parts of the body sustained at the same time. Motor vehicle accidents, the most frequent cause of head injuries, often result in multiple injuries. Therefore, the role of the physical therapist in promoting recovery of or compensation for lost function is essential. A recent development is the use of computer-assisted biofeedback to augment traditional physical therapy procedures (Gianutsos & Eberstein, 1987).

Occupational therapists evaluate patients' abilities to perform broad categories of tasks ranging from activities of daily living such as bathing, dressing, and feeding themselves to more complex or advanced tasks such as cooking, shopping, doing laundry, and driving a car. While they consider cognitive as well as physical aspects of these tasks, their focus is somewhat different from that of the neuropsychologist. The neuropsychologist looks at component cognitive skills that underly the abilities to perform many different tasks, while the occupational therapist focuses on specific tasks and the cognitive requirements of them. This difference carries over into the area of intervention. The neuropsychologist may provide general cognitive retraining to improve a skill such as visual scanning, which is needed to perform many different tasks. In contrast, the occupational therapist may teach patients to dress themselves or prepare meals, both of which require adequate visual scanning. Occupational therapists also include in their evaluations those features of a patient's environment that affect their ability to perform important tasks and include modifications of the environment in their interventions to a much greater extent than neuropsychologists typically do.

Speech therapists are, perhaps, best known for their work in treating verbal or expressive language deficits, but they also treat receptive disorders. Some speech therapists also address the social aspects of speech and language (pragmatics), and these merge with the area of social skills training, which is practiced by some behavioral psychologists.

Social workers may provide a number of services that can be encompassed under the term *case management*. These include evaluation of family, community, and financial factors influencing a patient's disability and rehabilitation. The social worker, as case manager, is often the person who finds many of the resources needed by patients and their families and coordinates their implementation. The social worker may also be the member of the rehabilitation team who provides counseling or psychotherapy for families of patients.

Hopefully, the major contributions of neuropsychologists to the rehabilitation team, in terms of assessment and cognitive retraining, are reasonably clear by now. There is one additional function, which is too often overlooked: In a field that is changing as rapidly as the rehabilitation of brain injury, it is essential that treatment techniques be evaluated. Which ones work, and which ones do not work? Which work better with one type of patient, and which work better with another type? The questions go on and on, and third-party payers are asking for more and better answers. The immense number of the factors, and the complex interaction of them, that result in the unique patterns of deficits and assets shown by individual brain-injured patients make it highly unlikely that large N studies of between group treatment effects will produce many useful answers to these questions. Instead, single-case experimental studies are needed. Gianutsos and Gianutsos (1987); Gray and Robertson (1989); Robertson et al. (1988); and Sohlberg and Mateer (1989), among others, provide excellent examples of the use of this methodology in brain-injury rehabilitation programs.

Behavioral psychologists may provide services in a number of different areas including improvement of medication compliance, increasing the frequency of adaptive behavior, and decreasing or extinguishing maladaptive behavior. In fact, a whole rehabilitation program may be based primarily on operant behavioral principles (Levenkron, 1987). Social skills training, which is needed by many brain-injured patients, particularly those with significant frontal lobe damage, is also among the techniques used by some behavioral psychologists (Dunn, 1987).

The inclusion of other professionals, sometimes on a part-time or consultant basis, in a rehabilitation program depends to some extent on the types of patients treated and on how broadly trained some of the other team members are. The services of a psychiatrist may be needed for severely depressed patients, for example, or one of the other physicians may treat them with psychiatric consultation. A special education teacher is called for if brain-injured children are treated and may be helpful with some other patients. A recreational therapist may provide education for patients in use of leisure time and assist with community reentry if the occupational therapist is not skilled in these areas. For patients with prospects of returning to employment a vocational rehabilitation specialist may assist with skill training, work habit training, and job hardening, counseling and placement. Finally, an optometrist or opthalmologist may be needed, on a consulting basis, to evaluate and correct some visual problems (Gianutsos & Matheson, 1987).

Illustrative Cases

The following two cases are presented to illustrate a number of the issues that have been discussed in this chapter. Both of these people were patients in a psychiatric hospital at the time they were first seen for neuropsychological evaluation.

Case 1

L. G. was a 23-year-old, white, right-handed female who was referred for neuropsychological evaluation to assist in clarifying diagnosis and plan treatment. Her affect was depressed, and her behavior was very childlike, with temper tantrums and self-destructive behavior when she did not get her own way. She was very deficient in even basic self-care skills. Her speech was described as "very immature," difficult to understand at times, with defective grammatical structure and apparent word-finding problems. She was unable to read above second or third grade level, recite the alphabet, or calculate even simple arithmetic problems. There was controversy over whether she had a "genuine" seizure disorder or whether her apparent seizures were "malingering" or "temper tantrums." Neurological examinations, including EEG studies, had been inconclusive. Although the history indicated that she had suffered a closed head injury in a rock climbing accident while in college 2 years earlier, few details of the injury had been obtained, and it had, for the most part, been ignored as a factor in understanding her behavior.

Neuropsychological evaluation resulted in a Halstead Impairment Index of 0.8, a Verbal IQ of 69, Performance IQ of 66, and a Full Scale IQ of 66 with evidence of more impairment of the left-cerebral hemisphere than of the right hemisphere. After it became clear that L. G. did, in fact, have evidence of significant brain damage, an EEG was obtained during the course of one sustained seizure. This resulted in a persistent effort to control the seizures with medication.

A rehabilitation plan was developed, which first used Bracy's (1989) and Gianutsos' (Gianutsos & Klitzner, 1981) CACR software to improve severely deficient attention and concentration. Later, Smith's (1984) software was used to improve language skills. For several months L. G. worked 1 hour a day 4 or 5 days a week with the therapist always present. Initial work was with programs designed to improve attention and concentration. A review of the patient's progress revealed that after a brief period of improvement, her reaction time on attention programs failed to show the continuing improvement that was expected, although she never made any errors. When this was explored with her, it became clear that she was very fearful about making errors in anything she did. Programs with variable speeds that forced her to make some errors at higher speeds were then introduced. Manipulation of the speed of these programs helped her increase her tolerance for making errors and learn adaptive responses to them. During the latter part of this period the therapist introduced a variety of language skill programs, and L. G.'s reading and spelling abilities improved dramatically.

A repeat neuropsychological evaluation about 9 months after the initial evaluation and just prior to L.G.'s discharge from the hospital showed a Halstead Impairment Index of 0.4, a Verbal IQ of 88, Performance IQ of 97, and a Full Scale IQ of 91. Her performance on Part B of the Trail Making Test, however, failed to improve. The therapist then realized that, although L.G.'s reading skill had improved, she had never relearned the sequence of the letters in the alphabet. She relearned this sequence and learned to alphabetize lists of 20 eight-letter words with no errors in about 2 weeks using the computer.

Following this evaluation L. G. was discharged from the hospital, and she was followed as an outpatient while continuing in the CACR Program 2-3 hours a day, 4 days a week. For the next year and a half she worked quite independently most of the time on assignments given to her by the therapist who spent 1-2 hours a week with her. Her language skills continued to improve, and she used a word processing program to write letters, which were generally at about "high school" level. She sometimes answered the phone in the office and wrote down messages reliably and accurately. Approximately 2 years after discharge from the hospital L. G. wrote an article about her rehabilitation, which was published, after only minimal editing, in an agency newsletter. Her progress with mathematical skills was less impressive, and the therapist decided that this was due, at least in part, to unresolved psychodynamic issues around money and independence.

L. G. now lives relatively independently in an apartment with another patient, but remains quite dependent on her sister, who lives near her, for many types of support. The nature of the relationship between L. G. and her sister remains problematic, and it has not been possible to intervene therapeutically in it. Another remaining problem is the difficulty in controlling seizures, along with periodic episodes of medication-induced toxicity. Largely because of these unresolved problems, future vocational prospects are uncertain. Prior to her head injury L. G. seemed likely to complete college successfully. Following the injury, and prior to her participation in the CACR program, she seemed destined to become a chronically psychiatrically disabled patient. Since her discharge from the psychiatric hospital, she has required only three or four brief hospitalizations in a general hospital to treat the complications of her seizure disorder. Her present cognitive abilities, while lower than the preinjury level, appear adequate to allow success in a community college or vocational school program if her remaining emotional problems can be resolved.

This case illustrates several points. An initial neuropsychological evaluation of a "psychiatric patient" revealed the important deficits resulting from a brain injury, which had been ignored as a factor in her psychiatric treatment and assisted in the development of a rehabilitation plan. A subsequent re-evaluation not only documented improvement in cognitive functioning after 9 months of treatment, but also revealed remaining deficiencies in skills and led to subsequent remediation of them.

The approach was generally aimed at restoration of function, and the major rehabilitation tool was a CACR program, but this would have been unsuccessful without the therapist's cognitive behavioral interventions around issues such as the patient's fear of making mistakes. Although probable intrapsychic and family dynamic issues were identified as blocking progress in one skill area and impeding increased independence, they remain unresolved. This patient was treated on an individual basis, and she might have benefited more from inclusion in group therapy with other similar patients.

Finally, the cost in terms of therapist time has been high: 5 hours a week for at least the first year and a half and 1-2 hours a week for another 2 years or so to date. This must be considered in the light of the probable cost of psychiatric hospitalization if she had not been treated this way. Assuming that she would have been a psychiatric inpatient for half of that time (638.75 days) at a cost of $300 a day, the bill would have been a staggering $191,625 compared to a possible $10,000 cost of the therapist's time. If overhead costs of 100% are added for the rehabilitation program, the cost of it was still about 10% of the cost of the projected psychiatric hospitalization without rehabilitation.

Case 2

O. M. was a 57-year-old, white, right-handed male with 16 years of education who had been hospitalized with a diagnosis of major depression. His depression had failed to respond to treatment with a variety of medications, and he was showing increasingly agitated behavior and suicidal ideation, with a number of ineffectual suicide attempts. Although his history revealed that he had suffered a posterior right-hemisphere cerebral infarct several years earlier, he was considered to have "recovered" from it without any significant effort at rehabilitation, and it had been ignored as a factor in his psychiatric condition. He was referred for neuropsychological evaluation to differentiate between depression and dementia.

On evaluation, O. M. had a Halstead Impairment Index of 1.0, a Verbal IQ of 112, a Performance IQ of 77, and a Full Scale IQ of 95 with evidence of the greatest impairment in the posterior portion of the right-cerebral hemisphere, including a left homonomous heminopsia. The functioning of the left hemisphere was generally intact, and auditory verbal memory was quite good.

On one of his early visits to the Psychology Service when O. M. was asked to read a banner on the wall which had 8-in.-high letters: "HAPPY BIRTHDAY PAUL," he responded, "PAUL." He reported that after spending 3 hours trying to read an article in the *Reader's Digest*, he was very distressed because he could not make any sense of what he had read and realized that he had failed to read most of the material on the left side of the page. He was also unable to find his way around the hospital by himself, even to go from his ward to the cafeteria, which was a short trip involving a direct route with only three turns.

A rehabilitation plan was developed using the Gianutsos (Gianutsos & Klitzner, 1981) CACR programs to improve attention and concentration and teach him visual scanning to compensate for his visual field defect. At the beginning of treatment O. M. was virtually unable to read because of his frustration over not being able to understand the material. He worked, with the therapist present, for 1 hour a day, 3-4 days a week for 3 months.

Attention, concentration, and visual scanning abilities improved steadily during this time. O. M.'s measured reading speed increased to about 100 words per minute with good comprehension, although he still failed occasionally to scan to the left side of the screen. Even though he had been an avid reader for most of his life prior to the cerebral infarct, it was a long time before he resumed reading on his own because of his memory of the frustration his earlier attempts had caused. When he did finally attempt to read on his own, he came to the psychology service one day to report that the evening before he had read the daily newspaper "from cover to cover." He was so pleased with his accomplishment that he then started over and "read it all again."

During O. M.'s early months in the program his therapist accompanied him from the ward to the Psychology Service and back every day because he could not find his way by himself. After several months the therapist helped him develop a "verbal map" (Jarvis & Hamlin, 1991) so that he could become more independent in this area, and he was eventually able to remember the sequence of steps without referring to the printed instructions.

As O. M.'s cognitive functioning improved, his depression began to lift and his suicidal ideation decreased, with no further suicide attempts. He was discharged to a nursing home, which was too far from the hospital to allow continued treatment in the rehabilitation program. The therapist made the most recent follow-up by phone with O. M.'s attorney about a year after discharge. The attorney indicated that O. M. was still reading, although he could not give further details about reading speed or comprehension. O. M. was leaving the nursing home regularly on his own to go shopping at a shopping center several blocks away. He had remembered how his therapist had helped him develop "verbal maps" to find his way around the hospital and described this to a nurse in the nursing home. The nurse had then helped him develop a "verbal map," which he used on his independent trips to the shopping center.

This is another case in which the effects of a psychiatric patient's earlier brain injury, from a cerebral infarct, were largely ignored in his treatment. A neuropsychological evaluation requested to differentiate between depression and dementia revealed focal deficits instead of dementia and lead to the development of a rehabilitation plan to address them. The approach was generally to teach the patient compensatory techniques, and CACR was a major tool in this patient's treatment, with a speed-reading program used for both assessment and retraining of reading and comprehension skills. In addition, the patient's difficulty in finding his way around was addressed through the use of the "verbal map" technique, which is a compensatory one. Follow-up after 1 year revealed that the patient had continued reading on his own and had been able to describe how he had been taught the "verbal map" technique so that he could use it in a new environment.

Conclusions

It is clear that neuropsychological evaluations now must address the question of planning for rehabilitation in addition to diagnosis. To be useful for rehabilitation planning, a neuropsychological evaluation must identify those areas of cognitive functioning that are spared as well as those that are impaired by brain injuries. Neuropsychological rehabilitation is the fastest growing area of both research and practice within the field of clinical neuropsychology today. Due to this, it may be at risk for an uncritical acceptance of fads such as "memory training" and the "computer panacea" notion. Several years ago, Gouvier, Webster, and Blanton (1986) sounded a warning that is just as timely today: "Professionals engaged in [cognitive rehabilitation] should exercise the utmost restraint in extolling the virtues of cognitive retraining or computerized practice exercises for brain injured patients" (p. 314).

Although the hope for a "memory training" technique to restore memory for brain-injured patients has not been, and may never be, achieved, domain specific procedural training (Schacter & Glisky, 1986; Glisky & Schacter, 1989) shows considerable promise as a procedure to assist some patients in returning to more productive lives. For others, teaching innovative compensatory techniques, providing new external aids to memory, and modifying environmental demands remain the most constructive approaches.

The increased availability and decreased cost of microcomputers has fostered a new cottage industry: the writing and marketing of software for CACR. To some it must appear that all one needs to restore brain-injured patients to their level of premorbid functioning is a computer and a package of CACR programs. Hopefully, this notion will not spread too far or last too long. The reality is that computers show considerable promise as tools to assist in the rehabilitation of some patients with some deficits. The treatment of deficits in attention and concentration, for example, will probably be facilitated by CACR. Memory will not be restored in this way. Even in those areas where CACR is a useful tool it will not replace human therapists. They are still needed to guide and support patients in their use of computers.

Whatever tools are used in cognitive rehabilitation, the prognosis for brain-injured patients will be improved if therapists' efforts are based on sound psychological principles. McGlynn (1990) has identified a number of behavioral principles and techniques that have potentially widespread applications. Meichenbaum's self-instructional technique has also been applied in a variety of ways (Lira, Carne, & Masri, 1983; Meichenbaum, 1973; Meichenbaum & Cameron, 1973; Meichenbaum & Goodman, 1971; Robertson et al., 1988; and Webster & Scott, 1983). The use of the Premack principle, which uses a more frequently performed activity as a reinforcer for a less frequently performed one, appears to have potential for increasing the participation of poorly motivated patients in some rehabilitation activities (McGlynn, 1990). The operant principles involved in the use of tokens, contingency contracting, and shaping have multiple applications, and modeling behavior is particularly important in treating deficits in executive functions and social skills.

Finally, neuropsychologists working in rehabilitation must be concerned with the whole person, not just the injury or the cognitive deficits. Sachs (1985) states clearly that the brain-injured person can only be understood and helped if one recognizes that the behavior seen following injury is a result of the complex ways people respond to changes:

> But it must be said from the outset that a disease is never a mere loss or excess—that there is always a reaction, on the part of the affected organism or individual, to restore, to replace, to compensate for and to preserve its identity, however strange the means may be: and to study or influence these means, no less than the primary insult to the nervous system, is an essential part of our role as physicians. (p. 4)

Concern with the whole person requires attention to behavioral or personality factors (Mooney, 1988); the person's age, education, work history, and social supports; as well as factors such as the nature and time of onset of the brain injury or disease (Jarvis, 1988a). All of these factors, and their interaction, must be considered in developing an individual rehabilitation plan.

Chapter 12

Forensic Issues

In recent years there has been a dramatic increase in the involvement of neuropsychologists in the forensic arena (Doerr & Carlin, 1991). Some have actively sought this expansion of their roles; while others may choose to avoid it, often because of concerns about the adversarial nature of the proceedings. It seems increasingly likely, however, that any neuropsychologist with an active practice will become involved in a forensic case at some point, whether by choice or otherwise (Bigler, 1986). For example, a recent case, which began with a fairly routine referral from a psychiatrist to determine whether or not his patient's depression "had an organic component," ended 2 years later with the neuropsychologist's testimony during a personal injury trial.

While recognizing this increase in the involvement of neuropsychologists in the forensic arena, it is important to be aware of an accompanying debate about its merits. On one side are those like Faust (1991) who claim that neuropsychologists have little, if anything, to contribute. On the other side are those like Barth et al. (1991) and Barth, Ryan, Schear, and Puente (1992) who, while acknowledging the need to proceed cautiously, contend that neuropsychologists have much to offer the courts. Given the present state of affairs, in which neuropsychologists are sometimes called into the forensic arena even when they have not sought an invitation, it seems wise to acquire an awareness of what is to be expected there.

The purpose of this chapter is to provide an orientation to the forensic arena and an introduction to the factors one must be aware of to participate successfully. The structure of the arena, or legal system, will be outlined, and the process and its rules will be described. The requirements for successful participation will be related, and a number of common pitfalls will be identified. The problem of dealing with possible malingering or exaggeration of deficits will receive special attention.

The Structure of the Legal System

Each state has its own court system, with trial courts and appeals courts. In addition, there is a federal system, which is also composed of both types of courts. There are also a number of administrative agencies at both state and federal levels, which operate much like trial courts. Trial courts produce decisions of both fact and law; that is, "what really happened" in the case at hand and which laws apply and how. Appeals courts only produce decisions about the law; they do not determine facts. Therefore, neuropsychologists are not involved in appeals court proceedings, although they may be effected by the resulting decisions. They may be involved in trials in either state or federal courts or in hearings before certain administrative agencies.

Trials may involve either charges under criminal laws or law suits under civil laws. Neuropsychologists are much less frequently involved in criminal trials. When they are, it is usually to provide testimony regarding the element of culpability or intent, which is called *mens rea* in the law, or about the defendant's competency to stand trial. Under most laws regarding serious crimes it is necessary to show that the person had a mental status, which made it possible to form the intent to commit the criminal act. Thus, a person who was psychotic and believed that the victim was "a demon who would steal my soul" if not eliminated, might be found not guilty by reason of insanity. Similarly, if a person's mental status is influenced adversely by chemicals, psychiatric disorder, or certain other factors such as significant cerebral dysfunction, a condition of "diminished capacity" may be found, and a less severe sentence may result. Finally, in order for a defendant to be tried, he/she must be competent at the time of the trial.

A civil trial involves a claim that the plaintiff was damaged by some action, or failure to act, of the defendant and that the plaintiff should be compensated for the damages. In order to receive compensation, the plaintiff must prove both liability on the part of the defendant and the nature and value of the resulting damages. A common example is a case in which the plaintiff claims that the defendant operated a motor vehicle in such a way that the plaintiff suffered a head injury resulting in cognitive losses and inability to return to work. The role of the neuropsychologist in such a case would be to assist in establishing the nature and "value" of the damages. He/she would not be involved in the determination of the defendant's liability, whether the defendant had been speeding or had failed to stop for a red light, for example, although liability must be proven in order for the plaintiff to receive compensation for damages. Thus, if it was shown at trial that it had been the plaintiff who had failed to stop for the red light, not the defendant, no compensation would be awarded to the plaintiff, regardless of the nature or severity of the resulting injuries.

The Legal Process

The legal process in which the neuropsychologist is involved begins with the first contact with one of the opposing attorneys and continues through the testimony at trial, although it may be aborted at any step. The detailed steps in the process of a civil suit over damages for personal injury will be described because this is the type of case in which neuropsychologists are most often involved.

The Initial Contact

The initial contact may be made by an attorney for either the plaintiff or the defendant. In either case, the attorney will ask whether the neuropsychologist has been contacted by the other party or has any other relationship with anyone involved in the case. If he/she has, the contact should end at that point. Otherwise, a period of negotiations regarding the neuropsychologist's involvement commences. (In the following discussion it will be assumed for the sake of simplicity that there are only two attorneys involved in a case:

one for the plaintiff and one for the defendant. In reality, some cases have multiple plaintiffs and/or multiple defendants, and each may be represented by a different attorney. In addition, in some cases either or both parties may be represented by large law firms, and different attorneys may handle different aspects of the case. Thus, the neuropsychologist will frequently deal with more than two attorneys.)

The first issue to be determined should be whether or not the neuropsychologist has the competence necessary to participate at various levels in the case. The attorney obviously wants to be able to put a competent expert witness on the stand at trial and may, consequently, ask about the neuropsychologist's training and experience. Occasionally an attorney may be considering several different neuropsychologists before making a choice and may ask for a copy of the neuropsychologist's curriculum vitae (CV). The CV supplied should provide enough detail to allow the attorney to evaluate competence in regard to the specific case.

The neuropsychologist must also assess his/her own competence to assist in each specific case. In order to do this one must obtain certain minimum information about the case such as certain demographic characteristics of the plaintiff and the nature of the injury. The most important characteristic of the plaintiff is age. If the party is a young child, and one has no experience evaluating children, it is necessary to decline the case. Less frequently, the plaintiff may not speak English or may have a sensory impairment such as deafness, which requires special skills on the part of the neuropsychologist in order to perform an adequate evaluation. In such cases, it is appropriate to offer a referral to a qualified neuropsychologist. In one case it turned out that a pediatric neuropsychologist who was bilingual in English and Spanish was needed. Since the neuropsychologist who was contacted by the attorney had neither of these qualifications, and did not know another neuropsychologist in the state who did, he was engaged by the attorney to search for and evaluate the qualifications of an appropriate expert. Similarly, if one is not competent to evaluate the type of injury involved, one should decline to participate.

It is wise, during the initial contact, to begin one's assessment of the attorney. Has the attorney worked with neuropsychologists before, and does he/she have a reasonable understanding of what a neuropsychologist can contribute to a case? Some attorneys may need, and most will appreciate, education about these issues. One should be prepared to provide reprints of articles and copies of books or professional brochures that present explanations in nontechnical language. Videotape presentations, if available, may be particularly instructive. These same materials may provide the basis for one's explanations to a judge or jury at trial.

One will typically get an early impression of the attorney's expectation of the neuropsychologist's role. Attorneys are advocates for their clients. It is their job to present the most favorable case possible for their clients. In contrast, the role of the neuropsychologist is to present, in an objective manner, data and opinions based on the data that will assist the court in determining the "facts" of the case. It is undoubtedly rare for an attorney to attempt to persuade a potential expert witness to present a less than objective opinion. However, if one is ever faced with an attorney who says, in essence, "I want you to perform an evaluation that will prove that my client suffered serious damages," one should, of course, decline participation.

Attorneys may not always supply all of the information that a neuropsychologist will find relevant to a case. An attorney representing a client who suffered a head injury in a motor vehicle accident may not even think of obtaining records of past psychiatric treatment, but the neuropsychologist should. Consequently, it is essential that the neuropsychologist inform the attorney about all of the relevant records that are needed in order to perform the most adequate evaluation possible and the possible consequences of not having them.

As indicated in chapter 10, a review of records is an essential step in establishing many facts in forensic cases. Unsupported information obtained from interviews with people who have an interest in the case is less credible than that obtained from official records and may be completely discredited if a witness for the opposing side presents records that contradict it. The neuropsychologist should ask the attorney to provide records that will supply all of the important types of information described in chapter 10. If some of these records reveal information that is unfavorable for the client's case, the attorney will welcome the opportunity to consider it at the earliest possible stage in the case.

If the attorney who initiates the first contact is representing the defendant, there may be some minor differences in the process. Frequently a defense attorney may not seek a neuropsychologist until after the plaintiff has been evaluated by another neuropsychologist. In that event, the first thing one should request is a copy of the other neuropsychologist's report and all of the data on which it is based. Sometimes the other neuropsychologist is reluctant to furnish such data, but the attorney can require that it be produced under the rules of discovery.

During the initial contact the neuropsychologist should also inform the attorney of the fees that will be charged, how often bills will be submitted, and the expectations for payment. Since most civil suits are not settled for several years, it is not always reasonable to wait until a case is settled for payment. Monthly billing is appropriate. One should also determine who will be responsible for payment. This is usually the attorney or an insurance company. Attorneys often represent plaintiffs on a contingency basis; that is, if the plaintiff wins the case, the attorney receives a percentage of the award. Although the issue will seldom arise, it is never appropriate for a psychologist to accept payment on a contingency basis.

The Evaluation

Preparation for a forensic evaluation requires consideration of several factors. First, one should review all available records regarding the patient's injury and history prior to seeing the patient. This will often yield suggestions that will help structure interviews with the patient and others. There may be differences between information given in an interview and that recorded in records. When there are, one should ask the patient about them, although it may be better to postpone such questions until a second interview conducted after the formal testing is completed to avoid increasing the patient's defensiveness during testing.

Preparation also requires consideration of which tests to use. The use of a widely accepted, reliable, and valid battery such as the Halstead Reitan Battery tends to increase credibility, and one should also consider what additional tests to use in order to provide the most thorough possible evaluation of the patient's complaints. If there are major complaints of memory problems, as there often are, additional memory testing is obviously needed. It is important to use only tests with which one is thoroughly familiar, not only with the administration, but also with the literature regarding issues such as reliability and validity. Bigler (1986, p. 529) has cautioned against using "unstandardized tests or unproven tests or any tests that are controversial in nature."

If the patient has been evaluated previously by a neuropsychologist employed by the opposing attorney, the tests used in that evaluation and the length of intervening time may also influence the choice of tests. It is useful to be able to compare the results of the two evaluations. If alternate forms of the tests used in the first evaluation are available, they are often a good choice. At other times, the same tests should be used, taking into consideration possible practice effects. Sometimes a review of the tests used earlier will reveal inadequate assessment of important areas of functioning, and different or additional tests will be appropriate.

Before beginning the evaluation, it is important to understand, and make certain that the patient/plaintiff understands, that the usual rules of confidentiality do not apply in this type of evaluation. It is necessary to explain that the report of the evaluation will be given to the attorney who employed the neuropsychologist and to have the patient sign a release of information allowing that. This should be done at the beginning of the evaluation.

As indicated in chapter 10, it is important to explain to the patient what the evaluation will be like and to encourage the patient's best efforts on tests. In addition, in forensic evaluations the possibility of malingering, or more often, exaggeration of deficits, must always be considered. It is important to address this issue at the beginning of the evaluation. Before testing begins, one can give the patient instructions such as the following:

> We are aware that people involved in litigation over injuries often are frustrated because some people do not believe their injuries are serious, and they sometimes have a natural tendency to exaggerate their deficits on testing. However, the tests administered are very sensitive to even subtle deficits, and they will show evidence of any exaggeration of deficits. Therefore, it is important that you put forth your best effort on all of the tests.

Complete and accurate recording of information obtained during the evaluation is important. There is typically a long period of time between the evaluation and testimony at trial. Delays of a year or two are common, and several years may elapse in some cases. Even if one can remember details of an interview or a patient's test behavior after 2 years, it may be difficult to convince a jury that the memory is accurate if there are no notes to support it.

It is also important to be able to identify the times when all information was obtained. In many forensic cases more than one evaluation is performed (Boyar, 1981). Bigler (1986) and Cullum, Heaton, and Grant (1991) have recommended this as one means of assessing possible deception. If one has performed more than one evaluation on the same patient, it is possible to mix up the records from two different evaluations while reviewing them at a later date. Jarvis and Hamlin (1984) indicate that this can lead to a loss of credibility if one is then asked how he/she can be certain that an event occurred on a specific date. Therefore, *every* sheet of paper in an evaluation record should include the name of the patient, the date of the testing or interview, and the name of the person who recorded the information.

Once testing is completed, it is essential that scoring of tests be accurate. "The presence of even a few minor computation errors, none of which alone would change the overall interpretation of the total data, in a voluminous record of a comprehensive neuropsychological evaluation may be used by an opposing attorney on cross examination to discredit an entire evaluation. For example, if the number of items 'passed' on a subtest of the WAIS is counted incorrectly, even if this would not change the scale score for that subtest, this may contribute to a picture of carelessness which can be exploited by an opposing attorney." (Jarvis & Hamlin, 1984, p. 214). Consequently, all scoring should be double-checked, ideally by a second person.

The Report

Psychologists usually assume that an evaluation will result in a written report. In forensic evaluations this is not always so. Weiner (1987) has identified certain types of situations in which a written report may not be wanted by the employing attorney. If the results of an evaluation do not support the attorney's theory of the case, the attorney might decide not to use the evaluation and might use a different strategy. Therefore, before a written report is prepared, attorneys may want to discuss the general nature of the findings with the psychologist.

The written report of a forensic evaluation will not only go to the attorney who employed the neuropsychologist; it will also be available to the opposing attorney as part of the discovery process if the neuropsychologist is listed as an expert witness; and it will become a part of the court record, entered as an exhibit. As such, it may be scrutinized by a number of people including both attorneys and other expert witnesses. It is essential that it be complete and accurate. It should include all of the elements described in chapter 13. It is particularly important that all sources of data be listed because one is frequently asked, "What sources of information did you rely on in forming your opinion, doctor?" (Sometimes, all of the records that would verify information, such as school records, may not be available at the time of the initial evaluation. In such cases, it is important to indicate in the report that one's conclusions are based on the information that was available at the time, such as the patient's self report. This makes it clear that conclusions may change if different information becomes available at a later date.)

It is also useful, particularly if one has examined a patient for the plaintiff's attorney, to anticipate that the opposing attorney may ask about the possibility of exaggeration of deficits. The section on "Validity of Conclusions" included in the report of Case 1 in chapter 13 illustrates one way this may be done. In general, the report of a forensic evaluation should be written so that it includes all of the key information that will be needed later to prepare for testimony at deposition and trial.

The Discovery Process

Discovery is a process through which the opposing attorneys are required to reveal to each other the evidence they plan to present at trial. As a result of this process, many cases are settled without a trial, and there are few surprises for either side when a case does go to trial. Copies of exhibits, such as reports furnished by expert witnesses are exchanged; interrogatories, which are written questions, may be submitted; and depositions, sworn testimony, may be taken.

The first encounter with the discovery process may be a request to furnish the test data on which the report of an evaluation was based. It is important to note that every request for information or opinion of any kind should be reported to the employing attorney, and the information or opinion should be given to that attorney, who will supply it to the opposing attorney, if it is required. Similarly, the neuropsychologist's requests for copies of records or interviews should be made through the employing attorney.

If a case proceeds beyond the initial stages of negotiation for a settlement, the neuropsychologist is likely to be required to give a deposition. The neuropsychologist may receive a subpoena requiring appearance at a specified time and place to be deposed. More commonly, the time and place will be negotiated by the attorneys and the deponant. Choose a time and place that are convenient and comfortable. Many neuropsychologists choose their office for convenience and because they feel comfortable in familiar surroundings. There may be a slight advantage to choosing a conference room adjacent to one's office. If the deposition is taken in the neuropsychologist's office the opposing attorney may take the opportunity to scrutinize the books on the shelves and ask questions about them that can be used in the deposition or on cross-examination at trial. It may be just as well to avoid this.

There will be a minimum of four people present at a deposition: the opposing attorney, who will question the witness, or deponant; the employing attorney, who will usually not ask any questions but may offer clarifications for the record; a court reporter, who will administer the oath and record the proceedings; and, of course, the deponant. The plaintiff may be present, and the attorney who will question the witness may be accompanied by a consultant who will advise the attorney, but will not ask any questions directly.

The procedure begins with the administration of the oath by the court reporter, just as in court. The witness will then be questioned by the opposing attorney. The attorney has at least three general goals in taking a deposition: (1) to learn as much about the opposing side's case as possible; (2) to learn as much about the witness as possible, strengths, weaknesses, how credible a witness the person will be at trial; and (3) to pin down the witness's testimony at trial. If court testimony differs from the testimony on deposition, the witness can be discredited.

The attorney begins questioning by asking about the witness's qualifications, often referring to the CV, which was produced earlier. There may be detailed questions about one's knowledge in a variety of areas. The attorney is probing for weaknesses. These are often followed by questions about the neuropsychologist's involvement in the case, including details of dates and times. There will be detailed questions about the procedures used in the evaluation and the conclusions reached. "Are you certain about that conclusion? Isn't it possible that...?"

If there has been another evaluation by a different neuropsychologist, there may be questions about agreement or disagreement between the two experts' conclusions. In one deposition the attorney went through the other neuropsychologist's entire report, point by point, asking, "On page one Dr. Smith said....Do you agree or disagree?" Both Doerr and Carlin (1991) and McMahon and Satz (1981) have provided lists of commonly asked questions, and Benjamin and Kaszniak (1991) have presented a list of suggestions, compiled from several different sources, for responding to various types of questions.

Certain types of questions may pose problems for a witness. Advance knowledge of what to expect should make it easier to deal with most of them. There may not appear to be any logic to the sequence in which the attorney asks questions. They may jump back and forth among several different areas. Don't be rattled by this; take each question as it is asked, pausing to be certain of the meaning before answering it. Control the tempo of the questions and answers; don't let the attorney control it by firing questions too rapidly. Answer questions succinctly and do not volunteer information. That is, don't suggest additional questions or information that the attorney may use. Do not try to answer any question you don't understand.

Attorneys will sometimes ask complicated compound questions. If this happens, ask that they be broken down and asked separately. Do not hesitate to say, "I don't understand the question," but don't help the attorney by rephrasing it. Be wary of hypothetical questions. They are often complicated questions of the form, "Now doctor, I want you to assume that a patient always did a and b and c, never did d or e or f, and only did g and h at night and never did g and h during the day. In your professional opinion could such a patient have a diagnosis of xyz syndrome if pqr syndrome had been ruled out by medical studies and if the patient didn't consume much alcohol?" Never try to answer such a question unless you are certain that you understand it *completely*, and do not hesitate to say, "I am unable to form an opinion about that."

Another type of question that must be approached cautiously is the one about what authoritative sources one relies on in forming opinions: "Doctor, are you familiar with Black's *Textbook of Neuropsychology* (a 3,000-page book), and don't you agree that it is an authoritative book?" Unless you have read and remember and agree with *everything* in the book, the answer to such a question should be a carefully qualified one.

Some questions are designed to "box the witness in" or place limits on the statements witnesses may make or the opinions they may offer later at trial without being discredited. The clue to recognizing such questions is the fact that they contain words like "all," "only," "ever," "never," and so on: "Is that the *only* thing you considered?" "Are those *all* of the signs you observed?" This is another type of question that requires a qualified answer such as, "To the best of my recollection at this time..."

Finally, do not be afraid to say, "I don't know." There is no expert witness in any field who knows the answer to every question that may be asked by an attorney.

The opposing attorney, who asked for the deposition and questioned the witness, is responsible for payment of the witness's fee for the deposition. Since the neuropsychologist will probably not have had any direct contact with this attorney before the deposition, the end of the deposition is a good time to ask to what address the attorney wants the bill sent.

During the deposition, the court reporter recorded everything that was said and will transcribe it. The witness will receive a copy of the transcript and an opportunity to correct any mistakes. This must be done prior to the date specified in the papers that accompany the transcript, or the transcript will be filed with the court without any changes. It is important to read the copy carefully, indicate any necessary changes, and return them to the court reporter on time because one's testimony at trial may be compared to the transcript and discredited if it differs on important points. Remember that the addition or omission of a single word like "not" can reverse the meaning of a statement. Keep in mind, however, that "editorial" changes are not allowed; only errors in transcription may be corrected.

The goals of the attorney taking a deposition were described earlier. The neuropsychologist should also keep in mind certain goals for the deposition. It provides an opportunity to evaluate the style of the opposing attorney, although in some cases the attorney's style may be different at trial, or a different attorney may handle the cross-examination at trial. At the least, it provides an opportunity to "practice" answering questions about the case, which may help reduce one's anxiety about that process. It also gives one at least a general idea of what the content of cross-examination may include at trial, although this, too, may be different, depending on what the attorney learns from the deposition.

A witness should critically review his/her performance in a deposition in two ways. One should study the transcript of the deposition, not only for accuracy, but also to determine how one can give better answers to questions, without, of course, changing the essence of the answer. It may be possible, for example, to identify ways in which one can explain something more clearly, or provide an illustration for the jury at trial. Second, there should always be a conference with the employing attorney following the deposition. The purpose of this is also a critical review of the witness's performance, with the advantage that the employing attorney is not only a more objective evaluator, but also an expert one.

Before the Trial

During the discovery process, a great deal of information is shared between the opposing attorneys. As the employing attorney obtains more information he/she may ask the neuropsychologist to review some of it. One may be asked to review material such as military records, preinjury medical records, or transcripts of other experts' depositions. Such reviews may require the submission of supplemental reports, which should be prepared as carefully as one's initial report, because they will be subjected to scrutiny by the opposing attorney and may be used at trial.

As the date for the trial approaches, there should be a pretrial conference between the employing attorney and the neuropsychologist. This should involve a discussion of the questions the attorney expects to ask and the answers the witness will give. Attorneys, understandably, do not like surprises during a trial, particularly from a witness they have called. The attorney may take the witness through a long list of possible questions, or if the two have worked together before or had earlier extensive discussions about the case, this aspect of the conference may be less detailed. The neuropsychologist should be prepared to suggest to the attorney specific questions that can help bring out important points. It may also be helpful to suggest questions that the attorney can use in the cross-examination of opposing expert witnesses. In the final pretestimony contact, usually by telephone after a jury has been selected in a jury trial, it is useful to inquire about the characteristics of the jurors to whom one will be speaking.

Testimony at Trial

The employing attorney will negotiate the scheduling of the appearance to testify with the expert witness. An attempt will be made to accommodate the witness's personal schedule, but it is important to recognize that the attorney may need to consider the schedules of many witnesses along with the schedule of the trial. The attorney will be presenting the "story" of the case, and an effective presentation of it requires that the elements of the "story" be presented in a logical sequence. Thus, one's testimony will be most effective if it is presented at the right time. Keep this in mind when negotiating the timing of testimony.

The neuropsychologist will be called to the witness stand by the employing attorney and sworn by the court. The employing attorney will ask questions about the witness's qualifications and then conduct the direct examination, which will be followed by the cross-examination by the opposing attorney. This may be followed by a redirect examination by the employing attorney. Infrequently, the judge may ask the witness questions at any point in the testimony.

Although it is the attorneys who question the witness, it is not the attorneys to whom one's responses should be addressed. A witness does not have to convince the attorney about the accuracy of his/her opinions. It is the "fact finder" who must be convinced, and to whom one's testimony should be addressed. In a jury trial the jury decides the facts, based on the evidence presented to it. On the basis of those facts and the law, which is given to them by the judge in the form of "instructions," the jury reaches a verdict for either the plaintiff or the defendant. Some trials are conducted by the judge, without a jury, and in them the judge is the "fact finder."

Some observers, including Kreutzer et al. (1990), have indicated that the most important role of the expert witness is to educate the jury, or judge, in a nonjury trial. There are several important implications of this: It is helpful to know who the jurors are. The employing attorney should have supplied information about their educational and occupational backgrounds, and this may provide some indication of the types of material they are likely to understand and what types of explanations they may need. It is important to face the jury when answering questions and observe their reactions. One may sometimes be able, for example, to pick up clues about their level of attention and understanding and use this to determine further the extent of detail and type of explanation or illustration that they can best use.

The first questions the employing attorney will ask are ones about the witness's professional background. These questions about education, training, experience, and publications are designed to demonstrate the neuropsychologist's qualifications as an expert witness. The judge, occasionally after additional questions by the opposing attorney, will then rule on whether the neuropsychologist will be accepted as an expert witness. An expert witness, unlike ordinary witnesses, is allowed considerable latitude in testimony and is allowed to offer opinions during testimony (Benjamin & Kaszniak, 1991).

This is followed by the direct examination, conducted by the employing attorney. Questions are generally broad in scope, allowing sometimes lengthy narrative responses. This is the neuropsychologist's opportunity to educate the jury about the neuropsychological aspects of the case. This is the part of testimony that can be prepared in advance with the greatest certainty. It is much like preparing a lecture for a class. Jargon should be avoided as much as possible. When technical terms are necessary, they should be explained as simply as possible. Quoting directly the patient's responses to questions can be helpful. A jury may pay little attention to a recitation of a patient's test scores, but may retain a vivid memory of a description of the implications that they have for everyday functioning: "This means that this former mathematics teacher can no longer balance her checkbook." Well-prepared visual aids such as charts, graphs, and even videotapes can be powerful teaching tools in the courtroom as well as in the classroom. Emphasize the strong points in the case, but recognize the weak points and identify them matter-of-factly.

Postol (1987, cited in Benjamin and Kaszniak, 1991) gave the following summary advice for expert witnesses: The expert's opinions must appear to be based on adequate knowledge, expressed in an unbiased manner, and meet the layperson's test of reasonableness—does it sound right and make sense (p. 27)?

The direct examination is followed by the cross-examination, conducted by the opposing attorney. It is this attorney's job to discredit the expert's testimony. The neuropsychologist's knowledge and skills may be challenged, doubts may be cast on the reliability of data, and opinions will certainly be questioned; in short, every attempt will be made to make the jury doubt what the expert presented on direct examination. It is difficult, but important, not to become defensive under such an attack. Confidence in one's knowledge, skills, data, and opinions should be conveyed by both the content and style of responses. A simple "I don't know" answer, when indicated, will convey this confidence and bolster overall credibility far more than a lengthy, evasive one, which ends up meaning the same thing.

The content of questions on cross-examination will be similar to the ones asked at the earlier deposition; some will be exactly the same. Problems will occur if the answers are different. This is why it is so important to check the transcript of the deposition for accuracy. It is the official record of what a witness said at that time. The same types of problem questions, such as lengthy, complicated, compound ones, may also be asked; and the earlier advice about handling them is still valid. If an expert says, "I don't understand the question," the jury may not understand it either. If that happens, jurors may well feel that the expert is more credible than the attorney who asked such an incomprehensible question. Brodsky (1991) has provided useful guidelines for dealing with testimony in general, and especially with the problems that may be encountered on cross-examination. A study of his book may be one of the best ways to prepare for cross-examination.

Redirect examination by the employing attorney may follow the cross-examination. This is usually relatively brief and aimed at repairing any damage done to the witness's testimony during cross-examination. It may provide an opportunity for the witness to explain or elaborate on answers given earlier.

Working With a Defense Attorney

The preceding discussion assumed that the neuropsychologist was employed by the plaintiff's attorney. There are some minor differences in cases on which one is employed by the defense attorney. First, in such a case the patient/plaintiff will usually have already been evaluated by another neuropsychologist. In this event, the tests used by the other neuropsychologist should be considered as part of the process of deciding which ones to use in the second evaluation, as described earlier.

The records reviewed should include not only the reports of any earlier evaluations, but also the data on which they were based, including all test forms and data, summary indices, notes recording interviews and patient behavior during testing, and records reviewed as part of the evaluation. One needs to evaluate not only the patient, but also any earlier evaluations of the patient.

One may start by examining the test data. First, consider whether the tests used constituted an adequate battery for the type of evaluation. Then, check scoring against the test instructions. Recalculate all scores and indices such as the Halstead Impairment Index. If T scores corrected for age, education, and sex were not used in the evaluation, they should be calculated using the procedures provided by Heaton et al. (1991). Using any corrected scores and indices, outline what conclusions one would reach on the basis of the data and compare them to the conclusions described in the report.

The next consideration should be the adequacy of the other aspects of the data base on which the report is based. This includes factors such as age, sex, medications, alcohol, and other drug use, as well as educational, occupational, military, medical, and psychiatric histories. Not only should all of these factors have been included, but the sources of the information about them must be evaluated. If the educational history, for example, was reported by the patient, a note should be made to obtain official school records for verification.

Finally, an additional section is needed in the report of a second, or subsequent, evaluation. This should compare the results/conclusions of the two evaluations. Both areas of agreement and disagreement should be described, and in the areas of disagreement, the reasons for the disagreement should be stated. These might include deficiencies in the earlier report such as incorrect scoring of tests or a failure to consider the patient's advanced age or history of prior head injuries. Another reason for differences may be the availability of more valid sources of information, such as official school records at the time of the second evaluation. Finally, a patient's condition may have changed over time, either as a result of further spontaneous recovery or intervening treatment. One must, of course, be careful to consider possible practice effects on certain tests as a possible explanation for some changes, as well as the possibility of attempted deception or malingering on the part of the patient.

Other Types of Civil Cases

There are at least two other types of civil cases in which neuropsychologists may be involved: civil commitment for involuntary treatment and appointment of a guardian. When the issue of civil commitment hinges on dangerousness, evidence regarding the patient's prior dangerous behavior is always the most compelling evidence, although neuropsychological evidence regarding the lasting effects of brain injury or disease may be relevant in an occasional case. When it hinges on the issue of grave disability, again, other behavioral evidence is more relevant, with neuropsychological evidence playing, at most, a supporting role. The issues in guardianship cases are similar to the ones in grave disability based civil commitment cases, and neuropsychological evidence is not likely to be primary. Several other types of civil cases in which psychologists may be involved are described by Weiner and Hess (1987), but neuropsychological issues are even less likely to be major factors in most of them.

Criminal Cases

Insanity pleas, issues of diminished responsibility, and questions regarding competency to stand trial may be involved in criminal cases. McMahon and Satz (1981) indicated, however, that they have never seen a case in which neuropsychological evidence was, by itself, sufficient to resolve these issues, and it is typically more relevant in the sentencing phase as evidence of a mitigating factor. It seems least likely to be sufficient in the first two types of issues because they both involve questions about the defendant's condition at the time of the crime. It may be somewhat more pertinent when the question is competency to stand trial, since the issue here is the defendant's present condition. Note, however, that the question is the specific ability to understand the nature of the charges, the consequences of being found guilty, and the ability to assist in one's own defense. A person can, of course, have very severe neuropsychological deficits and retain that ability. The laws regarding all of these issues in criminal cases vary from one jurisdiction to another, and it is essential that a neuropsychologist understand the laws that apply before undertaking an evaluation.

Administrative Hearings

Quasi-judicial administrative hearings are used to resolve cases including worker's compensation, some types of disability claims, and restriction or revocation of a license to practice an occupation or profession. The type of neuropsychological evaluation required is essentially the same as the one described in civil suits for damages. The hearing itself is less formal and is conducted by a hearing officer, who has a role similar to a judge in a nonjury civil trial. A written report may be accepted instead of testimony by the expert, and in such a case it is particularly important that the report be very thorough and written in language the hearing officer can understand, since it is the only opportunity to present one's data and conclusions.

Assessment of Malingering or Exaggeration of Deficits

The forensic arena is one in which adversaries contest every issue. Every claim, whether for compensation for damages or for release from responsibility for a crime, is contested by an opposing attorney, and one of the attacks that may be made is that the claimant or defendant is malingering or exaggerating deficits. Rogers (1988) has indicated that the possibility of malingering or deception should be considered in every case that involves a claim for damages. This, then, is an issue that the neuropsychologist must be prepared to address.

This issue is also extremely complicated and contains many questions and few, if any, definite answers. In addition to neuropsychological factors, motivational and psychiatric factors must also be considered. Traven and Protter (1984), for example, have pointed out that there is a continuum of malingering and malingering-like behaviors depending on the degree of conscious self-awareness. Cullum et al. (1991) also discuss the relationship of malingering to such psychiatric conditions as somatoform, conversion, and factitious disorders. It may be necessary to explain this complexity and uncertainty to some attorneys.

Most of the research in this area has focused on the ability of neuropsychologists to discriminate between the test records of brain-injured patients and those of "neurologically normal" subjects instructed to simulate brain injury. These are analog studies since they do not involve "real" malingerers. Pankratz (1988) and Cullum et al. (1991) have reviewed a number of studies of this type, which used single tests. There have been fewer analog studies using a comprehensive battery such as the Halstead-Reitan Battery. The one by Heaton, Smith, Lehman, and Vogt (1978) is the most carefully designed one, and it did not offer much optimism about neuropsychologists' ability to identify the simulators in a reliable manner. In sharp contrast, Goebel (1983) identified 94% of the simulators in his study, but the design was such that no useful conclusions can be drawn from the study.

Other studies have assessed the ability of neuropsychologists to identify simulated child (Faust, Hart, & Guilmette, 1988) and adolescent (Faust, Hart, Guilmette, & Arkes, 1988) malingerers with negative results. These studies prompted a response that was critical of the methodology from Bigler (1990), who noted, among other things, that the clinical information provided to the neuropsychologist "judges" did not include any data from tests specifically designed to detect malingering.

Another critical response was made by Schmidt (1989) who claimed that most, if not all, of the studies of neuropsychologists' ability to detect malingering are meaningless. Using the analogy of asking neuropsychologists to change a light bulb while standing on a four-legged chair with one false and two missing legs, he points out that in these studies only one of the legs, the test data, has been supplied to the psychologists who have been asked to detect malingering. The other three legs, that is, review of relevant records, interview data, and observations of patients' behavior, have not been available. Under these conditions, poor performance by the psychologists who are asked to detect malingering should not be surprising.

These criticisms, predictably, resulted in replies from Arkes, Faust, and Guilmette (1990) in which they argued that, "To say it's not so doesn't prove it isn't" (p. 248).

They generally dispute the relevance of most of Bigler's (1990) and Schmidt's (1989) arguments and dismiss the specialized tests for the detection of malingering mentioned by Bigler (1990) as having largely "anecdotal" support. They conclude that they have raised a serious doubt about the ability of neuropsychologists to detect malingering and call for additional research, the need for which can hardly be disputed.

Perhaps the most important general concern about studies of the ability to detect malingering is the fact that they have all been analog studies. Any such study can only assess the ability to detect *simulated* malingerers. This may be only slightly more useful than assessing the ability of physicians using a biochemical test for depression to detect subjects who are simulating depression. We have no way of knowing how real malingerers differ from people instructed to simulate malingering. Since *real* malingerers seldom confess to their malingering, it is difficult to conceive of a way to study their characteristics or evaluate their test performance directly.

It seems likely, then, that for the foreseeable future at least, that the ability of neuropsychologists to detect *real* malingerers will not be decided by a scientific test of statistical significance. Instead, it will be decided on a case-by-case basis in jury trials by jurors using the "layperson's test of reasonableness—does it sound right and make sense" (Benjamin & Kaszniak, 1991, p. 27). There are a number of things that can be done that not only meet that test, but also make psychological and neuropsychological sense.

First, it seems likely that relatively few of the people who claim deficits resulting from brain injuries are truly malingering, and most of them are probably so obvious that they are detected by attorneys who advise them to drop their claims. Exaggeration of real deficits is likely to be much more common. By the time a person who has suffered a brain injury resulting in cognitive deficits reaches a neuropsychologist, he/she has usually been required to submit to numerous medical tests, some of which may have been quite unpleasant, and describe his/her complaints to numerous other people, many of whom are clearly not supportive of the person's claims. By that time, the person may quite understandably feel, "Damn it, I know something is wrong with me, but no one believes me; I'm going to make sure this guy can see how much trouble I have," The statement for patients involved in litigation described earlier provides recognition of this and assures the patient that neuropsychological tests will not only detect real deficits, but also identify exaggeration of them. The use of this may both encourage patients to put forth their best efforts and help persuade a jury that they have done so.

The main key to meeting the tests of reasonableness and neuropsychological sense is consistency. All of the information about a case should lead to an integrated, consistent picture. The data obtained by the neuropsychologist from testing, interviews, and behavioral observations should be consistent with both the verified description of the event that caused the injury and the patient's description of symptoms. Neuropsychological data should be consistent with medical data (Pankratz, 1988). There should be consistency between them in terms of both severity and location of damage to the brain.

Consistency should exist within the data from a comprehensive battery such as the Halstead-Reitan Battery. Such a battery, containing groups of tests that measure common abilities, should yield a consistent picture of strengths and weaknesses when the results of different tests are compared. Bigler (1986) suggests that repeat testing may also be a useful way to search for consistency. More recently, Cullum et al. (1991) have elaborated on this point. They indicate that there should be consistency within the data from repeated testing, taking into consideration anticipated effects of factors such as spontaneous recovery and practice effects.

Finally, there should be consistency between the patient's statements about background factors and evidence about the same factors found in official records. If a person claims to have graduated from college with a degree in chemistry, college transcripts should confirm that. Similarly, statements about work history should be verified by official employment records. A person who exaggerates past accomplishments may not malinger or exaggerate deficits on testing, but is exaggerating the extent of the *loss* of abilities. That is, even if such a person's present abilities are accurately reflected by performance on neuropsychological tests, he/she is attempting deception by claiming that those limited abilities represent deficits that are the result of an injury for which a compensation claim is being made because the person's actual pre-injury level of functioning is exaggerated.

A number of specialized tests to detect malingering have been suggested. Lezak (1983) described a memory test, originally devised by Rey, which is presented to the subject as a *difficult* test requiring memorization of 15 items. In reality, the test is quite simple because of the way the items are grouped. The assumption behind the test is that malingerers will not realize how simple the test really is and will produce poorer performances than brain-injured people. The illusion of the test's difficulty may be weakened if it is given after other standard memory tests. Therefore, it may be more useful if it is presented earlier in the testing. Hiscock and Hiscock (1989) commented that one cannot be certain that a very poor performance on this test reflects attempted deception rather than a severe cognitive deficit, but comparison with performance on certain other tests should help resolve that question. Lee, Loring, and Martin (1992) present normative data for the performance of patients with neurological disorders on this test, which should also be helpful in interpretation.

Pankratz (1983, 1988), Binder (1992), and Binder and Pankratz (1987) have described a forced-choice testing technique which relies on the laws of probability. With this technique, which has also been called *symptom validity testing*, a specific claimed sensory or memory deficit is identified and a stimulus, which the patient claims to be unable to detect, is then presented randomly in one half of a large number of trials, and not presented in the other trials, with instructions to "guess" whether the stimulus was presented if he/she is not certain. If the person is truly unable to detect the presentation of the stimulus, the number of correct guesses will, of course, not differ significantly from 50%. If the patient's percentage of correct guesses is significantly greater than 50%, this is convincing evidence that he/she is actually able to perceive the stimulus presentation. Such patients may have a psychogenic, or unconscious, basis for their reported deficits and may benefit from an explanation of the test results in an effort to change their behavior. On the other hand, if the percentage of correct guesses is significantly less than 50%, the patient must have been able to detect the stimulus in order to give the wrong guesses, and this is evidence of attempted deception. The use of forced choice testing with claims of blindness, hearing loss, and tactile sensation loss has been reported by several different investigators (Binder, 1992).

Complaints of memory deficits are among the most common ones reported following brain injuries, and useful refinements and standardization of the forced choice testing technique have been reported in this area. In an early development, Binder and Pankrantz (1987) report a case of a patient who claimed severe memory loss. When she was asked to guess whether she had seen either a yellow pencil or a black pen, each presented randomly in 50% of 100 trials, her 37% performance was significantly below the chance level of 50%, and the suspicion of malingering was supported.

Hiscock and Hiscock (1989) suggest that the task used by Binder and Pankrantz (1987) was so obviously easy that it would be ineffective with many malingering patients. Consequently, they developed a seemingly more difficult test requiring recognition of numbers. In their test a 5-digit number, the target, was presented to the patient. Then, after a 5-second delay in the first block of trials, a 10-second delay in the second block off trials, and a 15-second delay in the third and final block of trials, the patient was shown another card, which contained both the target number and a different 5-digit number, the foil, and was asked to identify the target number. Although this task appears difficult, it was made quite easy because the target could be identified by the fact that it differed from the foil in either the first or last digit. The illusion of difficulty was also increased by telling the patient whether or not each response was correct and telling the patient that he had performed well after the first and third blocks of trials and, consequently, the task would be made more difficult on the next block by increasing the interval between the two presentations on each trial. In their 1989 report, Hiscock and Hiscock present data obtained from a suspected malingering patient, a severely demented patient, and a normal 5-year-old child using this test. Although the suspected malingerer's performance was at the chance level for the first block of trials, as was that of the demented patient, it declined to levels that were significantly below the chance level on the second and third blocks while the demented patient's performance did not differ significantly from the chance level on any trial.

The most recent refinement of the forced choice testing technique is the Portland Digit Recognition Test (PDRT) described by Binder (1992). This standardized test, available for purchase from Binder, is based on the earlier work of Hiscock and Hiscock (1989) and is very similar to the procedures described by them. The major difference is that the patient is required to count backward for 5 seconds between the presentation of the target number and the presentation of the test card, which contains both the target and the foil in the first block of trials, 15 seconds in the second block, and 30 seconds in the third block. In addition, normative data for normal subjects instructed to simulate brain dysfunction, patients with brain injuries who were not seeking compensation, and brain-injured patients who were seeking compensation are available for the PDRT. A thorough assessment of possible deception should include at least one of these specialized tests. When there are suspicious claims of memory loss, the PDRT seems to be the best one available at this time.

The inclusion of the MMPI has also been recommended because it may provide measures of "test taking attitude" (Binder, 1992; Cullum et al., 1991; Jarvis & Hamlin, 1984).

This may indicate, for example, that a person is "faking bad" on the MMPI. While such an indication may raise a suspicion about a patient's approach to other tests, it does not, by itself, necessarily mean that his/her performance on neuropsychological tests is invalid. When the MMPI is apparently valid, however, and there are no inconsistencies found elsewhere, the overall case for an absence of malingering or exaggeration of deficits is made stronger.

As indicated earlier, the report of a forensic evaluation can include a section indicating an assessment of the probable validity of the patient's performance and the conclusions reached. When all aspects of the evaluation are consistent and no evidence suggesting malingering or exaggeration of deficits is found, a high degree of confidence in the conclusions can be stated. When there are indications of attempts at deception found in the patient's reports of past history, inconsistencies in neuropsychological test data, data from tests for malingering, or the MMPI, the neuropsychologist should report them. When this occurs, the employing attorney may decide to change strategies, perhaps settling the case out of court, or a jury may have to make the final determination.

Concluding Comments

Participation in the forensic arena tests all of a neuropsychologist's knowledge and skills. Not only are all aspects of one's training and experience called on, but they must be applied in a generally unfamiliar arena according to a new set of rules. This carries with it an important set of responsibilities that have been summarized by Barth et al. (1992, pp. 535-536):

1. Regardless of who retains your services, remain unbiased in all aspects of assessment and testimony. Be sure to make this clear to all involved (patient and attorney) in the initial negotiations for your time and commitment to the case.

2. Use a comprehensive and standard neuropsychological assessment battery, and be sure to administer and score all tests in an accurate and traditional fashion.

3. Have the referring attorney provide all pertinent medical records concerning the injury, hospitalization, and treatment. A detailed patient history should also be obtained, to include previous neurologic, psychiatric, or medical disorders, substance use and abuse history, school and employment records, previous psychological, educational, and neuropsychological test results, and other available psychosocial information.

4. Be entirely familiar with all the data, including considering alternative explanations and interpretations, and review this information with the attorney prior to the deposition and the courtroom appearance.

5. Have an in-depth understanding of your patient's premorbid status, and recognize that some long-term impairments may be related to premorbid characteristics or variables apart from (yet perhaps related to) neurologic damage. Personality factors, depression, stress and pain may affect neuropsychological outcome.

6. Look for convergence and consistency in test results and consider all possibilities when such consistency is lacking.

7. Remember that in science and medicine, final results can rarely be explained by one simple phenomenon (e.g., clear-cut neurologic deficits, depression, pain, malingering). Take all variables into account, and consider each possibility from a probabilistic standpoint.

8. Proactively confront the issue of questionable motivation or malingering by reducing a patient's fear that his/her problems will not be adequately assessed through the neuropsychological evaluation. Describe the sensitivity of these test measures and warn the patient of the dangers of giving less than a best effort, which would consequently be noted in the neuropsychological report. Recognize also that there remains today considerable controversy about the accurate determination of malingering and that an obvious spectrum of motivational issues should be considered if malingering is suspected (i.e., a behavioral-motivational problem, depression, conscious malingering, unconscious malingering, or a factitious disorder).

9. Understand the literature...and its relationship to your case.

As indicated at the beginning of this chapter, any neuropsychologist may be called into the forensic arena without having planned for it. For those who are, it is hoped that this brief introduction to the clinical and legal issues involved will assist them. For those who consciously plan to enter the forensic arena, two additional pieces of advice are offered: First, this is no place for a "novice" to practice; become a very competent neuropsychologist before seeking forensic cases. Second, seek additional training in the legal aspects of the work; this chapter has provided only a brief introduction to these aspects.

Chapter 13

The Neuropsychological Evaluation Report

The report of a neuropsychological evaluation serves a number of important functions: It provides detailed clinical information regarding cognitive, behavioral, and emotional functioning in relationship to neurologic factors. It also provides a summary record of the services provided to the patient for hospital or agency administrative purposes, to meet the requirements of regulatory agencies, and to fulfill various legal requirements. It is the principal means of communicating the findings and recommendations of the evaluator to the referring person and to others who will implement the recommendations and make decisions about things such as eligibility for services and benefits for the patient. If the neuropsychologist is later required to testify about the evaluation, it will define the limits of the testimony and facilitate preparation for it. The importance of this was described in chapter 12. The purpose of this chapter is to outline the elements that are important in reports and to provide examples of reports that incorporate them. Matthews (1981) provides other examples of useful reports, albeit with quite different styles from the ones presented here.

Stylistic Issues

The clinical, administrative, and legal requirements of various settings will dictate to some extent the style of many reports. Regardless of these it is essential that a report be understandable by the reader if it is to be an effective communication tool. The reader of a neuropsychological report who cannot understand the arcane language used by neuropsychologists may come away impressed with the brilliance of the author, or may simply decide that neuropsychological evaluations are useless; it is more likely to be the latter. Another reader of the same report, whether or not impressed with the author's knowledge, might find the same report quite useful.

The point is that neuropsychologists are consultants and must be able to communicate with their referral sources, the readers of reports, in the consultees' language. Jarvis and Nelson (1967) indicate that this requires consultants to familiarize themselves with the culture and language of their consultees. If one is working consistently with the same types of referral sources, all physicians or all educators, for example, this is not likely to be a problem. When one shifts to a new referral source, however, it may be necessary to ask questions such as: What do attorneys need from me? How much do they understand about neuropsychology? and What language do I need to use to communicate with them?

There are at least three steps one can take to improve communication with referral sources and the resulting usefulness of neuropsychological reports. The first one is to familiarize oneself with the language, culture, and problems of the referral source by reading about them and talking to members of the potential referral group. The second is to provide basic, essential explanations to them of what neuropsychology is and what neuropsychologists can, *and cannot*, do to help them. It may be helpful in this regard to prepare suitable brochures or papers for them. The third is to ask for feedback about the usefulness of one's reports. This is probably done too rarely, but may be the most helpful step one can take.

Elements of the Report

The following elements should be included in most reports, although the sequence and organization will vary depending on specific requirements and preferences.

1. Patient identification.

2. Referral question(s).

3. Patient's history and background relevant to referral, including a description of the injury or illness.

4. Date(s) of testing and time required.

5. Sources of data.

6. Behavior during testing.

7. Medications at the time of testing.

8. Intellectual functioning and estimated changes.

9. General level of performance.

10. Pattern of performance: cognitive and behavioral strengths and weaknesses.

11. Personality-emotional factors.

12. Neurological implications.

13. Relevant environmental factors.

14. Recommendations and answer(s) to referral question(s).

Patient Identification

The patient identification should include, not only the patient's name, but also age, sex, handedness (lateral dominance), education, occupation, and marital status or family constellation. Age, sex, and lateral dominance have implications for interpretation of various aspects of test data, and inclusion of them in the identification provides evidence that they were considered as appropriate. Education and occupation may have implications for both interpretation of some data and recommendations for treatment, and family constellation may influence treatment.

Referral Questions

An explicit statement of the referral questions, which initiated the evaluation, is important because it determines, at least in part, the nature and extent of the evaluation procedures used and facilitates an assessment of the adequacy of the evaluation. For example, an evaluation to assess changes in functioning to help monitor progression of a neurological disease or progress in treatment may require less-extensive procedures than one designed to answer complex diagnostic questions or assist in planning a comprehensive rehabilitation program. At times it may be necessary to help the referring person define just what an appropriate referral question is and how it can best be addressed. If this is not done adequately and the referral questions are not stated explicitly, the referring person is not likely to be satisfied with the resulting report of the evaluation.

Relevant Background

The background factors that are relevant will depend to a certain extent on the referral questions in each case. Certain aspects of medical history, such as head trauma, neurological diseases, vascular and severe respiratory disorders, other systemic problems, and psychiatric disorders are among those that should always be noted. A history of alcohol and other drug use should be included, along with an indication of its reliability whenever this may be an issue, as it frequently is if substance abuse is suspected. Details of accidents, injuries, and suicide attempts are important; and results of previous psychological, neuropsychological, and medical tests should be included. Other information that may be relevant, depending on the questions involved, includes details of school performance; job performance; and evidence of the ability to function independently, care for oneself, and manage ones own affairs. Details of any apparent changes in these areas are particularly important.

Date of Evaluation and Time Required

Inclusion of the date(s) of testing is important to meet certain administrative and legal requirements for documentation and provides a reference point in cases that later involve retesting for any purpose. Information about the time required to complete testing provides evidence regarding the extensiveness of the evaluation, which can be an issue in some cases involving litigation. It also provides information about factors such as the patient's speed of performance and endurance compared to a similar group of patients, which may be clinically relevant.

Sources of Data

In some settings where many similar evaluations are performed for the same referral source there is a practice of describing the tests administered as "our standard neuropsychological battery," or a similar phrase. While this may be adequate for internal use, patients sometimes move and are seen by people in other settings who may not be familiar with the unique "standard neuropsychological battery" used in the setting from which an earlier report was received. Consequently, it is more helpful to list the specific tests used.

Other sources of data, discussed in chapter 10, should be described. The names of all people interviewed, along with the dates and lengths of interviews, should be indicated. When other records are reviewed, they should be described, and the sources of the records should be indicated. The source of a record may have a bearing on the credibility given to it in some cases. For example, a job performance evaluation provided by a patient may be viewed as suspect in comparison to one furnished by an employer in a case involving litigation.

Behavior During Testing

A report obviously cannot record all of the observations of the patient's behavior noted during testing; some selectivity is required. Behavior that has a bearing on the validity of test data is essential. A description of any behaviors that contribute to clarification of diagnosis will strengthen diagnostic inferences. In chapter 10 a number of types of behavior that have implications for everyday functioning and rehabilitation, including the way the patient relates to the examiner and the types of structure and reinforcement needed during testing, were described; these should be reported.

It is often useful to report examples of behavior that illustrate real life, or ecologically valid examples of deficits demonstrated by test data. For example, the implications of test data that show visual-spatial-perceptual deficits are much more clear if one also reports that the patient got lost while returning from the bathroom the third time after the examiner had accompanied him/her the first two times.

Medications

The medications being taken by the patient at the time of testing, and the doses, should be noted. The length of time they have been taken, particularly noting recent changes, and the serum levels of some medications such as anticonvulsants and lithium carbonate may also be important. In the case of inpatients, medications actually administered, as opposed to ordered by the physician, should be verified from the patient's chart, particularly in the case of prn orders for sedative-hypnotics.

It is more difficult to determine the doses of medications actually taken by outpatients, particularly confused or psychotic patients and those prone to abuse drugs. It is a good practice to have outpatients bring their bottles of medicine with them and to check their reports of how they are taking them against the instructions on the label. In extreme cases, if one suspects a discrepancy between the patient's report and the actual consumption, it may be helpful to reconcile the number of doses remaining in the bottle with the instructions and the date of the prescription. The significance of all of these factors is that they may have effects on that patient's performance on neuropsychological tests and, therefore, on the validity of the data (Heaton & Crowley, 1981).

In most cases it is advisable to have patients remain on prescribed medications at the time of testing. If performance deficits, which appear related to the medications, are observed, one can indicate this in the report and recommend repeat testing after withdrawal of the suspected medication, when medically feasible. If this is done, it may be possible to determine the effect of the medication on the patient's cognitive and behavioral functioning.

Intellectual Functioning

The amount of detail about intellectual functioning, which is included in reports, may be dictated, in some cases, by stylistic requirements; but, more importantly, it should be influenced by the needs of the referring person to whom the report is addressed. Some may only need a general statement regarding level of functioning; others, such as educators and rehabilitation specialists, may need more detailed data. In those cases it may be appropriate to include all of the WAIS subtest scores, for example.

An estimate of the extent to which present level of intelligence is likely to represent a change from an earlier level is obviously useful in terms of diagnosis, prognosis, and treatment. Lezak (1983) recommends using a patient's highest postinjury test scores as an estimate of premorbid level of functioning. Mortenson et al. (1991), however, have raised questions about the validity of this practice based on both empirical data and psychometric theory. Since assessment of the *changes* in functioning resulting from brain injury is often the most important issue in neuropsychological evaluations, other sources of data are needed.

The best data regarding this comes from comparison with earlier testing with the same or similar tests. This is seldom available, but school and military records sometimes include scores on achievement tests, which may yield "IQ equivalents" in addition to grades. The best one can often do is to compare the present level of functioning with the level that would have been expected in the past on the basis of the patient's educational and vocational history.

Level of Performance

The question of how much detailed information about the patient's level of performance on specific neuropsychological tests, and its resolution, are much the same as the preceding question. A neuropsychologically sophisticated rehabilitation specialist may need detailed information; other recipients of reports may need, and be able to use, much less. At a minimum, it is reasonable to provide a summary measure such as the Halstead Impairment Index or the Average Impairment Rating, with perhaps a brief phrase defining it. If the Halstead Impairment Index is used, it is usually helpful to indicate, also, the range of deficit of those scores which are in the impaired range; i.e., from "mild" to "severe."

Pattern of Performance

Although some reports describe the pattern of performance primarily in terms of test scores, it seems more instructive to focus primarily on the patient's pattern of cognitive and behavioral strengths and weaknesses, using test data illustratively. Thus, a statement such as "His remote memory is relatively intact compared to his recent memory, as illustrated by his adequate performance on tests such as the Information subtest of the WAIS compared to his severely impaired performance on the verbal memory portions of the Wechsler Memory Scale-Revised" is preferable to "He achieved a scale score of 11 on the Information subtest of the WAIS and only recalled six bits of information on the Logical Memory subtest of the Wechsler Memory Scale." Information about the pattern of the patient's strengths and weaknesses provides one of the foundations for treatment planning, and the more direct statement about the pattern of the patient's abilities seems more relevant.

Neurological Implications

The description of the neurological implications of a neuropsychological evaluation may be very important in cases involving diagnostic questions, but there can be some serious pitfalls in this area. First, some neuropsychologists, impressed by blind interpretations of data used in some research and teaching methods, including the approach used in this volume, may foolishly rely on it in clinical work, ignoring other critical information. Diagnostic statements should **never** be placed in clinical reports when they are based solely on blind interpretation of test data. Other sources of data such as interview information, behavioral observations, the patient's complete history, and medical data must also be considered; and all of these, along with test data, must yield a logical, consistent diagnostic picture.

Second, one must remember that all diagnostic statements are, in the final analysis, probability statements; and even a cursory review of the history of neuropsychology makes it clear that this is particularly true in this field. James A. Lewis, a neurologist who is familiar with the capabilities of neuropsychologists, has stated, "The report that reads: 'The patient has frontal lobe damage, as shown by...' will rightly be met with skepticism, if not frank hostility" (Lewis, 1986, p.101). A statement such as, "This pattern of performance is frequently seen in patients with frontal lobe damage." will not only evoke less skepticism and hostility, but is a more accurate reflection of the empirical evidence. A failure to heed either of these caveats will cause damage to the reputations of the individual neuropsychologist and the profession, and may jeopardize the treatment of the patients involved.

Personality Functioning

Inclusion of personality assessment in neuropsychological evaluations serves two purposes. First, it may help to clarify some diagnostic pictures such as the common question of differentiation between depression and dementia and questions about hysteria or malingering-like disorders.

Second, it helps provide an understanding of how the brain-injured person is coping with the effects of the injury. The inclusion of the MMPI in neuropsychological evaluations has become a widespread practice, and it often serves these purposes well. At times it is also helpful to use projective techniques to supply a different perspective on personality. The patient's behavior during testing and interviews with family members and others may provide some of the most revealing information, particularly about how the person is reacting to the brain injury. Case 2 in this chapter provides an example of this in the information supplied by the patient's wife about his reaction to his losses and how this affected their marriage. This also had implications for treatment, which had, unfortunately, not been seen prior to the neuropsychological evaluation.

Environmental Factors

The environment in which the patient lives or to which he/she will return has major implications for treatment. The most important aspects of the environment are the demands it places on the patient and the support it provides. In the first category are things such as the patient's job, educational program, and responsibility for management of the home and child care. Specific information about details of job responsibilities or school course load should be included, as should information about children in the home and the care they will require from the patient.

One of the most important aspects of the support available to the patient is the nature of living arrangements. A person living alone in an apartment will usually have less support available for coping with diminished abilities than one living with family members, for example. However, the attitudes of the people in the patient's environment (family members, employers, teachers, and others) toward the patient and the changes in the patient's behavior can have a major impact on both the type of treatment that is needed and the prognosis.

Recommendations and Answers to Referral Questions

All of the preceding sections of the report establish the basis for recommendations that are made. These should, obviously, address the referral questions that initiated the evaluation. At times it may not be possible to provide a complete answer to some referral questions. When this is the case, one should indicate it and state what further data, if this is known, would facilitate a more adequate answer. This may include a more complete history, work evaluation procedures, retesting at a later date, and various medical tests.

It is important for the neuropsychologist to remember that medical judgments are involved in the decision to order many of these tests, such as the balancing of risks and benefits with certain invasive procedures. The report, which says, "The patient should have…." will be received less warmly, to say the least, than the one that says "A…might help clarify the question of…." Similar caution is appropriate in recommending medications. A statement which reads, "An evaluation for possible treatment with antidepressant medication might be helpful," will often be viewed more favorably than one that recommends treatment with a specific antidepressant medication.

Among the most commonly requested recommendations are ones regarding patients' abilities to care for themselves, live independently, and work or function adequately in school. The hypotheses presented in chapter 8 are relevant in this regard. Teachers often need suggestions about both techniques for teaching brain-injured children and strategies for managing their behavior in the classroom. Similarly, nursing staff often need specific suggestions for managing problematic behavior of hospitalized patients. The techniques found useful by the examiner in eliciting the patient's cooperation and maximum effort during testing may provide a basis for these recommendations.

When recommendations are made for any of the psychologically based therapies such as psychotherapy, behavior therapy, or cognitive retraining, they should be as specific as possible, including, for example, suggestions regarding the type of reinforcers that are likely to be effective in a behavior therapy program and the issues that should be addressed in psychotherapy. Similarly, if cognitive rehabilitation is recommended, specific techniques that are likely to be helpful with the patient's deficits, as described in chapter 11, should be suggested.

The Final Step

After the report is completed, one additional step will often enhance its value. This is a discussion of it with the referring person and others who will be involved in implementing the recommendations to be certain that the referral questions have been answered and that the recommendations are understandable and feasible. This is particularly important in the case of referral sources with which one has not worked extensively in the past, and should be done whenever possible with the families of patients, especially when they will be involved in the patient's care and treatment. In forensic cases, it is essential to discuss the report with the referring attorney prior to deposition and trial so that neither the psychologist nor the attorney will experience any unnecessary surprises during those proceedings.

Sample Reports

The following two reports illustrate how the previously described elements are incorporated into reports for two different referral sources and different referral questions.

Case 1

We have completed our evaluation of Mr. Charles Robinson in response to your question of whether he has impairment of brain functioning as a result of a motor vehicle accident in February of 1981. Mr. Robinson is a 50-year-old, white, married, right-handed male with 12 years of education and a history of 20 years of employment as a truck driver for Allied Oil Supply as well as self-employment as an operator of a lawn mower repair business for several years.

Sources of Data

Interviews as Follows:

August 24, 1984: Mr. Robinson, 1$\frac{1}{2}$ hours; Jean and Herbert Smith, sister and brother-in-law of Mr. Robinson, 20 minutes.

August 31, 1984: Betty Robinson, wife, 1$\frac{1}{2}$ hours.

September 7, 1984: Herbert Smith, 30 minutes.

September 9, 1984: Betty Robinson, 15 minutes.

September 20, 1984: Allan Axe, Director of Human Resources, Allied Oil Supply, 30 minutes.

Review of records from: Doctors Nile, Mann, Pinester; and Mr. Carl Johns, Counselor.

September 7, 1984: The following tests were administered: Halstead-Reitan Battery, WAIS-R, Russell revision of the Wechsler Memory Scale, MMPI. (The MMPI was administered using tape-recorded questions, monitored by the examiner, due to the patient's poor reading skills.) Testing required 8 hours, with frequent breaks required due to Mr. Robinson's fatigue, which is somewhat longer than the time usually required to administer these tests to ambulatory outpatients.

History: Premorbid Level of Functioning

Mr. Robinson was born and raised in Clinton, New York. He attended public schools and, by his report, graduated from high school with "average" grades. (Official school records were not available at the time of this evaluation.) After graduation, he worked as a truck driver for a number of different employers until he went to work for Allied Oil Supply around 1960.

Prior to the injuries received in the February, 1981, motor vehicle accident, Mr. Robinson was a hard-working person of average intelligence with an excellent employment record. He had worked for 20 years for Allied Oil Supply as a driver, delivering supplies to oil rigs, reading invoices, checking merchandise against invoices, handling complaints from customers and writing credit memos; all of which presumably required an average intelligence; the ability to read, write, and perform arithmetic computations; and an ability to maintain satisfactory relations with customers. He performed these duties satisfactorily with no complaints from customers or his employer and no significant time lost from work.

In addition to this, he cared for a seriously ill mother until her death and operated his own lawn mower repair business evenings and weekends after her death. He also took care of the yard work at his home, which he owned. He is described by his wife as being considerate and loving toward her and a man who never drank more than "a half a beer" in the 20 years she knew him. Both he and his wife denied that he ever used other drugs.

At approximately 6:00 p.m. on February 2, 1981, Mr. Robinson was the restrained driver of a 1979 Ford pickup truck, which was struck head-on by another vehicle operated by a driver who was subsequently found guilty of driving under the influence of alcohol.

Mr. Robinson was unconscious at the scene of the accident and was taken by ambulance to Community Hospital where he was found to have compound fractures of the left arm and a fracture of the jaw as well as severe lacerations of his face and head. A CT scan immediately following hospital admission showed no skull fracture, but revealed a frontal/temporal hematoma. He gradually regained consciousness over a period of the next 3 days. No estimate of the period of posttraumatic amnesia is available. He remained in the hospital for 3 weeks, during which time a repeat CT scan showed that the hematoma was resolving satisfactorily. He was discharged to his home and the care of his family physician, Dr. Nile. He received essentially no rehabilitation services, but he has seen a chiropractor, Dr. Mann, for treatment of back pain about once every two weeks since then. Recently, he and his wife have begun seeing a counselor, Mr. Johns, for marital conflict.

There is no history of previous head injuries or seizures, surgery, or hospitalization for treatment of illness. He has no history of treatment for any psychiatric disorder prior to the accident.

He denied use of alcohol or other drugs, which was confirmed by his wife. He drinks, according to his wife's estimate, 10-12 cups of coffee a day and smokes about two packs of cigarettes a day. He was taking no medications at the time of this evaluation.

Behavioral Observations

At the time of my evaluation, Mr. Robinson presented as a right-handed, white man who appeared older than his age and very fatigued looking, although he stated that he had slept well the previous night but was always "tired." His grooming and hygiene appeared adequate except for his fingernails, which were very long, dirty, and had broken edges on both occasions when I saw him 2 weeks apart. His speech was dysarthric and slurred, and he had word-finding problems. He had difficulty maintaining concentration, and he appeared to fall asleep while I was talking with his sister and brother-in-law in his presence, which they stated he frequently does. He had difficulty remembering both remote and recently acquired information. For example, he was not certain of even the year of his injury and he had difficulty remembering my name under the following conditions:

1. I had talked to him on the phone 1 week prior to the interview, and I introduced myself to him by name at the beginning of the interview.

2. Fifteen minutes after the interview began I asked him my name and repeated it for him when he did not remember it.

3. Twenty minutes after that, he again did not remember my name, and I had him repeat it three times.

4. Finally, 20 minutes later, he remembered my name on inquiry.

Current Activities

Mr. Robinson said he did not return to work at Allied Oil Supply following the injury in 1981 because his supervisor visited him and said that he would not be able to do his job. He did, however, resume his work at his lawn-mower repair business, but he was no longer able to do this adequately. Both he and his wife, independently, reported that it took him three to four times as long as before the injury to perform routine tasks on this job. Consequently, this business went steadily down hill until it failed in June 1984. Mr. Robinson also stopped other productive activities that he used to perform, such as his yard work and typically, according to his wife, sits for long periods of time smoking and muttering, "I don't know what's happening—I don't know what to do—I don't know..." frequently without finishing sentences.

Mrs. Robinson also reported major changes in her husband's personality. She reported that he wears his clothes for a week at a time, not even taking them off when he goes to bed and only taking a bath when she fills the tub and insists that he bathe before going to see a doctor. She reports that he has been vulgar and abusive of her and made irrational accusations of her. For example, he has accused her of stealing money from the lawn-mower repair business, being glad that their daughter died, and not being as good in bed as his "girlfriend." She indicates that this has caused her much distress, forced her to sleep in a separate bedroom, and caused frequent severe, prolonged tension headaches, which only stopped when she recently moved to her mother's home in another city.

Intellectual Functioning

On the WAIS-R Mr. Robinson achieved a Verbal IQ of 78, a Performance IQ of 79, and a Full Scale IQ of 78, which places his current intellectual functioning in the Border-line range.

Neuropsychological Functioning, Level of Performance

On the Halstead-Reitan Battery Mr. Robinson achieved a Halstead Impairment Index of 1.0, which means that all of the tests that are most sensitive to brain damage were per-formed in the range that is characteristic of people with physically validated neuropathol-ogy. Even when Mr. Robinson's age and education are taken into consideration, his per-formance on all of these tests was in the moderately-to-severely impaired range with the single exception of his performance on the Category Test, which was only mildly impaired for a person of his age.

Neuropsychological Functioning, Pattern of Performance

Mr. Robinson's general cognitive functioning is severely impaired in all areas. He has significant deficits in attention and concentration demonstrated by his performance on the Seashore Rhythm and Speech Sounds Perception tests and the Digit Span Subtest of the WAIS and his inability to attend to ordinary conversation for more than a few min-utes at a time. His memory functioning, for both recent and remote events, is severely impaired for both verbal and nonverbal material. This was manifested by his severely impaired performance on all parts of the WMS-R; his low scores on the Information and Comprehension Subtests of the WAIS, which tap information learned long ago; and illus-trated by his difficulty in remembering my name even after numerous reminders.

He also has significant deficits in basic adaptive skills such as reading, spelling, and arithmetic. His functioning in these areas is clearly below the level he demonstrated on his job prior to his injury, and his present level of functioning would not allow him to perform these functions at the level required by that job. He has significant problems with communication, demonstrated by word-finding problems, dysarthria, and slurred speech, which would also prevent him from adequately carrying out his previous job duties.

On the Sensory Perceptual Examination, Mr. Robinson made numerous errors including consistent suppressions of stimuli to the left side of the body when both sides of the body were stimulated simultaneously, in spite of adequate perception of unilateral stimuli, in both tactile and auditory modalities; a predominance of left-sided errors of finger agnosia, dysgraphaesthesia, and dysteriognosis; and constructional dyspraxia. These may be related to problems in dressing and grooming, which his wife described.

Neurological Implications

Overall, these data are most consistent with static, bilateral damage to the brain with functions subserved by the frontal and temporal/parietal areas being most severely impaired. This is typical of a person 1 or more years after a closed head injury of the type caused by a motor vehicle accident which resulted in 12 or more hours of unconsciousness.

Personality and Emotional Functioning

The configuration of the validity scales on the MMPI indicates that Mr. Robinson responded to this test in a direct, honest manner, with no evidence of any attempt at deception. The profile on the clinical scales reflects a great deal of emotional distress with clinically significant depression. Mr. Robinson has severe feelings of inadequacy, helplessness, and hopelessness, but no suicidal ideation. His personal care has deteriorated to the point where his appearance and behavior have alienated him from most other people. The only remaining interpersonal relationships he has are those with his wife, sister, and brother-in-law, and his wife is so distressed by his behavior that she has recently separated from him.

Validity of conclusions

Prior to testing I gave him our standard instructions for patients involved in litigation. This is an explanation that we are aware that people involved in litigation over injuries often are frustrated because some people do not believe their injuries are serious, and they sometimes have a natural tendency to exaggerate their deficits on testing. However, the tests administered are very sensitive to even subtle deficits, and they will show evidence of any exaggeration of deficits. Therefore, it is important to put forth his best effort on all of the tests.

The following evidence supports the validity of the conclusions resulting from this evaluation:

1. There is no reason to believe that the data were influenced by medications since both Mr. Robinson and his family stated that he was not taking medicine. In fact he stated, "I don't believe in it." The fact that he continues in treatment with a chiropractor and a nonmedical counselor, neither of whom can prescribe medicine, supports this.

2. There is no reason to attribute his performance to a history of alcohol abuse, since both he and his family, independently, deny significant alcohol consumption. Furthermore, his best performance on testing was on the Category Test, which is usually quite impaired in alcoholics.

3. There is complete consistency between the pattern of the neuropsychological data and the history of a closed head injury.

4. There is a striking internal consistency within the neuropsychological data, which could not be faked by even a very sophisticated person. For example, the errors noted on the Sensory Perceptual Examination are consistent with the pattern of performance on the three trials of the TPT and the performance on the Seashore Rhythm Test.

5. I can find no inconsistencies among the data resulting from 8 hours of testing and over 4 hours of interviews, which would suggest any attempt at malingering or exaggeration of deficits.

6. Finally, while the profile on the clinical scales of the MMPI reflects a great deal of emotional distress, including depression, the profile on the validity scales reflects an open, honest approach to testing, which is not at all characteristic of people who are malingering or attempting to exaggerate their deficits ($L = 2$; $F - K = 5$).

Summary and conclusions

1. It is my opinion that Mr. Robinson has suffered, as a result of a closed head injury sustained in a motor vehicle accident, significant impairment of brain functioning manifested by deficits in most areas of adaptive cognitive functioning including memory, attention and concentration, easy fatigability, and problems with both receptive and expressive communication. Personality changes have also occurred resulting in a deterioration of interpersonal relations, including probably terminal marital problems. These cognitive losses and personality changes have resulted in an inability to function productively at gainful employment or, I fear perhaps, even to care for himself independently if he must live alone, now that his wife has left him.

2. I believe that Mr. Robinson should have available to him a comprehensive rehabilitation program that includes the following:

   a. Cognitive retraining of attention and concentration skills should be provided. This service is available on an outpatient basis, using computer training programs, from Neurological Rehabilitation Associates.

   b. Following this retraining, a reevaluation of memory functions should be performed to determine the residual memory deficits. These memory problems will probably not respond to retraining efforts, but the neuropsychologist at Neurological Rehabilitation Associates should be able to help Mr. Robinson develop compensatory techniques to help improve his functioning in this area.

   c. A speech and language evaluation should be performed to determine the type of speech therapy that is needed.

   d. Retraining of basic reading, writing, and arithmetic skills should also be provided. This can be done by the speech therapist or education specialist.

   e. An occupational therapy evaluation should be performed to identify the type of retraining that is needed in the area of activities of daily living such as hygiene and grooming.

    f. A psychiatric evaluation consultation may be useful to determine whether antide-
      pressant medication would be helpful.

    g. Group therapy with other brain-injured patients may help Mr. Robinson cope
      with his losses.

    h. Mrs. Robinson should be referred to a support group of the Colorado Head Injury
      Foundation to help her cope with her husband's behavior and understand the role
      she can play in his rehabilitation.

Please let me know if I can be of further assistance in your work with Mr. Robinson.

Discussion of Case 1

This is a case of a patient who was referred by an attorney who was handling the litigation over an injury resulting from a motor vehicle accident. Although the case was
eventually settled out of court, the report was written with the assumption that it might
go to trial and that the neuropsychologist would be called to testify. Consequently, many
details that are often asked for at trial are included in the report, such as the "Sources of
Data" and the premorbid history.

There is some disagreement over whether or not the "Validity of Conclusions" section
should be included in the report itself. The neuropsychologist must anticipate, and be
prepared to answer, questions about possible exaggeration of deficits or malingering. The
question is how this information is best supplied. It is often helpful to ask the attorney
one is working with whether or not he/she would prefer to have the information included
in the report, which will be available to the opposing attorney through discovery, or have
it communicated verbally. This is an issue of the strategy the attorney chooses to follow.
While it is appropriate to defer to an attorney about this, it is, of course, essential that the
neuropsychologist does not fall into the trap of letting an attorney suggest what the *content* of one's professional opinions will be.

Little emphasis was placed on the "Neurological Implications" section of the report
because examination of medical records made it clear that there had been a brain injury.
At trial, this evidence would be presented by the medical experts. Instead, the consistency of the neuropsychological evidence with the medical evidence was stressed.

A major value of a neuropsychological evaluation in a case of this type is to demonstrate how the patient's abilities to function on the job and in every day activities have
been affected by the brain injury. Consequently, a detailed picture of the patient's pre-
injury functioning was provided, and the neuropsychological deficits identified were
related to that functioning. Since the patient had worked for a small company that could
not provide a written job description, a manager of the company was interviewed to
obtain that information.

Little information was provided about actual test scores, although those could be
required during the discovery phase of the litigation. Keeping this raw data to a minimum in the report may reduce the tendency of some attorneys to ask during deposition or
trial about the "meaning" of each individual test score.

The detailed recommendations for rehabilitation were included to identify specific
treatment needs and to support the claim for the expense of such a program.

Case 2

Mr. Jason Bandur is a 41-year-old, white, right-handed man with a BS in Computer Science and an MBA, both from the University of Denver, who had a resection of a frontal meningioma in May 1989. He was referred by his physician, Dr. Glass, to determine whether he is able to return to his former job at this time.

Sources of Data

The following tests were administered on 8/8/90: Wechsler Adult Intelligence Scale-Revised (WAIS-R), Halstead-Reitan Neuropsychological Battery (HRB), Russell Revision of the Wechsler Memory Scale (RRWMS), Wide Range Achievement Test-Revised (WRAT-R), Rey Auditory Verbal Learning Test (RAVLT), MMPI, and Benton Judgment Of Line Orientation Test (JOLO). Testing required 6 hours. Mr. Bandur and his wife were interviewed together for 1 hour. In addition, I reviewed a copy of Mr. Bandur's job description, which he brought with him at my request.

Interview and Mental Status Examination

Mr. Bandur has worked as the marketing manager for Advanced Data Storage, Inc., supervising 100 sales people for 10 years. This job involves planning marketing campaigns, training sales people, checking sales reports and records, monitoring the performance of sales staff, and conducting sales meetings. He said his employer is eager for him to return to work, and he and his wife both said they feel he is able to return to work now. His wife says she "will not allow him to drive" because she is "concerned about liability." He denied any cognitive deficits at this time. The patient reported he was taking phenobarbitol, 30 mg, BID, which he has been taking since the surgery to prevent seizures.

The patient was alert and fully oriented. His mood was anxious and depressed. His affect was appropriate to thought content. Speech was coherent with no dysarthria or word-finding problems, but he spoke slowly and softly, often waiting for his wife to answer questions for him. There was no evidence of hallucinations or delusions.

During testing he frequently gave "I don't know" responses and required much encouragement to attempt an answer. He often said, "I can't do that" and on one of the major tests of cognitive functioning simply refused to continue when he encountered difficulty about halfway through the test. He said the test had "changed unfairly" which, of course, it had not.

After testing was completed, he asked me when he would find out whether he had "passed" the tests. When I told him that I would mail the report in 3 days, he was visibly upset and appeared on the verge of tears, apparently wanting an immediate answer.

Intellectual Functioning

On the WAIS-R he achieved a Verbal IQ of 101, a Performance IQ of 95, and a Full Scale IQ of 98. Scale Scores on Verbal Subtests ranged from 9 to 11, while on Performance Subtests the range was from 6 to 11. Overall, this places his intellectual functioning in the average range. However, on all of the Performance subtests, except one, he showed very defective ability to solve novel problems and identify essential elements in visual stimuli. On two of these subtests he gave up and refused to attempt the last, most difficult item. On item number 8 of the Block Design subtest he repeated the same design he had produced on number 7.

Overall, his intellectual functioning is in the normal range. However, considering his educational and occupational background, this probably represents a significant decline from an earlier level of functioning.

Neuropsychological Functioning—Level of Performance

On the HRB the patient achieved a Halstead Impairment Index of 0.7, indicating that most of the scores on those tests most sensitive to impaired brain functioning were in the impaired range. The average level of impairment was mildly-to-moderately severe.

Neuropsychological Functioning—Pattern of Performance

Attention and concentration were within normal limits, as were both verbal and non-verbal memory and learning of pairs of unfamiliar word associations on the RRWMS. However, analysis of performance on the RAVLT shows that he had increasing difficulty in learning new material as the complexity and unfamiliarity increased even slightly. Furthermore, although his retention was fairly adequate, retrieval from stored memory is deficient. The Aphasia Screening Test was performed within normal limits. The Sensory Perceptual Examination was within normal limits except for five errors on a test of fingertip number writing perception on the right hand. Visual-spatial-perceptual abilities are at least moderately impaired (JOLO), and visual scanning was very slow at times (Trail Making Test).

The most striking cognitive deficits were in abstraction, concept formation, and problem-solving abilities (Category Test). This was the test he refused to continue, claiming it had "changed unfairly." Had he completed it, making errors at the same rate on the remainder of the test, his score would have been as much as three standard deviations below the mean for people his age and education. Without even attempting half of the items the number of errors he made was well into the impaired range. It is very clear that concept formation and abstract problem solving beyond very simple, concrete problems are clearly beyond this man's ability at this time.

Personality

Performance on the MMPI produced a valid profile with evidence of clinically significant depression. In addition, observation of the patient's behavior during testing and of his interactions with his wife suggest that he is quite passive and dependent in his functioning at this time. He has a low frustration tolerance and easily becomes irritable. He appears to have low self-esteem and to lack confidence in his own abilities in spite of his claim that he feels he has no cognitive deficits and is ready to return to work. It appears likely that he will become more severely depressed when he either finds out that he cannot return to work or attempts to do so and encounters severe problems on the job.

The interaction between Mr. and Mrs. Bandur is a complicated one. On the one hand, they both indicated that they feel he is ready to return to his job now. However, Mr. Bandur clearly has many doubts about his own abilities, as manifested by his behavior during testing, and his wife "will not let him drive" because she is "concerned about liability." Although I did not explore this with them, I suspect that there may be some covert conflict between them about his true abilities to function, perhaps influenced by their financial burdens.

Summary and Recommendations

This is a 41-year-old, white, right-handed male whose current intellectual functioning is in the normal range. However, his deficient performance on those subtests of the WAIS that require the solution of novel problems suggests that this represents a significant decline from his premorbid level of functioning. Although memory is generally intact, he has increasing difficulty as the material to be learned increases even slightly in complexity, and he has difficulty in retrieval from stored memory. His most severe deficits are in concept formation and abstract problem solving beyond very simple, concrete problems.

This pattern of cognitive, behavioral, and emotional problems is typical of patients who have had surgical removal of a frontal meningioma. Considering the length of time since the surgery, it is unlikely that there will be any additional spontaneous recovery. Therefore, it is my opinion that, while he could probably perform routine, repetitive tasks adequately, he would not be able to handle his previous job, as he described it to me.

His visual-spatial-perceptual deficits and slow visual scanning abilities raise a question about his ability to drive safely, particularly in heavy traffic or unfamiliar surroundings. When Mrs. Bandur asked my recommendation about this, I told her that I recommend an evaluation of Mr. Bandur's ability to drive under these conditions by a professional driving instructor.

I believe it would be helpful for Dr. Glass to assess the response of both Mr. and Mrs. Bandur to the conclusion that Mr. Bandur would not be able to perform his former job adequately if he returned to work now to determine whether marital counseling would be helpful to them.

A psychiatric evaluation to determine whether Mr. Bandur would benefit from antidepressant medication may be helpful.

I recommend a vocational evaluation by the Western Assessment and Training Center to assist Mr. Bandur in identifying and preparing for suitable alternate employment.

Discussion of Case 2

This is a case of a patient who was referred by his primary care physician who, essentially wanted support for his opinion that the patient was not able to return to his former job. There was no litigation involved, and there was little chance that there would be in the future. Consequently, this report is less detailed in some respects than the report in Case 1.

Since the basic question was whether or not the patient could return to his former job, the responsibilities of that job were described in some detail. Under the circumstances of this noncontested case, a job description furnished by the patient seemed acceptable instead of requiring one furnished directly by the employer. Once again, neuropsychological data were described in terms of their relationship to job requirements.

Few actual test scores were provided because the physician was unlikely to be interested in them or to understand them. Instead, a fair amount of information about the patient's behavior during the interview and testing was supplied because this provided a vivid picture of the type of deficits that would interfere with job performance. Both the physician, the patient, and his wife would be able to appreciate this far better than test scores.

The usual section on "Neurological Implications" was omitted because the referring physician was thoroughly familiar with those aspects of the case, having made the initial diagnosis of a frontal meningioma, and cared for the patient since the surgery.

Although the initial referral question only asked whether the patient could return to his former job, additional recommendations were made. The issue of the patient's ability to drive safely was addressed because his wife raised it, and the patient's depression and the marital relationship were discussed because they were important factors that the referring physician had apparently not considered. Similarly, the issue of vocational rehabilitation needed to be addressed if the patient could not return to his former job, but detailed recommendations were not made because that seemed premature at the time of the report.

General Discussion of Reports

These two reports illustrate the relative importance of the elements described in the first part of this chapter in reports written for two different purposes. In other types of reports different emphases will be needed.

In a report written to answer a diagnostic question about dementia versus depression, for example, the section on "Neurological Implications" would be much more extensive, and reports addressed to more neuropsychologically sophisticated professionals might include considerably more detailed information about actual test scores. Reports that will be read and used by a variety of staff within an agency, hospital, or school should spell out recommendations for the details of treatment or education of the patient in terms that can be understood by those staff. A report on a patient who had a previous neuropsychological evaluation should indicate the nature and magnitude of changes that have occurred and their implications. Certain elements are essential in all reports. Beyond that, each report should be written to meet the unique needs of the recipient.

SECTION 3
ADDITIONAL INFORMATION

Chapter 14

Neurodiagnostic Procedures

Those studying neuropsychology need to know what our colleagues in neurology, neuroradiology and neurosurgery do in examining the nervous system. A knowledge of these procedures will contribute to an understanding of how the neurological examination and the neuropsychological assessment should be complementary. It will also illustrate what some of the indications are for more specialized neurological-radiological examination.

The Physical Neurological Examination

The physical neurological examination may be very extensive and concentrate on areas of suspected problems or, at other times, be a very brief "screening examination." The most superficial of such screening examinations has been described, perhaps facetiously, by one neurologist as consisting of simply an examination of the cranial nerves and testing for the Babinski reflex. On the other hand, the complete neurological examination may be an extremely thorough and time-consuming procedure. The following outline for a "routine" neurological examination is similar to one described by Steegmann (1962) and is typical of the complete neurological examination.

The neurologist usually begins by obtaining a neurological and medical history. Steegmann (1962) indicates that a number of points in the neurological history are particularly crucial.

Changes in state of consciousness are always assessed in the neurological examination. These conditions may range from the transitory clouding of consciousness seen in some seizures to the stupor or coma, which may accompany severe lesions of the central nervous system.

Headaches are given special attention, including a review of the duration, quality, location, and intensity of the pain, as well as various factors that may aggravate or relieve the pain. Dizziness and vertigo are evaluated with a focus on the factors that produce or alleviate them, as well as other related sensations and conditions such as tinnitus, nausea, and vomiting. Complaints of pain are assessed, with special attention to the nature of the pain, its frequency, duration, location, and intensity. Subjective reports of visual disturbances are recorded with attention to such factors as decreased acuity, sensitivity to light, blurring, or double vision. Similarly, disturbances of smell and taste are evaluated. Any history of convulsions is explored thoroughly with special attention to the presence of auras, loss of consciousness, and the nature and location of motor contractions. A history of vomiting is investigated to determine whether it was accompanied by nausea, pain, headache, or abdominal symptoms.

Motor weakness reported by the patient is evaluated to determine features of onset and course, location, severity, and duration of the weakness, and the conditions that relieve or exacerbate it. Bladder and bowel problems are explored to determine their specific nature, onset, and relationship to other factors. Difficulties in gait are considered, particularly to determine whether they are related to weakness or lack of coordination. Disturbances of speech are investigated to determine whether they are aphasic in nature or associated with problems in word knowledge, articulation, or memory. Related difficulties in chewing and swallowing are also frequently explored in connection with speech disturbances. Sleep patterns are examined to determine the duration of sleep, difficulty in sleeping, or excessive drowsiness. The focus here is often on changes in the sleep pattern. Autonomic functions, including sweating, sexual performance, urinary control, and digestive disturbances, are investigated. A brief mental status examination is almost always included and involves at least orientation, simple problem-solving, and memory.

A general medical and psychiatric history of both the patient and family members is typically obtained. A family history is particularly important when there is concern about convulsive disorders or hereditary conditions such as Huntington's chorea.

The equipment needed for the routine clinical neurological examination is fairly simple. It usually includes a flashlight, stethoscope, blood pressure cuff, ophthalmoscope, pins, cotton for testing tactile sensation, a percussion hammer, and tuning fork. Materials for testing sensations of temperature, taste, and smell are occasionally also included.

Many neurologists begin the actual physical examination by testing the 12 cranial nerves (olfactory, optic, trigeminal, facial, vestibulocochlear, glossopharyngeal, vagus, spinal accessory, oculomotor, trochlear, abducens, and hypoglossal). In a superficial examination the olfactory nerve may not be tested. When it is, this is done by asking the patient to identify the odor of substances such as oil of peppermint or ground coffee. The optic nerve is evaluated in several ways. A simple test of visual acuity may be done. The visual fields are mapped roughly by a direct confrontation technique similar to that used in the Sensory Perceptual Examination of the Halstead-Reitan Battery. If this leads to suspicion of visual field defects, more sophisticated techniques may be employed by the neurologist or by an ophthalmologist. Finally, the optic fundi are examined with an ophthalmoscope.

The 3rd, 4th, and 6th cranial nerves are functionally related and examined together. This consists of an examination of the external eyes and their positions, the pupils, and certain pupillary reflexes and eye movements under various conditions. The 5th cranial nerve is examined in both its motor and sensory divisions. In the former, mouth and jaw movements are evaluated; in the latter, sensations of various parts of the face are tested. The 7th cranial nerve is evaluated by having the patient perform various motor acts such as frowning, closing the eyes tightly, or elevating the eyebrows. Taste sensation may also be tested using four basic substances: sweet, sour, bitter, and salt.

The most common testing of the 8th nerve is a fairly crude test of auditory acuity. If decreased acuity is noted, further testing with a tuning fork may be done to determine whether the decrease in acuity is of a conduction deficit or nerve deficit type. More definitive evaluation of hearing loss requires a specialized audiometric examination. The 9th and 10th nerves are assessed by observing the position and movement of the palate and tongue. The 11th nerve is tested by having the patient move his shoulders up toward the ears against resistance to the examiner's hands on the patient's shoulders, and by having the patient turn his head to one side against resistance to the examiner's attempt to pull the chin back. The 12th cranial nerve is evaluated by examination of the position and movement of the patient's tongue and by having the patient repeat certain words or phrases that require complex tongue movement and coordination. At some point in the neurological examination, the neurologist typically observes the size and shape of the head, and skull tenderness or pain.

The extent of the examination of the patient's motor system will vary considerably from one assessment to another, depending on the nature of the patient's complaint and the observations made in the first general portions of this examination. These include a general inspection of the patient's ability to carry out certain simple motor tasks such as walking, sitting down, and squatting. This includes an assessment of the patient's station and gait. The term *station* refers to the way in which a person stands, and the term *gait* refers to the way in which he/she walks. General muscle tone, range of motion, and strength are evaluated. When specific problems are suspected, assessment of strength is very thorough and complex, including testing of many different muscle groups. Grading of strength is typically done by the neurologist on a relatively crude 6-point scale. More refined testing of muscle function requires utilization of the specialized techniques of electromyography.

When most people think of a neurological examination, they probably think of the testing of reflexes. This is because the examination of reflexes is done more frequently than some other parts of the neurological examination. Both deep reflexes, which are produced by tapping a tendon or muscle, and superficial reflexes, which are elicited by stimulation of a sensory area, are tested. The speed and strength of the reflex is assessed and usually graded on a relatively crude 4-point scale. Differences in reflexes on the two sides of the body are given special attention, as is the presence of any pathological reflex such as Babinski's sign.

The neurologist always makes at least a superficial assessment of the patient's coordination and may test coordination more specifically by having the patient carry out certain complex actions such as finger to nose or heel to shin maneuvers. The presence of any abnormal movements such as tics, tremors, or choreiform movements is always noted.

As with the motor examination, the extent of the sensory examination may vary considerably, depending on the patient's complaint and other clinical findings. A complete sensory examination involves assessment of sensations of pain, temperature, touch, position, and vibration. Once again, the neurologist is particularly concerned with differences in these sensations on different sides and different parts of the body.

Overall, the neurological examination is a process that often proceeds in a successive screening manner. A history is always obtained and this dictates to some extent the nature and extent of the physical examination. The results of the various parts of the physical examination determine the extent to which other portions of the examination are carried out, and the overall results of the physical examination determine to some extent the use of other more specialized tests.

It should be clear from this brief description of the typical neurological examination that there are certain limitations and values inherent in this procedure. A major limitation is posed by the skill of the neurological examiner. Many portions of the examination require subjective judgments and grading. These are most obvious in the motor examination and the assessment of reflexes, where relatively crude rating scales are typically employed. The cooperation of the patient also poses another major limitation. Certain portions of the examination, such as the sensory examination, obviously cannot be carried out adequately on an unconscious patient. The patient must also have sufficient comprehension to cooperate with certain portions of the examination. He/she must, for example, be able to report accurately the sensations experienced during the sensory examination. The ability to do this will be influenced by factors such as intelligence, psychiatric condition, and general willingness to participate and cooperate.

Compared to other diagnostic procedures, the clinical neurological examination has a major value in that it is noninvasive and therefore produces no risk to the patient. For the most part, the examination involves little discomfort to the patient and is relatively inexpensive when compared to other specialized procedures described next.

Specialized Neurological Assessment Procedures

Just as the neuropsychologist should understand the nature of the clinical neurological examination, he/she should also be familiar with neurophysiological and specialized neuroradiological diagnostic methods. The decision to utilize any of these specialized techniques is dictated by a number of factors. The most prominent among these are the indications from the neurological history and the clinical examination. The different procedures yield information about different parts of the nervous system and have various reliabilities and validities associated with them.

The simplest, most readily available, and most widely utilized of these techniques is the ordinary X-ray of the skull or spine. This procedure is inexpensive and has no morbidity/mortality rate or discomfort for the patient. It is most useful in identifying the nature and extent of damage to the skull or spine due to trauma, but has the lowest hit rate for identifying other types of neuropathological processes (Filskov & Goldstein, 1974).

The EEG is also widely available, relatively inexpensive, has no morbidity or mortality, and little discomfort for the patient. The EEG is most typically indicated when there is a history or suspicion of a seizure disorder and is often useful in identifying the anatomical focus of the seizures through analysis of bioelectrical activity by cerebral region. It is also a relatively weak technique for identifying other types of neuropathological processes. It is useful to determine brain death and plays a role in the diagnosis of narcolepsy.

Neurologists, ophthalmologists, and audiologists have applied computer technology to improve the power of electroencephalographic examinations. Kandel et al. (1991) have reviewed the diagnostic use of visual evoked potentials. In this procedure, EEG recordings are made from the occipital area while the patient is presented with visual stimuli. These may be flashes of light or patterned visual material. A lengthy series of stimuli (for example, 64 flashes of light at a rate of one per second) is presented to the patient while EEG recordings are made. A computer averages the responses and the resulting average response pattern is presented via an oscilloscope. Various characteristics of the response pattern (particularly wave latency) are measured and recorded by the computer, and a permanent tracing is made for further measurement and study. Similar techniques have been utilized to study brain stem auditory responses (Kandel et al., 1991) and somatosensory evoked responses from stimuli applied to the limbs. Evoked potential studies are noninvasive, create little discomfort for the patient, and can be performed relatively quickly.

Electromyography (EMG) and nerve conduction studies, which are often done in conjunction with each other, do not have any morbidity or mortality rates associated with them, although they do entail a mild to moderate degree of discomfort for the patient. EMG studies typically involve insertion of small needle electrodes into various muscles in order to assess electrical function of the muscles. In nerve conduction studies one typically applies an electrical current to a proximal peripheral nerve and measures the conduction speed to a distal recording electrode. These studies are used to differentiate between neuropathic and myopathic disorders and to determine the extent of progression or rehabilitation in various conditions.

Examination of cerebrospinal fluid obtained through a lumbar puncture is widely available and inexpensive. There can be some degree of discomfort to the patient with this procedure, possible postprocedure headache, and some risk of infection, as would be expected with any invasive procedure. Increases in intracranial pressure may be noted by measurement. The appearance of the spinal fluid may indicate the presence of blood cells or xanthochromia. Unless caused by needle trauma, red blood cells demonstrate hemorrhage; white suggest infection. Ordinarily, the spinal fluid should be clear and colorless, and any deviation from this appearance should lead to a strong suspicion of a lesion in the nervous system. Microscopic examinations of the spinal fluid may identify the presence of infection, such as meningitis or syphilis, and the study of the complex chemistry of the spinal fluid may contribute to diagnoses such as multiple sclerosis.

The procedures described above can all be carried out in an office or clinic setting. Angiography, however, is a more seriously invasive procedure and is usually carried out in a hospital setting. This involves the introduction of a radiopaque substance into an artery through a catheter. The femoral artery is often utilized. Serial X-rays of the skull are then taken as the radiopaque substance circulates through the cerebrovascular system. There is a low morbidity/mortality rate associated with angiography. This procedure is extremely valuable in visualizing any abnormalities or lesions of the vascular system. It may also demonstrate space occupying lesions, which distort the structure of the vascular system. Transfemoral angiography may soon be replaced by MRA (magnetic resonance angiography).

Since the advent of CT and MRI, pneumoencephalography is seldom performed any more. Pneumoencephalography is an invasive technique with a low morbidity/mortality rate. This procedure requires the removal of spinal fluid through a lumbar puncture and the injection of air with subsequent examination of the air-filled ventricular and subarachnoid spaces. This technique is most useful for visualizing distortions of the ventricular system resulting from space occupying lesions, cerebral atrophy, or hydrocephalic conditions (ventricular dilatation). A common complication of pneumoen-cephalography is a severe postprocedure headache.

Other neurological diagnostic vistas have been opened up by the expansion of computer technology. The best known of these is computed tomography (CT) (or computed axial tomography— CAT). In the head CT scan procedure, the brain is X-rayed using a discrete beam from many different angles originating in an arc around the head and at varying depths and levels. This is often done both with and without the injection of a contrast medium into the vascular system of the brain. The computer then reconstructs pictures of different "slices" (lateral-horizontal) through the brain. These may be viewed by the radiologist on a TV screen and permanent photographs of them made for further study. The technical details and history of this procedure have been described by Gordon, Herman, and Johnson (1975) (also see Kandel et al., 1991). This technique is quite accu-rate for the detection of many types of lesions as small as one centimeter in size. As do all other radiographic techniques, it relies on the difference in density between normal brain tissue and abnormal brain tissue to detect lesions. Since some lesions are identical in density to normal brain tissue, they may be missed by this neuroradiological tech-nique. Furthermore, chemical and metabolic disorders cannot be detected on CT scans. Artifacts may result from patient movement, and it is sometimes necessary to sedate patients in order to eliminate movement. Additionally, one can expect some risk of ana-phylactic shock when a contrast medium is introduced into the vascular system.

Magnetic Resonance Imaging (MRI) is a noninvasive procedure that produces higher-quality images of "slices" (lateral-horizontal, coronal, or sagittal) of the brain. Although a mathematics and physics background is very handy when trying to understand or describe this technology, it basically involves creating a strong electromagnetic field around the patient's head, which aligns the spin axes of hydrogen nuclei along that field. A radio wave is then passed through the area of the brain being studied causing the spin of the nuclei to tip in a "gyroscope-like" motion. When the radio wave is turned off, the spinning nuclei return to their previous orientation, thus releasing energy, which can be measured using a radio receiver. These energy releases or "relaxation" times vary depending upon tissue conditions, which when monitored and subjected to mathematical formuli can be forged into extremely detailed computerized pictures of the brain with astounding resolution (Kandel et al., 1991). Given its noninvasive nature and accurate depiction of neural structure and pathology, MRI technology is considered superior to CT for most diagnostic situations. The exceptions may be in early head trauma or certain psychiatric conditions where there may be excessive movement of the head while in the machine's gantry (Uzzell, 1989). In these cases, CT scans are currently superior in reduc-ing movement artifact.

Positron Emission Tomography (PET) scans and Single Photon Emission Computed Tomography (SPECT) scans combine CT technology with nuclear medicine to create technicolor CT type pictures, which demonstrate glucose use and blood flow in various regions of the brain. In this procedure, the patient must ingest radioactively tagged glu-cose, which when exposed to an X-ray negative, will show areas of the brain in which there is glucose uptake and use. During these procedures, the patient is often asked to perform certain cognitive and perceptual tasks that require glucose utilization and will show up on the X-ray negative, thus potentially charting functional/anatomical correlations. The PET technology is complicated and expensive since a cyclotron is necessary to produce the radioactive tag used in this procedure. Furthermore, the cyclotron must be located at the PET scan site since the radioactive material must have a very short half-life. The SPECT scan uses only a single photon, and for this reason, the radioactivity tagged glucose has a longer half-life and can be shipped from a cyclotron center, thus reducing the overall cost. The drawback to the SPECT scan is that its lower "power" creates problems in resolution when making pictures. This is, however, being addressed by the use of multiple camera heads to create simultaneous pictures from several different angles. SPECT scanners are presently available in most large medical centers and university hospitals, but PET scanners are still being used mostly in experimental processes (Kandel et al., 1991).

From the preceding discussion it should be clear that each of these techniques has its own particular advantages and disadvantages. Skull X-rays, angiograms, pneumoencephalograms, CT scans, and MRI all give the physician a "picture" of the brain, which may be invaluable in cases where surgical intervention is indicated. Examination of the cerebrospinal fluid indicates abnormalities of intracranial pressure, changes in the chemistry of the fluid, and the presence or absence of disease organisms. EEG techniques disclose the pattern of electrical activity of the brain and may lead to identification of locations of lesions. One should note, however, that of the procedures described, only PET and SPECT scans can give some direct evidence of functional integrity.

The neuropsychological examination, on the other hand, is a noninvasive procedure, which may suggest the presence of lesions before they can be detected by other techniques, and has the major advantage of showing the effect that a lesion has on the patient's cognitive and behavioral functioning. Most importantly, the neuropsychological evaluation identifies areas of strength as well as those of impaired functioning, which is essential in planning treatment and rehabilitation.

Neurological and neuropsychological techniques should be complementary rather than competitive. Neurophysiological and neuroradiological techniques (as well as the physical neurological exam) can be essential in pinpointing the location of lesions and in facilitating surgical and other medical intervention. Neuropsychological techniques are vital in identifying the functional effects of lesions and in describing the areas of relatively intact functioning that are important in planning rehabilitation and treatment.

REFERENCES

Acker, M. B. (1986). Relationships between test scores and everyday life functioning. In B. P. Uzzell & Y. Gross (Eds.), *Clinical neuropsychology of intervention* (pp. 85-117). Boston: Martinus Nijhoff.

American Psychiatric Association. (1987). *Diagnostic and statistical manual of mental disorders* (3rd ed.—rev.). Washington, DC: Author.

Arkes, H. R., Faust, D., & Guilmette, T. J. (1990). Response to Schmidt's (1988) comments on Hart, Guilmette, and Arkes (1988). *Professional Psychology: Research and Practice, 21*(1), 3-4.

Bales, J. (1990). Validity of assessment debated in courtrooms. *APA Monitor, 21*(10), 7.

Barth, J. T., & Boll, T. J. (1981). Rehabilitation and treatment of central nervous system dysfunction: A behavioral medicine perspective. In C. Prokov & L. Bradley (Eds.), *Medical psychology: Contributions to behavioral medicine* (pp. 242-266). New York: Academic Press.

Barth, J. T., Gideon, D. A., Sciara, A. D., Hulsey, P. H., & Anchor, K. N. (1986). Forensic aspects of mild head trauma. *Journal of Head Trauma Rehabilitation, 1*(2), 63-70.

Barth, J. T., & Macciocchi, S. N. (1986). Dementia: Implications for clinical practice and research. In S. B. Filskov & T. J. Boll (Eds.), *Handbook of clinical neuropsychology* (Vol. 2, pp. 398-425). New York: Wiley.

Barth, J. T., Ryan, T. V., & Hawk, G. L. (1991). Forensic neuropsychology: A reply to the method skeptics. *Neuropsychology Review, 2*(3), 251-266.

Barth, J. T., Ryan, T. V., Schear, J. M., & Puente, A. E. (1992). Forensic assessments and expert testimony in neuropsychology. In S. Hanson & D. Tucker (Eds.), *State of the art reviews: Physical medicine and rehabilitation* (Neuropsychological assessment), Philadelphia: Hanley and Belfus, 6(3), 531-546.

Baum, B., & Hall, K. M. (1981). Relationship between constructional praxis and dressing in the head injured adult. *The American Journal of Occupational Therapy, 35*(7), 438-442.

Benedict, R. H. B. (1989). The effectiveness of cognitive remediation strategies for victims of traumatic head injury: A review of the literature. *Clinical Psychology Review, 9*, 605-626.

Benjamin, G. A. H., & Kaszniak, A. (1991). The discovery process: Deposition, trial testimony, and hearing testimony. In H. O. Doerr & A. S. Carlin (Eds.), *Forensic neuropsychology: Legal and scientific bases* (pp. 17-32). New York: Guilford.

Bennett, T. (1988). Use of the Halstead-Reitan neuropsychological test battery in the assessment of head injury. *Cognitive Rehabilitation, 6*(3), 18-24.

Benton. A. L. (1963). *The Revised Visual Retention Test.* New York: Psychological Corporation.

Benton, A. L. (1992). Clinical neuropsychology: 1960-1990. *Journal of Clinical and Experimental Neuropsychology, 14*(3), 407-417.

Benton, A. L., Varney, N. R., & Hamsher, K. deS. (1978). Visuospatial judgement. *Archives of Neurology, 35*, 364-367.

Ben-Yishay, Y., Ben-Nachum, Z., Cohen, A., Gerstman, L., Gordon, W., Gross, Y., Hofien, D., Piasetsky, E., & Rattok, Y. (1978). *Working approaches to remediation of cognitive deficits in brain damage.* Supplement to the 6th Annual Workshop for Rehabilitation Professionals, New York.

Ben-Yishay, Y., Piasetsky, E. B., & Rattok, J. (1987). A systematic method for ameliorating disorders in basic attention. In M. J. Meier, A. Benton, & L. Diller (Eds.), *Neuropsychological rehabilitation* (pp. 165-181). New York: Guilford Press.

Berg, E. A. (1948). A simple objective technique for measuring flexibility in thinking. *Journal of General Psychology, 39*, 15-22.

Berg., L. (1984). Focal infections. In L. P. Rowland (Ed.), *Merritt's textbook of neurology* (7th ed., pp. 72-78). Philadelphia: Lea & Febiger.

Bernard, L. C. (1990). Prospects for faking believable memory deficits on neuropsychological tests and the use of incentives in simulation research. *Journal of Clinical and Experimental Neuropsychology, 12*(5), 715-728.

Bigler, E. D. (1986). Forensic issues in neuropsychology. In D. Wedding, A. Horton, & J. Webster (Eds.), *The clinical neuropsychology handbook: Behavioral and clinical perspectives* (pp. 526-547). New York: Springer.

Bigler, E. D. (1990). Neuropsychology and malingering: Comment on Faust, Hart, and Guilmette (1988). *Journal of Consulting and Clinical Psychology, 58*(2), 244-247.

Binder, L. M. (1986). Persisting symptoms after mild head injury: A review of the postconcussive syndrome. *Journal of Clinical and Experimental Neuropsychology, 8*(4), 323-346.

Binder, L. M. (1992). *Portland Digit Recognition Test manual.* Portland, OR: Author.

Binder, L. M., & Pankrantz, L. (1987). Neuropsychological evidence of a factitious memory complaint. *Journal of Clinical and Experimental Neuropsychology, 2*, 167-171.

Boll, T. J. (1986). Nontraditional and threshold considerations in neuropsychological assessment. In S. B. Filskov & T. J. Boll (Eds.), *Handbook of clinical neuropsychology* (Vol. 2, pp. 103-120). New York: Wiley.

Boll, T. J., Heaton, R., & Reitan, R. M. (1974). Neuropsychological and emotional correlates of Huntington's chorea. *The Journal of Nervous and Mental Disease, 158*(1), 61-69.

Boyar, J. T. (1981). Nonorganic factors on neuropsychological examination: Utility of repeat neuropsychological measures. *Clinical Neuropsychology, 3*(4), 15-17.

Bracy, O. J. (1984). *Cognitive rehabilitation: A process approach*. Paper presented at the Texas State Occupational Therapy Conference, Houston, TX.

Bracy, O. J. (1989). *Computer software for cognitive rehabilitation*. Indianapolis, IN: Psychological Software Services.

Bracy, O. J., Bracy, N. P., Dacquisto, V. S., & Owens, S. G. (1990). *Computer assisted memory notebook*. Indianapolis, IN: NeuroScience Publishers.

Bracy, O. J., Lynch, W., Sbordone, R., & Berrol, S. (1985) Cognitive retraining through computers: Fact or fad? *Cognitive Rehabilitation, 3*(2), 10-25.

Braunling-McMorrow, D., Lloyd, K., & Fralish, K. (1986). Teaching social skills to head injured adults. *Journal of Rehabilitation, 52*(1), 39-44.

Brodsky, S. L. (1991). *Testifying in court: Guidelines and maxims for the expert witness*. Washington, DC: American Psychological Association.

Brooks, N. (1984). Cognitive deficits after head injury. In N. Brooks (Ed.), *Closed head injury: Psychological, social, and family consequences* (pp. 44-73). New York: Oxford University Press.

Burns, R. A. (1984). Stroke in young adults. In L. P. Rowland (Ed.), *Merritt's textbook of neurology* (7th ed., pp. 177-181). Philadelphia: Lea & Febiger.

Butters, N., Sax, D., Montgomery, K., & Tarlow, S. (1978). Comparison of the neuropsychological deficits associated with early and advanced Huntington's disease. *Archives of Neurology, 35*, 585-589.

Caplan, B. (1987). *Rehabilitation psychology desk reference*. Rockville, MD: Aspen Publishers.

Chelune, G. J., & Moehle, K. A. (1986). Neuropsychological assessment and everyday functioning. In D. Wedding, A. Horton, & J. Webster (Eds.), *The clinical neuropsychology handbook: Behavioral and clinical perspectives* (pp. 489-525). New York: Springer.

Conoley, J. C., & Kramer, J. J. (1989). *10th mental measurements yearbook*. Lincoln, NB: Buros Institute of Mental Measurement.

Council on Scientific Affairs (1988). Magnetic resonance imaging of the central nervous system. *Journal of the American Medical Association, 259*(8), 1211-1222.

Cullum, C. M., Heaton, R. K., & Grant, I. (1991). Psychogenic factors influencing neuropsychological performance: Somataform disorders, factitious disorders, and malingering. In H. O. Doerr & A. S. Carlin (Eds.), *Forensic neuropsychology: Legal and scientific bases* (pp. 141-174). New York: Guilford.

Cullum, C. M., Steinam, D. R., & Bigler, E. D. (1984). Relationship between fluid and crystallized cognitive functions using Category Test and WAIS scores. *International Journal of Clinical Neuropsychology, 1*(3), 172-174.

Cummings, J. L., Tomiyasu, U., Read, S., & Benson, D. F. (1984). Amnesia with hippocampal lesions after cardiopulminary arrest. *Neurology, 34*, 679-681.

DeFilippis, N. A. (1993). *Category Test: Computer Version Research Edition*. Odessa, FL: Psychological Assessment Resources.

DeFilippis, N. A., & McCampbell, E. (1979). *Manual for the Booklet Category Test*. Odessa, FL: Psychological Assessment Resources.

Diller, L., & Gordon, W. A. (1981). Interventions for cognitive deficits in brain-injured adults. *Journal of Consulting and Clinical Psychology, 49*(6), 822-834.

Dixon, C.E., Taft, W.C., & Hayes, R.L. (1993). Mechanisms of mild traumatic brain injury. *Journal of Head Trauma Rehabilitation, 8*(4), 1-12.

Dodrill, C. B. (1981). Neuropsychology of epilepsy. In S. B. Filskov & T. J. Boll (Eds.), *Handbook of clinical neuropsychology* (pp. 366-398). New York: Wiley.

Dodrill, C. B. (1986). Psychosocial consequences of epilepsy. In S. B. Filskov & T. J. Boll (Eds.), *Handbook of clinical neuropsychology* (Vol. 2, pp. 338-363). New York: Wiley.

Doerr, H. O., & Carlin, A. S. (Eds.). (1991). *Forensic neuropsychology: Legal and scientific bases.* New York: Guilford.

Dunn, M. (1987). Social skills and rehabilitation. In B. Caplan (Ed.), *Rehabilitation psychology desk reference* (pp. 345-364). Rockville, MD: Aspen Publishers.

Eisner, J., & Kreutzer, J. S. (1989). A family information system for education following traumatic brain injury. *Brain Injury, 3*(1), 79-90.

Fahn, S. (1984). Huntington's disease and other forms of chorea. In L. P. Rowland (Ed.), *Merritt's textbook of neurology* (7th ed., pp. 517-520). Philadelphia: Lea & Febiger.

Faust, D. (1991). Forensic neuropsychology: The art of practicing a science that does not yet exist. *Neuropsychology Review, 2*(3), 205-232.

Faust, D., & Guilmette, T. J. (1990). To say it's not so doesn't prove that it isn't: Research on the detection of malingering. Reply to Bigler. *Journal of Consulting and Clinical Psychology, 58*(2), 248-250.

Faust, D., Hart, K., & Guilmette, T. J. (1988). Pediatric malingering: The capacity of children to fake believable deficits on neuropsychological testing. *Journal of Consulting and Clinical Psychology, 56*, 578-582.

Faust, D., Hart, K., Guilmette, T. J., & Arkes, H. R. (1988). Neuropsychologists' capacity to detect adolescent malingerers. *Professional Psychology: Research and Practice, 19*, 508-515.

Faust, D., Ziskin, J., & Hiers, J. B. (1991). *Brain damage claims: Coping with neuropsychological evidence.* Los Angeles: Law and Psychology Press.

Filskov, S.B., & Goldstein, S.G. (1974). Diagnostic validity of the Halstead-Reitan neuropsychological battery. *Journal of Consulting Psychology, 42*, 382-388.

Georgemiller, R., & Hassan, F. (1986). Spatial competence: Assessment of route-finding, route learning, and topographical memory in normal aging. *Clinical Gerontologist, 5*, 19-37.

Gerbench, S. G., Priest, J. D., Boen, J. R., Staub, C. P., & Maxwell, R. E. (1983). Concussion incidences and severity in secondary school varsity football players. *American Journal of Public Health, 73*, 1370-1375.

Gianutsos, J. G., & Eberstein, A. (1987). Computer-augmented feedback displays: Treatment of hemiplegic motor deficits as a paradigm. In B. Caplan (Ed.), *Rehabilitation psychology desk reference* (pp. 365-384). Rockville, MD: Aspen Publishers.

Gianutsos, R., & Gianutsos, J. (1987). Single-case experimental approaches to the assessment of interventions in rehabilitation. In B. Caplan (Ed.), *Rehabilitation psychology desk reference* (pp. 453-470). Rockville, Maryland: Aspen Publishers.

Gianutsos, R., & Klitzner, C. (1981). *Computer programs for cognitive rehabilitation.* Bayport, NY: Life Science Associates.

Gianutsos, R., & Matheson, P. (1987). The rehabilitation of visual perceptual disorders attributable to brain injury. In M. J. Meier, A. Benton, & L. Diller (Eds.), *Neuropsychological rehabilitation* (pp. 202-241). New York: Guilford Press.

Gilandes, A. J., & Touyz, S. W. (1983). Forensic neuropsychology: A selective introduction. *Journal of Forensic Science, 28,* 713-725.

Gilewski, M. J., & Zelinski, E. M. (1988). Memory Functioning Questionnaire (MFQ). *Psychopharmacology Bulletin, 24*(4), 665-670.

Glisky, E. L., & Schacter, D. L. (1989). Extending the limits of complex learning in organic amnesia: Computer training in a vocational domain. *Neuropsychologia, 27*(1), 107-120.

Goebel, R. A. (1983). Detection of faking on the Halstead-Reitan neuropsychological test battery. *Journal of Clinical Psychology, 39,* 731-742.

Golden, C. J. (1977). The validity of the Halstead-Reitan Battery in a mixed psychiatric and brain damaged population. *Journal of Consulting and Clinical Psychology, 45,* 1043-1051.

Golden, C. J. (1978). *Diagnosis and rehabilitation in neuropsychology.* Springfield, IL: Thomas.

Golden, C. J., Osman, D. C., Moses, J. A., & Berg, R. A. (1981). *Interpretation of the Halstead-Reitan neuropsychological battery.* New York: Grune & Stratton.

Goldstein, G. (1987). Neuropsychological assessment for rehabilitation: Fixed batteries, automated systems, and non-psychometric methods. In M. J. Meier, A. Benton, & L. Diller (Eds.), *Neuropsychological rehabilitation* (pp. 18-40). New York: Guilford Press.

Goldstein, S. G., Daysack, R. E., & Kleinknecht, R. A. (1973). Effect of experience and amount of information on identification of cerebral impairment. *Journal of Consulting and Clinical Psychology, 41,* 30-34.

Gordon, R., Herman, G. T., & Johnson, B. A. (1975, October). Image reconstruction from projections. *Scientific American, 233*(4), pp. 56-68.

Gouvier, D. W., Uddo-Crane, M., & Brown, L. M. (1988). Base rates for post-concussional symptoms. *Archives of Clinical Neuropsychology, 3,* 273-278.

Gouvier, D. W., Webster, J. S., & Blanton, P. D. (1986). Cognitive retraining with brain injured patients. In D. Wedding, A. Horton, & J. Webster (Eds.), *The clinical neuropsychology handbook: Behavioral and clinical perspectives* (pp. 278-324). New York: Springer.

Grant, D. A., & Berg, E. A. (1948). A behavioral analysis of degree of impairment and ease of shifting to new responses in a Weigl-type card sorting problem. *Journal of Experimental Psychology, 39,* 404-411.

Grant, I. (1987). Alcohol and the brain: Neuropsychological correlates. *Journal of Consulting and Clinical Psychology, 55*(3), 310-324.

Gray, J. M., & Robertson, I. (1989). Remediation of attentional difficulties following brain injury: Three experimental single case studies. *Brain Injury, 3*(2), 163-170.

Gronwall, D., & Wrightson, P. (1975). Cumulative effects of concussion. *Lancet, 2,* 995-997.

Guilmette, T. J., Faust, D., Hart, K., & Arkes, H. R. (1990). A national survey of psychologists who offer neuropsychological services. *Archives of Clinical Neuropsychology,* 5(4), 373-392.

Halstead, W. C. (1947). *Brain and intelligence: A quantitative study of the frontal lobes.* Chicago: University of Chicago Press.

Hamlin, D. H., & Jarvis, P. E. (1987). *Neuropsychological services in state mental health systems* (Study #85-541). Washington, DC: National Association of State Mental Health Program Directors.

Hart, T., & Hayden, M. E. (1986). The ecological validity of neuropsychological assessment and remediation. In B. P. Uzzell & Y. Gross (Eds), *Clinical neuropsychology of intervention* (pp. 21-50). Boston: Martinus Nijhoff.

Hartman, D. E. (1988). *Neuropsychological toxicology.* New York: Pergamon.

Hathaway, S. R., & McKinley, J. C. (1942). A multiphasic personality schedule (Minnesota): III. The measurement of symptomatic depression. *Journal of Psychology, 14,* 73-84.

Hayes, R. L., Jenkins, L. W., & Lyeth, B. C. (1992). Neurotransmitter mediation mechanisms of traumatic brain injury: Acetycholine and excitatory amino acids. *Journal of Neurotrauma, 9* (Supplement 5), 173-187.

Heaton, R. K. (1980). *A manual for the Wisconsin Card Sorting Test.* Odessa, FL: Psychological Assessment Resources.

Heaton, R. K. (1993). *WCST: Computer Version-2 Research Edition.* Odessa, FL: Psychological Assessment Resources.

Heaton, R. K., Chelune, G. J., & Lehman, R. A. W. (1978). Using neuropsychological and personality tests to assess the likelihood of patient employment. *Journal of Nervous and Mental Diseases, 166,* 408-416.

Heaton, R. K., Chelune, G. J., Talley, J. L., Kay, G. G., & Curtiss, G. (1993). *Wisconsin Card Sorting Test manual: Revised and expanded.* Odessa, FL: Psychological Assessment Resources.

Heaton, R. K., & Crowley, T. J. (1981). Effects of psychiatric disorders and their somatic treatments on neuropsychological test results. In S. B. Filskov & T. J. Boll (Eds.), *Handbook of clinical neuropsychology* (pp. 481-524). New York: Wiley.

Heaton, R. K., Grant, I., Anthony, W. Z., & Lehman, A. W. (1981). A comparison of clinical and automated interpretation of the Halstead-Reitan battery. *Journal of Clinical Neuropsychology,* 3(2), 121-141.

Heaton, R. K., Grant, I., & Matthews, C. G. (1986). Differences in neuropsychological test performance associated with age, education, and sex. In I. Grant & K. M. Adams (Eds.), *Neuropsychological assessment in neuropsychiatric disorders: Clinical methods and empirical findings* (pp. 100-120). New York: Oxford University Press.

Heaton, R. K., Grant, I., & Matthews, C. G. (1991). *Comprehensive norms for an expanded Halstead-Reitan battery.* Odessa, FL: Psychological Assessment Resources.

Heaton, R. K., Nelson, L. M., Thompson, D. S., Burks, J. S., & Franklin, G. M. (1985). Neuropsychological findings in relapsing-remitting and chronic-progressive multiple sclerosis. *Journal of Consulting and Clinical Psychology*, *53*, 103-110.

Heaton, R. K., & Pendleton, M. G. (1981). Use of neuropsychological tests to predict adult patients' everyday functioning. *Journal of Consulting and Clinical Psychology*, *49*, 807-821.

Heaton, R. K., Smith, H. H., Lehman, R. A. W., & Vogt, A. T. (1978). Prospects for faking believable deficits on neuropsychological testing. *Journal of Consulting and Clinical Psychology*, *46*, 892-900.

Heinrichs, R. W. (1990). Current and emergent applications of neuropsychological assessment: Problems of validity and utility. *Professional Psychology: Research and Practice*, *21*, 171-176.

Hevern, V. W. (1980). Recent validity studies of the Halstead-Reitan approach to clinical neuropsychological assessment: A critical review. *Clinical Neuropsychology*, *3*, 20-23.

Hiscock, M., & Hiscock, C. K. (1989). Refining the forced-choice method for the detection of malingering. *Journal of Clinical and Experimental Neuropsychology*, *11*(6), 967-974.

Jarvis P. E. (1988a). Neuropsychology in Colorado: Some data and some questions. *Colorado Psychological Association Bulletin*, *7*, pp. 1, 4.

Jarvis P. E. (1988b). In search of an adequate neuropsychological evaluation. *Colorado Psychological Association Bulletin*, *7*, pp. 3, 6.

Jarvis, P. E. (1990). The importance of patient friendliness in CACR programs and some tips for improving it. *Cognitive Rehabilitation*, *8*(4), 24-28.

Jarvis, P. E.,& Barth, J. T. (1979). The neglect of physical-neurological factors in community mental health practice: A proposal for a better balance. *Clinical Neuropsychology*, *1*, 20-23.

Jarvis, P. E., & Barth, J. T. (1984). *Halstead Reitan test battery: An interpretive guide*. Odessa, FL: Psychological Assessment Resources.

Jarvis, P. E., DeFilippis, N., & Hamlin, D. (in press). The Category Test and the BCT: Equivalent tests but different instructions? *The International Journal of Clinical Neuropsychology*.

Jarvis, P. E., & Hamlin, D. H. (1984). Avoiding pitfalls in compensation evaluations. International *Journal of Clinical Neuropsychology*, *6*(3), 214-216.

Jarvis, P. E., & Hamlin, D. H. (1991). The use of verbal maps to help people with right-cerebral hemisphere lesions compensate for perceptual-spatial deficits. *Journal of Rehabilitation*, *57*(3), 51-53.

Jarvis, P. E., & Nelson, S. (1968). Familiarization, a vital step in mental health consultation. *Community Mental Health Journal*, *11*, 343-348.

Jarvis P. E., & Vollman R. R. (1983). Beyond the obvious: Two cases illustrating the need to consider both physical-neurological and psycho-social factors in assessment. *Clinical Neuropsychology*, *5*(3), 109-111.

Jubelt, B., & Harter, D. H. (1984). Viral infection. In L. P. Rowland (Ed.), *Merritt's textbook of neurology* (7th ed., pp. 79-115). Philadelphia: Lea & Febiger.

Kandel, E. R., Schwartz, J. H., & Jassell, T. M. (1991). *Principles of neural science* (3rd ed.). New York: Elsenier.

Katz, R., & Nagy, V. T. (1984). CATS: Computerized aphasia treatment system. *Cognitive Rehabilitation*, 2(4), 8-11.

Katzman, R. (1984a). Delirium and dementia. In L. P. Rowland (Ed.), *Merritt's textbook of neurology* (7th ed., pp. 1-5). Philadelphia: Lea & Febiger.

Katzman, R. (1984b). The Dementias. In L. P. Rowland (Ed.), *Merritt's textbook of neurology* (7th ed., pp. 508-514). Philadelphia: Lea & Febiger.

Kaufman, David M. (1981). *Clinical neurology for psychiatrists*. New York: Grune & Stratton.

Kløve, H. (1963). Clinical neuropsychology. In F. M. Forster (Ed.), *The medical clinics of North America*. New York: Saunders.

Kreutzer, J. S., Harris-Marwitz, J., & Myers, S. (1990). Neuropsychological issues in litigation following traumatic brain injury. *Neuropsychology*, 4, 249-259.

Kreutzer, J. S., Hill M. R., & Morrison, C. (1987). *Cognitive rehabilitation resources for the Apple II computer*. Indianapolis: Neuroscience Publishers.

Kreutzer, J. S., Leininger, B. E., Sherron, P. D., & Groah, C. H. (1990). Managing psychosocial dysfunction. In P. Wehman & J. S. Kreutzer (Eds.), *Vocational rehabilitation for persons with traumatic brain injury* (pp. 35-69). Rockville, MD: Aspen.

Kreutzer, J. S., Wehman, P., Morton, M. V., & Stonnington, H. H. (1988). Supported employment and compensatory strategies for enhancing vocational outcome following traumatic brain injury. *Brain Injury*, 2(3), 205-223.

Lawton, M. P. (1988). Scales to measure competence in everyday activities. *Psychopharmacology Bulletin*, 24(4), 609-613.

Lee, G. P., Loring, D. W., & Martin, R. C. (1992). Rey's 15-item visual memory test for the detection of malingering: Normative observations on patients with neurological disorders. *Psychological Assessment*, 4(1), 43-46.

Levenkron, J. C. (1987). Behavior modification in rehabilitation: Principles and clinical strategies. In B. Caplan (Ed.), *Rehabilitation psychology desk reference* (pp. 383-416). Rockville, MD: Aspen Publishers.

Lewis, J. A. (1986). Neurological diagnostic tests. In S. B. Filskov & T. J. Boll (Eds.), *Handbook of clinical neuropsychology* (Vol. 2, pp. 81-102). New York: Wiley.

Lezak, M. D. (1983). *Neuropsychological assessment* (2nd ed.). New York: Oxford University Press.

Lezak, M. D. (1987a). Assessment for rehabilitation planning. In M. J. Meier, A. Benton, & L. Diller (Eds.), *Neuropsychological rehabilitation* (pp. 41-58). New York: Guilford Press.

Lezak, M. D. (1987b). Relationships between personality disorders, social disorders, social disturbances, and physical disability following traumatic brain injury. *Journal of Head Trauma Rehabilitation*, 2(1), 57-69.

Lira, F. T. Carne, W., & Masri, A. M. (1983). Treatment of anger and impulsivity in a brain damaged patient: A case study applying stress inoculation. *Clinical Neuropsychology*, 5(4), 159-160.

Long, C.J., & Hunter, S. E. (1981). Analysis of temporal cortex dysfunction by neuropsychological techniques. *Clinical Neuropsychology, 3*(1), 16-23.

Long, C. J., & Klein, K. (1990). Decision strategies in neuropsychology II: Determination of age effects on neuropsychological performance. *Archives of Clinical Neuropsychology, 5,* 335-345.

Luria, A. R. (1963). *Restoration of function after brain injury.* New York: Macmillan Co.

Luria, A. R. (1966). *Higher cortical functions in man.* New York: Basic Books.

Luria, A. R. (1973). *The working brain.* New York: Basic Books.

Lyle, O. E., & Gottesman, I. I. (1977). Premorbid psychometric indicators of the gene for Huntington's disease. *Journal of Clinical and Consulting Psychology, 45*(6), 1011-1022.

Lynch, W. J. (1983a). Cognitive retraining using microcomputer games and commercially available software. *Cognitive Rehabilitation, 1*(1), 19-22.

Lynch, W. J. (1983b). The use of a word processor in language rehabilitation. *Cognitive Rehabilitation, 1*(6), 20-23.

Mahurin, R. K., DeBettignies, B. H., & Pirozzolo, F. (1991). Structured assessment of independent living skills: Preliminary report of a performance measure of functional abilities in dementia. *Journal of Gerontology, 40*(2), 58-66.

Marsh, N. V., & Knight, R. G. (1991). Relationship between cognitive deficits and social skill after head injury. *Neuropsychology, 5*(2), 107-117.

Matthews, C. G. (1981). Neuropsychology practice in a hospital setting. In S. B. Filskov & T. J. Boll (Eds.), *Handbook of clinical neuropsychology* (pp. 645-685). New York: Wiley.

Matarazzo, J. D. (1972). *Wechsler's measurement and appraisal of adult intelligence* (5th ed.). Baltimore: Williams and Wilkins.

Mayes, S. D., Pelco, L. E., & Campbell, C. J. (1989). Relationships among pre- and post-injury intelligence, length of coma and age in individuals with severe closed-head trauma. *Brain Injury, 3*(3), 301-313.

McCampbell, E., & DeFilippis, N. A. (1979). The development of a booklet form of The Category Test: A preliminary report. *Clinical Neuropsychology, 1,* 33-35.

McFie, J., & Thompson, J. A. (1972). Picture Arrangement: A measure of frontal lobe function? *British Journal of Psychiatry, 121,* 547-572.

McGlynn, S. M. (1990). Behavioral approaches to neuropsychological rehabilitation. *Psychological Bulletin, 108*(3), 420-441.

McMahon, E. A., & Satz, P. (1981). Clinical neuropsychology: Some forensic applications. In S. B. Filskov & T. J. Boll (Eds.), *Handbook of clinical neuropsychology* (pp. 686-701). New York: Wiley.

Meichenbaum, D. (1973). A self-instructional approach to stress management: A proposal for stress inoculation training. In C. Spielberger & I. Sarason (Eds.), *Stress and anxiety* (Vol. 1, pp. 237-263). New York: Wiley.

Meichenbaum, D., & Cameron, R. (1973). Training schizophrenics to talk to themselves: A means of developing attentional controls. *Behavior Therapy, 4,* 515-534.

Meichenbaum, D., & Goodman, J. (1971). Training impulsive children to talk to themselves: A means of developing self-control. *Journal of Abnormal Psychology, 77,* 115-126.

Meier, M. J., Benton, A., & Diller, L. (1987) *Neuropsychological rehabilitation.* New York: Guilford Press.

Meyer, V. (1961). Psychological effects of brain damage. In H. J. Eysenck (Ed.), *Handbook of abnormal psychology* (pp. 529-565). New York: Basic Books.

Moehl, K. A., & Long, C. J. (1989). Models of aging and neuropsychological test performance decline with aging. *Journal of Gerentology: Psychological Sciences, 44*(6), 176-177.

Mooney, G. F. (1988). Relative contributions of neurophysical, cognitive, and personality changes to disability after brain injury. *Cognitive Rehabilitation, 6*(5), 14-20.

Mortenson, E. L., Gade, A., & Reinisch, J. M. (1991). A critical note on Lezak's "best performance method" in clinical neuropsychology. *Journal of Clinical and Experimental Neuropsychology, 13*(2), 361-371.

Niemann, H., Ruff, R. M., & Baser, C. (1990). Computer-assisted attention retraining in head-injured individuals: A controlled efficacy study of an outpatient program. *Journal of Consulting and Clinical Psychology, 58*(6), 811-817.

O'Connor, M., & Cermak, L. S. (1987). Rehabilitation of organic memory disorders. In M. J. Meier, A. Benton, & L. Diller (Eds.), *Neuropsychological rehabilitation* (pp. 260-279). New York: Guilford Press.

Oltman, J. E., & Freidman, S. (1961). Comments on Huntington's chorea. *Diseases of the Nervous System, 21,* 313-319.

Pankrantz, L. (1983). A new technique for the assessment and modification of feigned memory deficits. *Perceptual and Motor Skills, 57,* 367-372.

Pankrantz, L. (1988). Malingering on intellectual and neuropsychological measures. In R. Rogers (Ed.), *Clinical assessment of malingering and deception* (pp. 169-194). New York: Guilford.

Parente, R., & Anderson-Parente, J. K. (1990). Vocational memory training. In J. S. Kreutzer & P. Wehman (Eds.), *Community integration following traumatic brain injury* (pp. 157-168). Baltimore: Brooks.

Parsons, O. A. (1987). Neuropsychological consequences of alcohol abuse: Many questions—some answers. In O. A. Parsons, N. Butters, & P. E. Nathan (Eds.), *Neuropsychology of alcoholism: Implications for diagnosis and treatment* (pp. 153-175). New York: Guilford Press.

Parsons, O. A., Butters, N., & Nathan, P. E. (1987). *Neuropsychology of alcoholism: Implications for diagnosis and treatment.* New York: Guilford Press.

Parsons, O. A., & Farr, S. P. (1981). The neuropsychology of alcohol and drug use. In S. B. Filskov & T. J. Boll (Eds.), *Handbook of clinical neuropsychology* (pp. 320-365). New York: Wiley.

Pendleton, M. G., & Heaton, R. K. (1982). A comparison of the Wisconsin Card Sorting Test and the Category Test. *Journal of Clinical Psychology, 36*(2), 392-396.

Pendleton, M. G., Heaton, R. K., Lehman, R. A. W., & Hulihan, D. (1982). The diagnostic utility of the Thurston Word Fluency Test in neuropsychological evaluations. *Journal of Clinical Neuropsychology, 4*(4), 307-317.

Peyser, J. M., & Poser, C. M. (1986). Neuropsychological correlates of multiple sclerosis. In S. B. Filskov & T. J. Boll (Eds), *Handbook of clinical neuropsychology* (Vol. 2, pp. 364-397). New York: Wiley.

Plum, F., & Posner, J. B. (1962). Delayed neurological deterioration after anoxia. *Archives of Internal Medicine, 110*, 56-63.

Poser, C. M., Alter, M., Sibley, W. A., & Scheinberg, L. C. (1984). Multiple sclerosis. In L. P. Rowland (Ed.), *Merritt's textbook of neurology* (7th ed., pp. 593-610). Philadelphia: Lea & Febiger.

Posner, M. I., & Rafal, R. D. (1987). Cognitive theories of attention and the rehabilitation of attentional deficits. In M. J. Meier, A. Benton, & L. Diller (Eds.), *Neuropsychological rehabilitation* (pp. 182-201). New York: Guilford Press.

Povlishock, J. T. (1985). The morphopathologic responses to experimental head injuries of varying severity. In D. F. Becker & J. T. Povlishock (Eds.), *Central nervous system trauma status report* (pp. 443-452). Richmond, VA: Byrd.

Prigatano, G. P., Parsons, O., Wright, E., Levin, D. C., & Hawryluk, G. (1983). Neuropsychological test performance in mildly hypoxic patients with chronic obstructive pulmonary disease. *Journal of Consulting and Clinical Psychology, 51*(1), 108-116.

Prockop, L. D. (1984). Disorders of cerebrospinal and brain fluids. In L. P. Rowland (Ed.), *Merritt's textbook of neurology* (7th ed., pp. 199-226). Philadelphia: Lea & Febiger.

Reitan, R. M. (1955a). Certain differential effects of left and right cerebral lesions in human adults. *Journal of Comparative and Physiological Psychology, 48*, 474-477.

Reitan, R. M. (1955b). The distribution according to age of a psychologic measure dependent upon organic brain functions. *Journal of Gerontology, 10*, 338-340.

Reitan, R. M. (1959a). *The effects of brain lesions on adaptive abilities in human beings.* Seattle: University of Washington.

Reitan, R. M. (1959b). *Manual for administration of neuropsychological test batteries for adults and children.* Unpublished Manuscript.

Reitan, R. M. (1972). *Neuropsychological interpretations of underlying neurological disorders.* Seattle: University of Washington.

Reitan, R. M. (1975). Assessment of brain-behavior relationships. In P. McReynolds (Ed.), *Advances in psychological assessment* (Vol. 3, pp. 186-242). San Francisco: Josey-Bass.

Reitan, R. M. (1979a). *Manual for administration of neuropsychological test batteries for adults and children.* Tucson, AZ: Reitan Neuropsychological Laboratory.

Reitan, R. M. (1979b). *Neurological correlates of neuropsychological measures.* Tucson, AZ: Reitan Neuropsychological Laboratory.

Reitan, R. M. (1984). *Aphasia and sensory-perceptual deficits in adults.* Tucson, AZ: Neuropsychology Press.

Reitan, R. M., & Boll, T. J. (1971). Intellectual and cognitive functions in Parkinson's disease. *Journal of Consulting and Clinical Psychology*, *37*, 364-369.

Reitan, R. M., & Davidson, L. A. (1974). *Clinical neuropsychology: Current status and applications*. Washington, DC: Winston and Sons.

Reitan, R. M., & Tarshes, E. L. (1959). Differential effects of lateralized brain lesions on the Trail Making Test. *Journal of Nervous and Mental Disorders*, 129, 257.

Reitan, R. M., & Wolfson, D. (1985). *Halstead-Reitan neuropsychological test battery: Theory and clinical interpretation*. Tucson, AZ: Neuropsychology Press.

Reitan, R. M., & Wolfson, D. (1988a). The Halstead-Reitan neuropsychological test battery and REHABIT: A model for integrating evaluation and remediation of cognitive impairment. *Cognitive Rehabilitation*, *6*(3), 10-17.

Reitan, R. M., & Wolfson, D. (1988b). *Traumatic brain injury: Vol. II. Recovery and rehabilitation*. Tucson, AZ: Neuropsychology Press.

Reitan, R. M., & Wolfson, D. (1993). *Halstead-Reitan neuropsychological test battery: Theory and clinical interpretation* (2nd ed.). Tucson, AZ: Neuropsychology Press.

Rimel, R. W., Giordani, B., Barth, J. T., Boll, T. J., & June, J. A. (1981). Disability caused by minor head injury. *Neurosurgery*, *9*, 221-228.

Robertson, I., Gray, J., & McKenzie, S. (1988). Microcomputer-based cognitive rehabilitation of visual neglect: Three multiple-baseline single-case studies. *Brain Injury*, *2*(2), 151-163.

Roediger, H. L. (1990). Implicit memory retention without remembering. *American Psychologist*, *45*(9), 1043-1056.

Romanczyk, R. G., & Tyc, V. (1988). Cognitive rehabilitation and the use of computer technology: Significant stride or grand illusion? *Behavior Therapist*, *11*(1), 17-19.

Ross, L. Thrasher, M., & Long, C. J. (1990). Decision strategies in neuropsychology: Vol. I. Determination of lateralized cerebral dysfunction. *Archives of Clinical Neuropsychology*, *3*, 273-285.

Russell, E. W. (1975). A multiple scoring method for the assessment of complex memory functions. *Journal of Consulting and Clinical Psychology*, *43*(6), 800-809.

Russell, E. W., Neuringer, C., & Goldstein, G. (1970). *Assessment of brain damage: A neuropsychological key approach*. New York: Wiley.

Sacks, Oliver (1985). *The man who mistook his wife for a hat and other clinical tales*. New York: Summit.

Saunders, R. L., & Harbaugh, R. E. (1984). The Second impact in contact-sports head trauma. *Journal of the American Medical Association*, *252*(4), 538-539.

Sbordone, R. J. (1987). A neuropsychological approach to cognitive rehabilitation within a private practice setting. In B. Caplan (Ed.), *Rehabilitation psychology desk reference* (pp. 323-342). Rockville, MD: Aspen Publishers.

Sbordone, R. J. (1990). Psychotherapeutic treatment of the client with traumatic brain injury. In J. S. Kreutzer & P. Wehman (Eds.), *Community integration following traumatic brain injury* (pp. 139-153). Baltimore: Brooks.

Sbordone, R. J., Seecof, M., & Hall, S. B. (1983). *Digit-Digit Attention Test* [Computer Program]. Fountain Valley, CA: Robert J. Sbordone, Inc.

Schacter, D. L., & Glisky, E. L. (1986). Memory remediation: restoration, alleviation, and the acquisition of domain-specific knowledge. In B. P. Uzzell & Y. Gross (Eds.), *Clinical neuropsychology of intervention* (pp. 257-282). Boston: Martinus Nijhoff.

Scheinberg, L. C., & Smith, C. R. (1987). Signs and symptoms of multiple sclerosis. In L. C. Scheinberg & N. J. Holland (Eds.), *Multiple sclerosis: A guide for patients and their families* (2nd ed., pp. 43-52). New York: Raven Press.

Schmidt, J. P. (1989). Why recent researchers have not assessed the capacity of neuropsychologists to detect malingering. *Professional Psychology: Research and Practice, 20,* 140-141.

School Health and Sports Medicine Committee (1990). *Guidelines for management of concussion in sports.* Denver, CO: Colorado Medical Society.

Sena, D. A. (1985). The effectiveness of cognitive retraining for brain injured individuals. The International *Journal of Clinical Neuropsychology, 7,* 62.

Sena, D. A. (1986). The effectiveness of cognitive retraining for brain-impaired patients. *Journal of Clinical and Experimental Neuropsychology, 8,* 142.

Sena, H. M., & Sena D. A. (1986a). A comparison of subject characteristics between treatment and nontreatment patients. *Archives of Clinical Neuropsychology, 1,* 74.

Sena, H. M., & Sena D. A. (1986b). A quantitative validation of the effectiveness of cognitive retraining. *Archives of Clinical Neuropsychology, 1,* 74.

Shipley, W. C. (1946). *Institute of living scale.* Los Angeles: Western Psychological Services.

Smith, J. (1984). *Cognitive rehabilitation* [Computer program]. Dimondale, MI: Hartley Courseware.

Sohlberg, M. M., & Mateer, C. A. (1989). *Introduction to cognitive rehabilitation.* New York: Guilford Press.

Spreen, O., & Strauss, E. (1991). *A compendium of neuropsychological tests.* New York: Oxford University Press.

Steegmann, A. T. (1962). *Examination of the nervous system: A student's guide.* Chicago: Year Book Medical Publishers.

Story, T. A., & Sbordone, R. J. (1988). The use of microcomputers in the treatment of cognitive-communicative impairments. *Journal of Head Trauma Rehabilitation, 3*(2), 45-54.

Taylor, R. (1990). Relationships between cognitive test performance and everyday cognitive difficulties in multiple sclerosis. *British Journal of Clinical Psychology, 29,* 251-252.

Teasdale, G., & Mendelow, D. (1984). Pathophysiology of head injuries. In N. Brooks (Ed.), *Closed head injury: Psychological, social, and family consequences* (pp. 4-36). New York: Oxford University Press.

Thompson, L. L., Heaton, R. J., Matthews, C. G., & Grant, I. (1987). Comparison of preferred and nonpreferred hand performance on four neuropsychological tests. *The Clinical Neuropsychologist, 1*(4), 324-334.

Travin, S., & Protter, B. (1984). Malingering and malingering-like behavior: Some clinical and conceptual issues. *Psychiatric Quarterly, 56*(3), 189-197.

Trenerry, M. R., Crosson, B., DeBoe, J., & Leben, W. R. (1989). *Stroop Neuropsychological Screening Test manual*. Odessa, FL: Psychological Assessment Resources.

Uzzell, B. P. (Ed.). (1989). *Neuropsychology, 3*(4).

Vicente, P. J. (1980). Neuropsychological assessment and management of a carbon monoxide intoxication patient with consequent sleep apnea: A longitudinal case report. *Clinical Neuropsychology, II*(2), 91-94.

Vogenthaler, D. R. (1987). Rehabilitation after closed head injury: A primer. *Journal of Rehabilitation, 53*(4), 15-21.

Vogenthaler, D. R., Smith, K. R., & Goldfader, P. (1989). Head injury, an empirical study: Describing long-term productivity and independent living outcome. *Brain Injury, 3*(4), 355-368.

Walsh, K. W. (1985). *Understanding brain damage: A primer of neuropsychological evaluation*. New York: Churchill Livingstone.

Wechsler, D. (1945). A standardized memory scale for clinical use. *Journal of Psychology, 19*, 87-95.

Wechsler, D. (1955). *Manual for the Wechsler Adult Intelligence Scale*. New York: The Psychological Corporation.

Wechsler, D. (1981). *WAIS-R manual*. New York: The Psychological Corporation.

Wechsler, D. (1987). *WMS-R Manual: Wechsler Memory Scale Revised*. New York: The Psychological Corporation.

Webster, J. S., & Scott, R. R. (1983). The effects of self-instructional training on attentional deficits following head injury. *Clinical Neuropsychology, 5*, 69-74.

Wehman, P., & Kreutzer, J. S. (Eds.) (1990). *Vocational rehabilitation for persons with traumatic brain injury*. Rockville, MD: Aspen.

Wehman, P., Kreutzer, J., Sale, P., West, M., Morton, M. V., & Diambra, J. (1989). Cognitive impairment and remediation: Implications for employment following traumatic brain injury. *Journal of Head Trauma Rehabilitation, 4*(3), 66-75.

Weiner, I. B. (1987). Writing forensic reports. In I. B. Weiner & A. K. Hess (Eds.), *Handbook of forensic psychology* (pp. 511-528). New York: Wiley.

Weiner, I. B., & Hess, A. K. (1987). *Handbook of forensic psychology*. New York: Wiley.

Wheeler, L., Burke, C. J., & Reitan, R. M. (1963). An application of discriminant functions to the problem of predicting brain damage using behavioral variables. *Perceptual and Motor Skills, 16*, 417.

Wilkinson, D. A. (1987). CT scan and neuropsychological assessment of alcoholism. In O. A. Parsons, N. Butters, & P. E. Nathan (Eds.), *Neuropsychology of alcoholism: Implications for diagnosis and treatment* (pp. 76-102). New York: Guilford Press.

Wilson, B. A. (1987). *Rehabilitation of memory*. New York: Guilford Press.

Yahr, M. D. (1984). Parkinsonism. In L. P. Rowland (Ed.), *Merritt's textbook of neurology* (7th ed., pp. 526-536). Philadelphia: Lea & Febiger.

Yalom, I. D. (1983). *Inpatient group psychotherapy*. New York: Basic Books.

APPENDIXES

Appendix A

Glossary

This glossary includes definitions of many of the technical terms used in this Guide as well as a number of other terms that the psychologist may encounter in both the neuropsychological and neurological literature and in reports of neurological examinations.

Absence Seizures. Form of epilepsy in children characterized by a short altered state of consciousness (petit mal seizures).

Acalculia. Inability to perform simple mathematical calculations due to cerebral dysfunction.

Abscess. Circumscribed infection which is characterized by a buildup of pus surrounded by a thick wall of cells.

Afferent Fibers. Neuronal pathways which carry information upward toward the cerebral cortex from peripheral areas of the nervous system.

Agnosia. Inability to recognize sensory stimulation due to cerebral dysfunction.

Agraphia. Inability to write due to cerebral dysfunction.

Akinesia. Inability to move due to cerebral dysfunction.

Alexia. Inability to read due to cerebral dysfunction.

Amygdala. One of the structures of the limbic system which is located at the base of the temporal lobe.

Aneurysm. The weak wall of a vein or artery which dilates and fills with blood. Such defective vascular areas may burst, causing hemorrhages of the adjacent tissue.

Angiography. A radiological procedure to enhance pictures of the cerebral vasculature by taking X-rays of the head following the introduction of a radiopaque contrast material to a major artery.

Angular Gyrus. A convolution of the cerebral cortex in the area of the parietal lobe which is intimately involved in the production of speech.

Anomia. Inability to name common items and figures due to cerebral dysfunction.

Anterior Commissure. Neuronal pathways, which connect the temporal lobes.

Anterograde Amnesia. Usually referred to as a loss of memory for events which follow cerebral trauma such as head injuries (post traumatic amnesia).

Aphasia. Inability to or deficit of communication due to cerebral dysfunction.

Apraxia. Inability to initiate planned movements due to cerebral dysfunction.

Arachnoid Space. One of the three layers of the meninges which is filled with fibrous tissue and acts as the conduit for cerebrospinal fluid to travel around the brain.

Arteriosclerosis. Disease of the vascular system characterized by a build up of fatty deposits on the inner walls of veins and arteries, restricting blood flow throughout the brain.

Astereognosis. Inability to tactilely recognize simple and familiar objects and shapes due to cerebral dysfunction.

Astrocytoma. Type of neoplasm which arises from astrocyte cells. These tumors are usually unencapsulated and intracerebral.

Ataxia. Muscular incoordination associated with cerebellar dysfunction.

Atrophy. Shrinkage of (brain) tissue due to loss of neuronal processes.

Axon. The portion of a neuron which transmits energy from the cell body to the receptors of other neurons.

Basal Ganglia. Nuclei associated with the forebrain (amygdala, caudate nucleus, claustrum, globus pallidus, and putamen).

Bilateral. Referring to both sides of the body or both cerebral hemispheres.

Bitemporal Hemianopsia. Visual field loss in both temporal areas which is caused by damage to the optic chiasm.

Brain Scan. Method of identifying neurological disturbances such as cerebrovascular accidents and neoplasms by injecting a radioisotope material into an artery and scanning the head with a Geiger counter to determine where the radioisotopes are collecting (in collections of blood, highly vascularized tumors, arteriovenous malformations, etc.).

Brain Stem. Thalamus, hypothalamus, basal ganglia, midbrain, and hindbrain.

Broca's Area (Aphasia). A portion of the left frontal lobe located near the motor strip, which is intimately involved in the production of speech. Disruption of this area can cause a Broca's aphasia which is characterized by deficits in expressive speech.

Central Sulcus (Fissure of Rolando). A large fissure that separates the frontal and parietal lobes.

Cerebellum. A large structure that mediates motor coordination located in the posterior part of the brain below the occipital lobes.

Cerebrovascular Accident (CVA). Ischemic disorder or disruption of blood flow in the brain due to an occlusion of a portion of the vascular system from a thrombus or embolus, or a hemorrhage.

Cerebrospinal Fluid (CSF). A clear fluid produced by the choroid plexis in the ventricles and circulated around the brain and spinal cord through the subarachnoid space.

Cingulate Bodies. Tissue found in the limbic system above the corpus callosum.

Computed Axial Tomography (CAT or CT Scan). State of the art, computer assisted X-rays measuring densities of sections of the brain.

Computed Tomography (CT Scan). Computerized representation of cross sections of the brain based upon multiple X-rays of tissue density.

Concussion. A head injury which is usually characterized by a loss of consciousness.

Conduction Aphasia. An expressive aphasia which is characterized by an understanding of language, yet an inability to repeat words correctly.

Constructional Dyspraxia. Difficulty in reproducing (drawing) simple, geometric designs and objects.

Contrecoup. An effect in closed head injury which is characterized by damage to brain tissue at a location opposite the site of impact due to the brain's bouncing off the walls of the cranium.

Contralateral. Referring to the opposite side of the body or brain.

Contrast Study (X-ray). Injection of a radiopaque dye into an artery, or air into the spinal column, followed by X-rays of the brain to highlight the cerebrovascular system or ventricle, respectively.

Contusion. Injury to the vascular system which produces hemorrhaging and associated swelling.

Corpus Callosum. Intracerebral tissue connecting the right and left hemispheres.

Cortex. The outer area or layer of brain tissue which is comprised of sulci and gyri.

Cranial Nerves. Twelve pairs of nerves that emanate from the brain and carry sensory and motor signals to and from the periphery of the central nervous system.

Cyst. A sac of fluid usually associated with an infectious disorder.

Decerebrate (Rigidity). Injury to the brain stem and/or cerebellum causing extension of limbs.

Decorticate (Rigidity). Injury to the thalamus, internal capsule and white matter causing flexion of the limbs.

Degenerative Disease. Loss of neurons and cerebral atrophy, the most common of which is referred to as primary neuronal degeneration, or Alzheimer's disease.

Dementia. Deterioration of mental functions characterized by cognitive decline and memory impairment.

Dendrites. Receptor structures of a neuron which are characterized by branch-like projections.

Dura. The outermost layer of the meninges.

Dysarthria. Difficulty in articulation.

Dyscalculia. Difficulty in performing simple arithmetic calculations.

Dyskinesia. Difficulty in movement.

Dyslexia. Difficulty in reading.

Dysnomia. Difficulty in naming common objects and shapes.

Dysphasia. Difficulty in speech/communication.

Efferent Fibers. Neuronal pathways which carry information downward from the cerebral cortex to the peripheral areas of the nervous system.

Electroencephalography (EEG). A method of recording bioelectrical discharge from the cortex of the brain through extradermal electrode placement.

Electromyogram (EMG). A method of recording bioelectrical discharges from muscle groups.

Embolus. An object such as an air bubble or blood clot, which can become lodged in a vessel or artery causing an occlusion of blood flow.

Encapsulated. An enclosure or covering, usually associated with the outer area of a neoplasm.

Encephalitis. Infection of the central nervous system.

Encephalomalacia. Softening of brain tissue.

Encephalopathy. Degeneration of the brain.

Ependymal Cells. Cells that comprise the inner layer of the ventricle walls.

Epilepsy. Significant seizure disorder including classifications such as tonic-clonic, absence, and partial complex seizures.

Evoked Potentials. Measurement of the latency and wave form of visual and auditory signals.

Extracerebral (Extrinsic). Outside of the cerebral hemisphere, usually referring to neoplasms or cerebrovascular disruptions located between the skull and brain.

Extrinsic. See extracerebral.

Fissure. Large sulcus or groove located in the cerebral cortex.

Frontal Lobes. The two largest areas of the brain anterior to the central sulcus (or Fissure of Rolando).

Gerstmann Syndrome. Disorder that is characterized by dyscalculia, dysgraphia, finger agnosia, and right-left confusion.

Glial Cells. Connective tissue of the brain.

Glioblastoma (Multiforma). Neoplasm arising from glial cells.

Glioma. See glioblastoma.

Gray Matter. Cells and connective tissue in the internal areas of the brain.

Gyrus (Gyri). Convolutions that comprise the surface of the brain.

Halstead-Reitan Neuropsychological Test Battery. This battery currently consists of eight tests. The Halstead Impairment Index is computed from the scores derived from the first five of these tests:

Category Test—a complex test that requires a number of higher order functions, including new problem solving, judgment, abstract reasoning, concept formation, and mental efficiency. It is also a test of learning ability utilizing nonverbal material and includes a memory component.

Tactual Performance Test—a complex test requiring the ability to sustain adequate strength and speed of movement. It also requires tactile perception, problem solving, incidental memory, and new learning ability in the absence of visual cues.

Seashore Rhythm Test—a test requiring the ability to discriminate between different patterns of nonverbal sounds. It also requires the ability to sustain attention and concentration as well as eye-ear-hand coordination.

Speech Sounds Perception Test—a test requiring the ability to discriminate between different patterns of verbal sounds. Attention, concentration, and ear-eye-hand coordination are also required.

Finger Oscillation Test—a test requiring simple motor speed with some degree of coordination.

Aphasia Screening Test—a test that taps a number of areas of potential dysfunction including dysnomia, dyslexia, spelling dyspraxia, dyscalculia, dysgraphia, right-left confusion, dysarthria, and constructional dyspraxia.

Sensory Perceptual Examination—a test that examines tactile, auditory, and visual perception.

Trail Making Test—a test requiring problem solving, perception, motor speed and coordination, and the ability to maintain attention on two aspects of a stimulus situation.

Hematoma. A buildup or pool of blood usually associated with the meninges of the brain.

Hemiparesis. Weakness affecting one side of the body.

Hemiplegia. Paralysis affecting one side of the body.

Hemorrhage. Bleeding.

Hippocampus. Anterior temporal lobe structure, which is actively involved in memory function.

Homonymous Hemianopsia. Loss of vision in one half of the visual field of both eyes (right temporal and left nasal, or right nasal and left temporal).

Hypothalamus. Structure dorsal to the thalamus which is involved in many behaviors such as sleeping, sexual activity, eating, and emotions.

Ideokinetic Apraxia. Inability to carry out a motor activity without a reference object.

Infarct. Dead (brain) tissue associated with an occlusion of the vasculature.

Intracerebral (Intrinsic). Within the cerebral hemispheres, usually referring to neoplasms or cerebrovascular disruptions.

Ipsilateral. The same side of the body.

Ischemia. Lack of blood flow to an area of the brain or other organ.

Intracranial Pressure (ICP). Level of pressure within the skull and cerebrospinal fluid system.

Korsakoff's Syndrome. Deterioration of the brain and cognitive abilities (particularly in memory) caused by chronic and severe alcohol abuse.

Laceration. A tear or cut.

Lateral Fissure (Sylvian Fissure). The deep sulcus or groove separating the temporal and parietal lobes.

Lesion. Tissue damage.

Limbic System. Interconnected structures in the brain (hippocampus, cingulate gyrus, septum, amygdala, olfactory bulb, mammillary bodies, and fornix), which are involved in emotional responses.

Lumbar Puncture. Insertion of a needle into the spinal column to remove cerebrospinal fluid for analysis and to determine level of intracranial pressure.

Magnetic Resonance Imaging (MRI). Computerized imagery based on the analysis of the magnetic properties of the substance of the brain and which resembles the pictures gathered from CAT scans.

Medulla Oblongata. Structure of the brain below (and connected to) the pons and above the spinal cord.

Medullablastoma. Neoplasm of the medulla oblongata.

Meninges. Membranes that provide the venous drainage system of the brain, comprised of the dura mater, pia mater, and arachnoid.

Meningioma. Neoplasm arising in the meninges.

Meningitis. Infection of the meninges.

Metastatic Neoplasm. Tumors that develop from abnormal cells which have migrated from another area of the body.

Motor Neuron. Neurons that emanate from the spinal cord and extend to muscles.

Myelin Sheath. Encompassing the axons of many nerves.

Neoplasm. A tumor.

Neuron. A nerve cell in the brain, which is comprised of a cell body, axon, and dendrites.

Neurotransmitter. A chemical substance that is released into the synaptic space between neurons to facilitate the chemical/electrical transmission of information between cells.

Occipital Lobes. Posterior portion of the brain next to the parietal and temporal lobes.

Oligodendroglia. Glial cells that serve a support function in the brain.

Oligodendroglioma. A neoplasm that arises from oligodendroglia.

Optic Chiasm. The area in which the optic nerves separate and cross over to the contralateral cerebral hemisphere. It is located in the basal portion of the brain, near the pituitary.

Papilledema. Swelling of the optic disc due to increased intracranial pressure.

Paraphasia. Usually referred to as a communication deficit characterized by the substitution or addition of incorrect words into sentences.

Parietal Lobe. Portion of the brain that is posterior to the central sulcus and rostral to the temporal lobe.

Parkinson's Disease. A disorder that primarily involves the motor functions of the cerebellum and is characterized by tremors and gait deficits.

Peripheral Nerves. Those nerves that lie outside of the central nervous system (brain and spinal cord).

Pia Mater. The portion of the meninges that lies directly above the brain.

Plasticity. Ability of the brain to compensate and change in response to brain injury.

Pneumoencephalography. Also referred to as "air studies" since it is characterized by the removal of some cerebrospinal fluid through a lumbar puncture and the replacement of that fluid with air. X-rays are then taken of the head after the air has traveled to the ventricles and through the arachnoid space. Such a procedure is designed to enhance the view of the ventricles and midline so that atropy, intracranial pressure, and the indirect results of neoplasms may be seen.

Pons. Large oblong structure in the area of the brain stem and comprised of motor fibers.

Positron Emission Tomography (PET Scan). Sophisticated computer assisted X-ray procedure which is similar to the CAT scan and assesses the uptake and utilization of glucose within the brain.

Postcentral Gyrus. Convolution of the cerebral cortex which is located just posterior to the central sulcus and is involved in the mediation of sensory activity.

Precentral Gyrus. Convolution of the cerebral hemisphere which is located just anterior to the central sulcus and involved in the mediation of motor activity.

Ptosis. A drooping eyelid associated with damage to the oculomotor cranial nerve.

Reticular Activating System (Formation). The portion of the brain stem which mediates level of systemic arousal.

Roentgenography. X-ray photographic techniques.

Shear/Strain. The stretching or breaking of the axons and/or dendrites of nerves as a result of head trauma.

Single Photon Emission Computed Tomography (SPECTScan). Similar procedure to PETScan measuring cerebral blood flow and glucose uptake and utilization, with less precise resolution.

Stereognosis. The tactile recognition of objects and shapes.

Strabismus. Lateral deviation of one eye.

Stroke. General classification for disorders of the brain that are characterized by a disruption of blood flow.

Sulcus. A groove or space between the gyri of the cerebral cortex.

Synapse. The space between the terminal end of the axon and another cell body where neurotransmitters are released to carry signals from one nerve to another.

Temporal Lobes. Areas of the brain located dorsal to the parietal lobes (separated from the parietal lobe by the lateral sulcus).

Thalamus. Structures of the brain located to each side of the third ventricle and involved in some gross aspects of sensation.

Thrombus. A blood clot that lodges in an artery or vessel, creating an occlusion.

Tinnitus. Ringing in the ears or the perception of noise in the head.

Transient Ischemic Attacks (TIA). Having to do with short periods of insufficient blood supply to selected portions of the brain (usually involving small vasculature).

Unencapsulated. See encapsulated.

Unilateral. Refers to one side of the body.

Ventricles. Four spaces within the brain through which cerebrospinal fluid circulates.

Vesicles (Synaptic). Small structures at the terminal point of an axon that contain the neurotransmitter substances.

Visual Agnosia. An inability to recognize common objects and shapes.

Wernicke's Aphasia. Inability to communicate verbally due to the impairment of receptive abilities.

White Matter. Connecting tissue within the brain.

Xanthrochromia. The discoloration of cerebrospinal fluid due to the presence of blood cells.

Appendix B

Medical Terminology Abbreviations

ADL	Activities of daily living
AEB	As evidenced by
AKA	Also known as
AMA	Against medical advice
ant	Anterior
A/P	Anteroposterior
A & P	Auscultation and percussion
art	Artery
ASCVD	Arteriosclerotic cardiovascular disease
ASHD	Arteriosclerotic heart disease
AV	Arteriovenous
bid	Twice a day
BP	Blood pressure
$\bar{c}$	With
CA	Cancer
CAT scan	Computerized Axial Tomography
CBS	Chronic Brain Syndrome
CC	Chief complaint
CHI	Closed head injury
CNS	Central nervous system
C/O	Complains of
COLD	Chronic obstructive lung disease
COPD	Chronic obstructive pulmonary disease
cran	Cranial
CSF	Cerebrospinal fluid

CT	Computed tomogram
CVA	Cerebrovascular accident
D/C	Discontinue
diff	Differential
DUI	Driving under influence
DWI	Driving while impaired
DX	Diagnosis
ECT	Electroconvulsive therapy
EEG	Electroencephalogram
EKG	Electrocardiogram
EOM	Extraocular movements
ER	Emergency Room
ETOH	Ethyl alcohol
Fx	Fracture
GI	Gastrointestinal
HA	Headache
H & P	History and physical
HEENT	Head, eyes, ears, nose, throat
hs	At bedtime
Hx	History
ID	Identification
I & D	Incision and drainage
I & O	Intake and output
ICU	Intensive Care Unit
IEP	Individual education plan
ILS	Independent living skills
IM	Intramuscularly
IV	Intravenously
Kcal	Calorie
Kg	Kilogram
lac	Laceration

Lat	Lateral
LD	Learning disability
Li	Lithium
LLE	Left lower extremity
LLQ	Left lower quadrant
LOC	Loss of consciousness
LOS	Length of stay
LP	Lumbar puncture
LUE	Left upper extremity
LUQ	Left upper quadrant
LV	Left ventricle
LYTES	Electrolytes
Med	Medial
mEq	Milliequivalents
MG	Milligram
MI	Myocardial infarction
mj	Marijuana
mod	Moderate
MRI	Magnetic resonance imaging
MS	Mental status
MSE	Mental status examination
NAD	No apparent distress
NG	Nasogastric
NKA	No known allergy
NKDA	No known drug allergies
NOS	Not otherwise specified
NP	Nasopharyngeal
NPO	Nothing by mouth
NTE	Not to exceed
N/V	Nausea and vomiting
OBS	Organic Brain Syndrome

occip	Occipital
o, d	Right eye
Op	Operation
OPD	Outpatient department
OR	Operating room
o, s	Left eye
OT	Occupational Therapy
OTC	Over the counter (non Rx items)
O, u	Both eyes
PA	Posteroanterior
P & A	Percussion and auscultation
para	Paraplegic
pc	After meals
PE	Physical Examination
PEG	Feeding tube
PERLA	Pupils equal and react to light and accommodation
PET	Positron Emmission Tomography
PMH	Past medical history
PMI	Past medical illness
po	By mouth
post	Posterior
prn	As needed
PT	Physical Therapy
PTA	Post-traumatic amnesia
q	Every
qam	Every morning
qd	Daily
qh	Every hour
q2h, etc.	Every two hours, etc.
qhs	Every night
qid	Four times a day

qod	Every other day
QPM	Every evening
quad	Quadriplegic
RBC	Red blood count
RDS	Respiratory distress syndrome
RLE	Right lower extremity
RLQ	Right lower quadrant (abdomen)
R/O	Rule out
ROM	Range of motion
ROS	Review of systems
RT	Recreational Therapy
RTC	Return to clinic
RTW	Return to work
RUE	Right upper extremity
RUQ	Right upper quadrant (abdomen)
RV	Right ventricle
Rx	Prescription
$\overline{s}$	Without
SOB	Shortness of breath
S/P	Status post
SPECT	Single Photon Emission Computed Tomography
Sx	Symptoms
thromb	Thrombosis
tid	Three times a day
Tx	Treatment
U/A	Urinalysis
URI	Upper respiratory infection
UTI	Urinary tract infection
VR	Vocational Rehabilitation
vs	Vital signs
V/P	Ventriculo/peritoneal

w/	With
WBC	White blood count
WD	Well developed
WNWN	Well nourished
WNL	Within normal limits
W/O	Without
W/U	Workup
x	Times

Appendix C

Neuroanatomical Illustrations

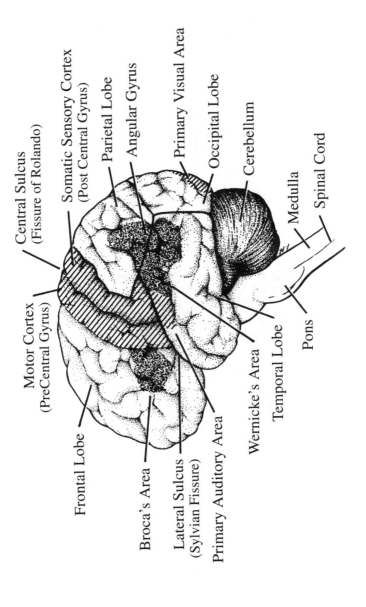

Figure C-1. Lateral view of the brain.

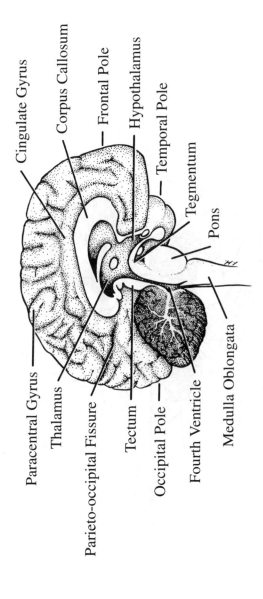

Cingulate Gyrus

Corpus Callosum

Frontal Pole

Hypothalamus

Temporal Pole

Tegmentum

Pons

Paracentral Gyrus

Thalamus

Parieto-occipital Fissure

Tectum

Occipital Pole

Fourth Ventricle

Medulla Oblongata

Figure C-2. Medial view of internal structures of the brain.

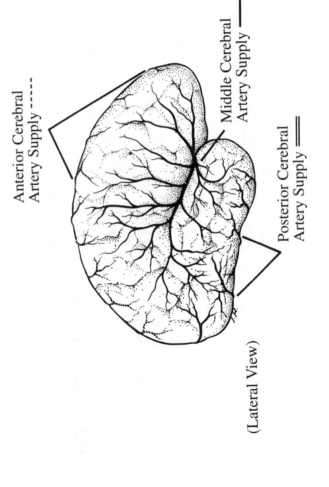

Anterior Cerebral
Artery Supply -----

Middle Cerebral
Artery Supply ——

Posterior Cerebral
Artery Supply ══

(Lateral View)

Figure C-3. Lateral view of cerebrovascular system.

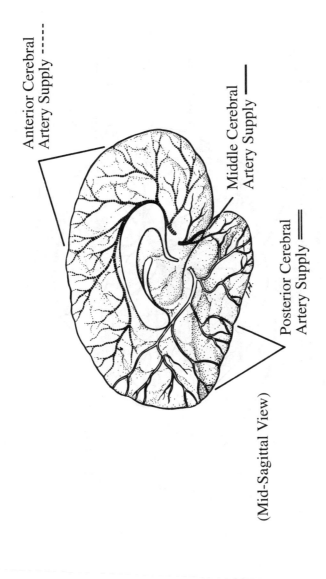

Anterior Cerebral
Artery Supply - - - - -

Middle Cerebral
Artery Supply ——

Posterior Cerebral
Artery Supply ═══

(Mid-Sagittal View)

Figure C-4. Medial view of cerebrovascular system.

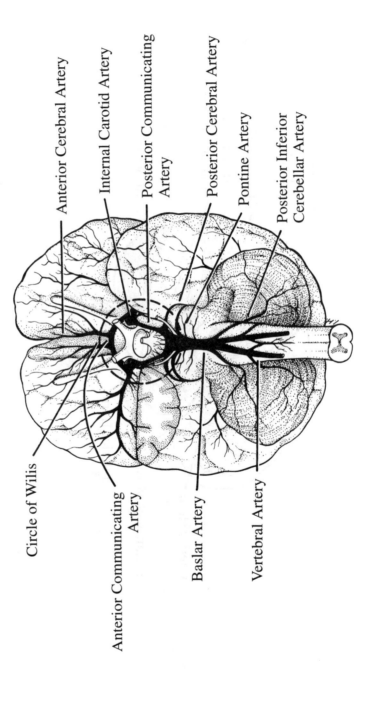

Figure C-5. Caudal view of cerebrovascular system.

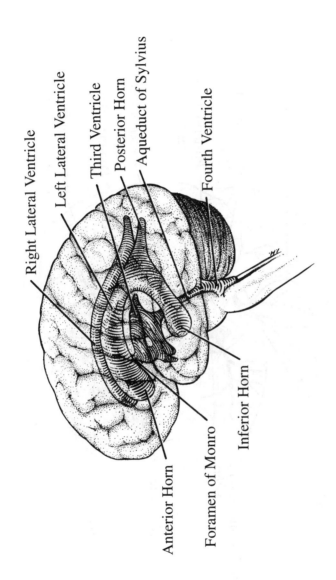

Right Lateral Ventricle

Left Lateral Ventricle

Third Ventricle

Posterior Horn

Aqueduct of Sylvius

Fourth Ventricle

Anterior Horn

Foramen of Monro

Inferior Horn

Figure C-6. Ventricular system.

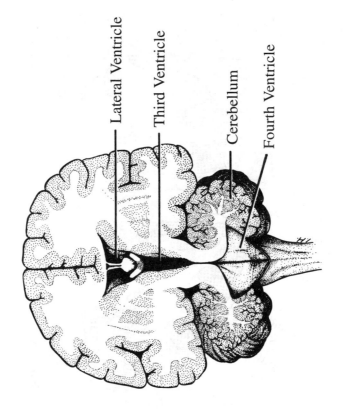

Figure C-7. Ventricular system.

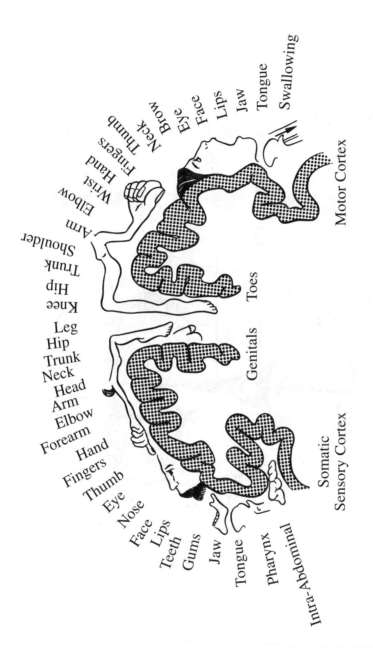

Figure C-8. Functional locations on sensory and motor strips.

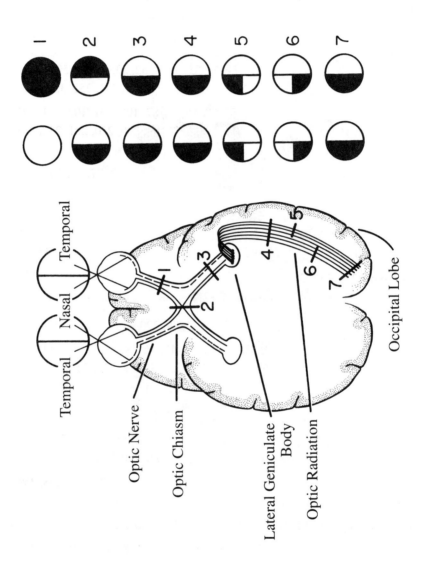

Figure C-9. Optic tracts and visual field deficits.

INDEX